PRIMAL BODY, ~~PRIMAL~~

"For those of us who suffer from life-altering illnesses, *Primal Body, Primal Mind* is a clean slice through the cultural fog of bad nutrition and worse science in which we've been lost for a generation. If you wonder—especially out loud, to doctor after doctor—why it still hurts, then open this book and start reading. You have found your champion, and she comes bearing answers. Did I mention five stars? This book is fabulous."

LIERRE KEITH, AUTHOR OF *THE VEGETARIAN MYTH*

"If you want to *really* know about how your brain and body work, read this book!"

THOM HARTMANN, AUTHOR OF *THE EDISON GENE: ADHD AND THE GIFT OF THE HUNTER CHILD*

"Nora Gedgaudas has loaded *Primal Body, Primal Mind* with the information and resources essential for anyone who hopes to survive the 21st century in mental and physical health."

JULIA ROSS, AUTHOR OF *THE DIET CURE* AND *THE MOOD CURE* AND EXECUTIVE DIRECTOR OF THE RECOVERY SYSTEMS CLINIC

"I consider Nora's work to be the definitive statement on the nutritional needs of the brain. It is required reading for all of my patients and for anyone with an interest in maintaining their own vitality throughout their life."

GLEN ZIELINSKI, D.C., D.A.C.N.B., ASSISTANT PROFESSOR OF CLINICAL NEUROLOGY AT CARRICK INSTITUTE FOR GRADUATE STUDIES

"As an investment advisor, I stress the importance of health to my clients and subscribers. Why is that? Because a clear mind and strong body are the first step to creating and keeping your wealth, whether it is personal or financial. Yes, we can understand how our mind and bodies function! Yes, we can feed ourselves the nutritious food that makes us powerful! Nora Gedgaudas's *Primal Body, Primal Mind* teaches you essential knowledge you need to survive and *thrive* in the 21st century."

CATHERINE AUSTIN FITTS, FOUNDER AND MANAGING MEMBER OF SOLARI INVESTMENT ADVISORY

"These days, hormones are a hot topic. In *Primal Body, Primal Mind,* Gedgaudas focuses on those hormones that are commonly imbalanced and problematic to the American population, contributing to symptoms such as weight gain, low energy, poor mood, and even premature aging. In clear and simple terms Nora describes the root of these problems and outlines solutions that are effective and easy to apply. This is the book you want to read."

JANET R. LANG, D.C., AUTHOR, EDUCATOR, AND
FOUNDER OF RESTORATIVE ENDOCRINOLOGY

"Nora Gedgaudas lights a path toward dietary discretion and natural health that obliterates much of the standard dietary doctrine along the way. Larger truths have a tendency to be simple. It is so here as well."

SIEGFRIED OTHMER, PH.D., COAUTHOR OF *ADD: THE 20-HOUR SOLUTION* AND CHIEF SCIENTIST AT THE EEG INSTITUTE

"*Primal Body, Primal Mind* covers a wide range of health topics but ties them all back to one central idea: physically, we are virtually identical to our Paleolithic ancestors. We may drive minivans and listen to modern jazz on iPods, but our bodies and brains haven't really evolved past the Stone Age. Overall, an excellent read and an excellent resource."

TOM NAUGHTON, COMEDIAN, FORMER HEALTH
WRITER, AND CREATOR OF *FAT HEAD*

"It's a health plan so easy even an unga bunga caveman can do it! Gedgaudas uses humor, science-based facts, and common sense to debunk many of the myths we have been told about weight and health control in the 21st century. In the world of healthy high-fat, low-carb nutrition research and education, this is yet another book to complement your healthy lifestyle change."

JIMMY MOORE, AUTHOR OF *LIVIN' LA VIDA LOW CARB*

"Nora explores where our dietary requirements originated and how they affect our mood and vulnerability to diseases and explains the complex issues of nutrient assimilation, digestion gluten sensitivity, and celiac disease. Find out if you're a fat burner or a sugar burner, learn the bad news about gluten, soy, milk proteins, and the nutritional bases for depression, ADHD, and other common disorders. This book is so much more than another 'what to eat' book."

JULIE HOLLAND, M.D., AUTHOR OF *THE POT BOOK*
AND *WEEKENDS AT BELLEVUE*

PRIMAL BODY, PRIMAL MIND

Beyond the Paleo Diet for Total Health and a Longer Life

NORA T. GEDGAUDAS, CNS, CNT

Healing Arts Press
Rochester, Vermont • Toronto, Canada

Healing Arts Press
One Park Street
Rochester, Vermont 05767
www.HealingArtsPress.com

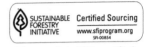

SUSTAINABLE FORESTRY INITIATIVE — Certified Sourcing — www.sfiprogram.org — SFI-00854

Text stock is SFI certified

Healing Arts Press is a division of Inner Traditions International

Note to the reader: This book is intended as an informational guide. The remedies, approaches, and techniques described herein are meant to supplement, and not to be a substitute for, professional medical care or treatment. They should not be used to treat a serious ailment without prior consultation with a qualified health care professional.

Library of Congress Cataloging-in-Publication Data

Gedgaudas, Nora T.
  Primal body, primal mind : beyond the paleo diet for total health and a longer life / Nora T. Gedgaudas.
      p. cm.
  Summary: "Combining your body's Paleolithic needs with modern nutritional and medical research for complete mind-body wellness"—Provided by publisher.
  Originally published: 2009.
  Includes bibliographical references and index.
  ISBN 978-1-59477-413-3
  1. Dietetics. 2. Diet therapy. 3. Health. 4. Nutrition. I. Title.
  RM216.G34 2011
  615.8'54—dc23

2011014048

Printed and bound in the United States by Lake Book Manufacturing
The text stock is SFI certified. The Sustainable Forestry Initiative® program promotes sustainable forest management.

10   9

Text design and layout by Virginia Scott Bowman
This book was typeset in Garamond Premier Pro and Gill Sans with Avant Garde and Gill Sans as display typefaces

To send correspondence to the author of this book, mail a first-class letter to the author c/o Inner Traditions • Bear & Company, One Park Street, Rochester, VT 05767, and we will forward the communication, or contact the author at **www.PrimalBody-PrimalMind.com**.

*For Lisa, without whose tireless dedication
and support this book would not have been possible.
Also, this book is for all those in my life who
have relentlessly supported me, my heart, and my work.
You have my eternal love and gratitude.*

*And finally, for our ancestors, who hold an important
key for all of us to the future of our survival.*

■ ■ ■

"The writer is fully aware that his message is not orthodox; but since our orthodox theories have not saved us we may have to readjust them to bring them into harmony with Nature's laws. Nature must be obeyed, not orthodoxy."

WESTON A. PRICE,
NUTRITION AND PHYSICAL DEGENERATION (1939)

Cautionary Note and Disclaimer

I am not a physician; I am a nutritional therapist and cannot and do not prescribe. The information provided here is for educational purposes only. Any decision on your part to read and use this information is your personal choice. The information in this book is not meant to be used to diagnose, prescribe for, or treat any illness. Please discuss any changes you wish to make to your medical treatment with a qualified, licensed health care provider.

Although millions of people have been able to transition to a very-low-carbohydrate diet without documented harm, there are some people for whom a low-carb diet must be approached with some caution.

If you are taking medication to control your blood sugar or blood pressure, you may need to quickly reduce the dosage and may need to discontinue this medication altogether if you significantly restrict your carbohydrate intake. **This is best done under the supervision of an experienced and qualified licensed health care provider.**

Although the diet advocated in this book stresses the consumption of only moderate levels of protein and is not a "high-protein diet," for anyone who has serious kidney disease, any increase in dietary protein can potentially be a problem. If you have kidney disease, you should consult your doctor before making any changes to your diet.

If you have gallbladder attacks or gallstones, you should exercise extreme caution where increasing dietary fat is concerned, and you may first need to resolve this issue with your trusted and knowledgeable licensed natural health care provider before embarking on any major dietary change.

Anyone who has any other serious illness such as unstable cardiovascular disease, cancer, or liver disease needs to exercise caution if making dietary changes. You should consult your physician for guidance.

Finally, if you are pregnant or lactating, you **should not** overly restrict protein (or fat) intake. Also, young children and teens have much more demanding nutrient needs and should not have their protein or fat intake overly restricted. There is still no dietary carbohydrate (sugar or starch) requirement for such individuals, but know that radical changes to your existing diet if you are pregnant—other than eliminating junk foods—may not be advisable and should be approached only under the guidance of a qualified and knowledgeable health care professional.

Contents

PART ONE
Primal Body

PART TWO

Primal Mind

PART THREE

Paradise Lost

———■———

■ ■ ■

■ ■ ■

Illustration Permissions

1.2 Changes per capita availability of dietary fats in the United States; data borrowed from *Coronary Heart Disease: The Dietary Sense and Nonsense* by George V. Mann, M.D.

1.3 U.S. dietary fats table and cooking sources; data borrowed from Coronary Heart Disease: The Dietary Sense and Nonsense by George V. Mann, M.D.

1.5 Cartoon by Sidney Harris; by permission from Sidney Harris, ScienceCartoonsPlus.com

1.6 The prehistoric food pyramid the U.S. Department of Agriculture (and other vested interests) didn't want you to see; created by Kirk Kristlibas, Avalonik Society Media

1.7 Cartoon by Cox & Forkum; reprinted with permission from CoxandForkum.com

2.1 Omega-3s vanish in the feedlot; by permission from *Pasture Perfect* by Jo Robinson

3.1 Cartoon by Jack Ohman

7.1 Cartoon by Sidney Harris; by permission from Sidney Harris, ScienceCartoonsPlus.com

8.2 Framingham Heart Study data—thirty-year observation; borrowed from *Coronary Heart Disease: The Dietary Sense and Nonsense* by George V. Mann, M.D.

8.3 Cartoon by Sidney Harris; by permission from Sidney Harris, ScienceCartoonsPlus.com

8.4 Comparison of cholesterol eaten per day in patients with coronary heart disease and healthy subjects; data borrowed from *The Cholesterol Myths* by Uffe Ravnskov, M.D., Ph.D.

10.1 The prostaglandin pathways: conversion of essential fatty acids to prostaglandins; re-created by permission from Sally Fallon

15.1 Cartoon by Cox & Forkum; by permission from CoxandForkum.com

16.1 Cartoon by Sidney Harris; by permission from Sidney Harris, ScienceCartoonsPlus.com

18.1 Cartoon by Cox & Forkum; by permission from CoxandForkum.com

21.1 Cartoon by Sidney Harris; by permission from Sidney Harris, ScienceCartoonsPlus.com

22.1 Image courtesy of *Science,* "Calorie Resriction Delays Disease Onset and Mortality in Rhesus Monkeys," 32, no. 5937: 201–4.

24.1 Cartoon by Sidney Harris; by permission from Sidney Harris, ScienceCartoonsPlus.com

25.1 Cartoon by Jack Ohman

26.1 Mental illnesses associated with increasingly severe neuronal magnesium deficiency; illustration by permission from George Eby, www.George-Eby-Research.com

29.1 Cartoon by Jack Ohman

30.1 Cartoon by Sidney Harris; by permission from Sidney Harris, ScienceCartoonsPlus.com

Foreword

Mark Steinberg, Ph.D.

In this life, health of mind and body is the big prize. Toward that end, Nora Gedgaudas's *Primal Body, Primal Mind* takes us a long way.

This book is a nutritional treasure map leading to optimal wellness, the way nature intended. The author has outlined and detailed a thorough documentation of nutritional principles and has linked them directly to evolutionary history. More important, she has provided direct guidelines for shopping and eating in ways that will eliminate a host of physiological and mental disorders and restore followers to the natural condition of health and wellness that accrues from eating as we were biologically designed to. Since applying the principles outlined in this book, I have lost forty pounds and enjoy much improved health and well-being.

Primal Body, Primal Mind is loaded with understandable explanations and solutions tied to everyday actions and changes that anyone can make. It is a journey into the realm of biology, politics, and self-care that you will never get from formal academic education. As well as being a gem of nutritional and dietary sense, *Primal Body, Primal Mind* offers comprehensible insights into the biochemistry of behavior and consumerism. Gedgaudas's approach to the (Paleolithic) dietary habits that have sustained humans without pills or potions for millennia stands in stark and welcome truth against the nonsense so relentlessly peddled for our allegiance and dollars.

Gedgaudas teaches things that your mother should have, and she does so without nagging or sermonizing. Her writing is eloquent, factual, and straightforward, and she provides many practical tips, including websites and other resources. Her arguments and data are scientifically documented, and the manuscript is well organized and easily referenced.

Reading Gedgaudas's jewel might make you a bit sheepish about how you've been duped by so many commercial interests, including the diet and publishing industries. Quickly, however, you will be grateful for her leadership out of the wilderness of illness and digestive trickery that so easily nickel-and-dimes us away from truly feeling good and maintaining ourselves and a high quality of life.

In reading *Primal Body, Primal Mind,* it becomes obvious that Gedgaudas cares for herself and for others. I know this firsthand, since Nora is a colleague engaged in the clinical practice of EEG neurofeedback. As a neuropsychologist with thirty-five years of experience and the author of two popular books on brain training, mental fitness, and living healthfully, I endorse Nora's reputation and expertise in the clinical care of people by using the scientific techniques about which I have written. She is among the elite of professionals who can restore health and promote growth by harnessing nature's principles with effective care.

I recommend *Primal Body, Primal Mind* to my patients and friends, and I believe that this is "must reading" for anyone serious about health care and self-care.

MARK STEINBERG, PH.D., is a licensed psychologist and a clinical neuropsychologist as well as an NBC medical consultant. He is the author of *ADD: The 20-Hour Solution* and *Living Intact: Challenge and Choice in Tough Times.*

Foreword

▪ ▪ ▪ ▪ ▪ ▪ ▪ ▪ ▪ ▪ ▪

Brent Pottenger

We can't opt out of nutrition. We have to eat. We have to drink. We have to do something about it. But the modern nutritional landscape can be complex and contradictory beyond belief.

One-size-fits-all is a size that fits no one.

Ever since we scientized nutrition, our health states have declined, unfortunately. Decisions about what to eat and drink have morphed from habits of culture—of heritage—to calculated choices based on reduction-ist nutritional theories, with little consideration for how human beings reached modernity in the first place. Just in the past few decades, for instance, scientific research on what human beings should consume to fuel their metabolism has produced countless conclusions that contra-dict one another: traditional whole foods like eggs have bounced between heaven ("eggs are good for you") and hell ("eggs are bad for you"), mak-ing stops in dietary purgatory along the way ("more evidence is needed to determine the health effects of eggs"). With all this white noise con-founding things, it is no wonder that people feel frustrated with food. This trend is unsustainable, and it does not translate into healthy people in the end. Perhaps incorporating insights from the philosophy of science could help us solve our nutritional scientific challenges. When we do this, an important theme emerges: at some point, you have to self-experiment with your personal diet to figure out what works and what does not work for your body, because each person displays biochemical individuality as a result of varying genomic backgrounds and microbiomic makeups.

However, not all self-experimentation starting points are created equal.* Science and history have some important things to say if we approach them the right way. And since you have to start somewhere, some nutritional, scientific, and philosophical tools may help you progress along your personal health journey. To start, modern medicine espouses the slogan "First, do no harm" to emphasize the importance of respecting conservative approaches to healing before resorting to drastic, riskier measures. Applying this warning to human nutritional practice seems wise because it challenges everyone to analyze the assumptions underlying their recommendations, theories, and hypotheses. In practice, there are many ways to answer the question What is the safest guide for deciding which foods and drinks to start self-experimenting with? Personally, I answer this question, with the intention of doing as little harm as possible, by suggesting that looking at traditional cultures' dietary practices is the best place to begin tinkering with foods and drinks. Why? Across the globe and throughout human history, populations consuming diets consistent with their ancestral traditions have averted the *diseases of civilization,* such as diabetes and heart disease, that are harming more and more people in contemporary societies. Notably, examining traditional diets provides a large-scale evolutionary experiment with far more enrollees than we could ever herd into a formal clinical trial to test with a double-blind, placebo-controlled intervention experiment. In his noted book *The Logic of Scientific Discovery,* Sir Karl Popper, a philosopher of science who worked extensively on the problem of induction (reasoning from the specific to the general), famously concluded, "The majority of the problems of theoretical philosophy, and the most interesting ones, can be re-interpreted . . . as problems of method" (Popper 2002). Amid the malaise of conflicting information about human diet available today, a logical method for investigating and understanding nutritional science is to have people self-experiment with diets that are consistent with their ancestral heritage, followed by appropriate responses to physiological feedback, such as inflammation or allergies, to stumble (semiblindly) upon modern diets that are safe, enjoyable, and practical, all at the same time.

To start, some may refute the notion of individuality when it comes

---

*Please see Seth Roberts's work on self-experimentation (www.sethroberts.net).

to dietary guidelines, but this type of inductive reasoning does not hold up to scientific scrutiny. Each human being expresses what Dr. Roger Williams termed biochemical individuality. Williams captured this sentiment beautifully when he said, "Nutrition is for real people. Statistical humans are of little interest" (Bland 1998). What this amounts to biologically is the reality that each person processes and assimilates nutrients differently. In part, these differences result from genomic and microbiomic diversity.

With the attention that the Human Genome Project has received recently, people are more aware than ever that genes contribute to individual differences among people (Pollack 2010). Yet, perhaps more important, the emerging Human Microbiome Project shows that people contain ten times as many nonhuman microorganismal cells in their bodies than they do human ones, and this has potentially far-reaching implications for human nutritional considerations, disease prevention, and healing interventions (Peterson et al. 2009; Candela et al. 2010; Turnbaugh et al. 2009). Whenever people consume foods and drinks for energy, these nutrients interact with both human and nonhuman cells in concert within their body. On the one hand, the interactions that these nutrients have with human cells can influence genetic expression. In modern scientific parlance, these dynamics fall under the category of nutrigenomics, a subcategory of epigenetics, or even more broadly, functional genomics. These effects, while key to determining our phenotypes, could be trumped by the multidirectional interactions between our diets and our microbiomes. In short, we aren't who we thought we were when it comes to gene–environment interplay. By definition, a microbiome is all the nonhuman microorganisms (and their genetic material) that live in and on a person's body. Given this (hopefully) symbiotic relationship, these microorganisms also consume the foods and drinks that we intake during mealtimes. In response to the environments that these meals produce within our digestive system, microorganisms extract and assimilate nutrients for their own use and benefit. In this way, these microorganisms are intimately linked to our dietary intake habits because they depend on us for energy sources to run their metabolic machinery.

Thus, if each person displays microbiomic individuality because his or her body harbors unique compositions of microorganisms, then it follows logically that this would enhance biochemical individuality even further, over and above the variability associated with human genomics alone (Qin et al. 2010). For example, populations of people living in Japan have developed, through lateral gene transfer, the ability to digest seaweed (Hamilton 2010). This type of evolutionary event illustrates concretely how deeply our dietary practices are connected to our microbiomes and how groups of people adapt to their ecological niches in fascinating ways. The new frontier for this nutritional science field could be termed "epimicrobiomics"—a domain where scientists seek ways to alter microbiomic expression in people's bodies by prescribing specific dietary recommendations involving prebiotics (foods and drinks that "feed" beneficial microorganismal growth and maintenance in our digestive system), probiotics (foods and drinks that contain beneficial microorganisms), and/or synbiotics (which combine prebiotics and probiotics synergistically). All these rapidly advancing areas of inquiry seem promising, but when it comes to nutritional scientific philosophy, the most important message that genomics and microbiomics have to share is the working conjecture that each individual has a distinctive genomic background and microbiomic makeup and has distinct nutritional needs that must be met for optimal well-being.

As a reader of this book, you're beginning a personalized cartographic (mapmaking) exercise, with Nora serving as your insightful guide. To begin, I have to admit a caveat: I'm a big Nora Gedgaudas fan. After all, an author who names a chapter of her book after my ancestor Francis M. Pottenger Jr., M.D., is going to hold a special place in my book.* So, I'm biased positively toward what Nora has to say. Everything is subjective, anyway.

I happen to think that what Gedgaudas communicates in *Primal Body, Primal Mind* provides self-experimenting *bricoleurs* with an array of logical health conjectures to evaluate, assess, and then, perhaps, test on their own bodies via "$n = 1$ (patient-of-one)" clinical trials. When you read books as an *epistemocrat* (someone who holds his or her own knowledge in great suspicion), you simply reflect on and judge them for what the authors intended to accomplish; a single book cannot be all things to all people. Nora, in my opinion, accomplishes what she set out to tackle with this book.

Nora's sharp. And she writes with a memorable, enjoyable punch.

---

*Please see the Price-Pottenger Nutrition Foundation's website (www.ppnf.org) to learn more about Francis M. Pottenger Jr.

She understands things like the thought-experiment that it's naive to think most plants are our safe, edible friends. From an evolutionary perspective, it seems we'd be wise to be extra careful about the roles of plants in our diets (they may require special preparation and/or cooking, for instance, to be consumed safely); because they've evolved under selection pressures as *immobile* organisms, that is, without the ability to run away or fight back physically, plants protect themselves from herbivores and omnivores by producing, holding, and releasing toxins (such as tannins and lectins) throughout their bodies. Most animals, on the other hand, have evolved "fight-or-flight" capacities and thus, if we catch them successfully, seem safer to eat because their tissues probably contain fewer poisons than plant cells do.

Nora also embraces a meta-rule formation for individualized health. This is the process of making our own rules to guide our choices, such as "Don't consume anything that causes a negative physiological reaction," reminding us to *listen to our own body* every step of the way as we deduce, for ourselves, what works and what doesn't work in our patient-of-one case. And we must always remember a potent psychological concept that my astute friend Professor Aaron Blaisdell, of the University of California, Los Angeles, introduced me to called "overshadowing" (hat tip to Pavlov), which occurs when the initial stimulus is so strong that it blocks the perception of a second, downstream effect. For example, when people drink a soda, the initial stimulus from the sugar is so great that it overshadows the energy crash and feelings of poor health that follow shortly after consumption. In this way, overshadowing inhibits people from responding appropriately to the poisons they ingest and inhibits their ability to learn via conditioning degrade as a result. Nora hopes to shed light on this type of overshadowing to help people really listen to their body in ways they never did before.

Nora's ray of light starts all the way back in the Ice Age, and then she works her way forward to the present, searching our ancestry for hypotheses about our physiology. From these inquiries, Nora discusses Pottenger's research because she's concerned about our future generations. In his studies, Pottenger witnessed the degradation of health in successive generations when his cats were fed improper (processed and sugary) diets. Since the Industrial Revolution, it seems, as people have consumed more and more nonreal, processed foods, human beings have experienced a degradation in health and a concurrent rise in *diseases of civilization* that parallel the problems Pottenger observed in his research. Nora hopes that we are not too many generations into our modern metabolic syndrome woes, because Pottenger's experiments also showed that it takes a few generations of proper nutrition to restore animals to vibrant health.

Given our current health care and medical predicaments, what does Nora suggest? Well, within the **"eat real foods"** domain, she gracefully nudges folks toward good lipids from pastured meats, fish, butter, yogurt, coconuts, avocados, and a few other key sources; moderate, quality protein, primarily from animal sources and some nuts; and low-carbohydrate intake, mainly from nonstarchy vegetables and some fruit (seasonally). That's a starting glimpse of her well-developed and thoughtful human diet discussion; I'll leave the rest for you to peruse in her book.

Nora also feels that the destruction of our soil and the changes in the types and quality of our foods today suggest that supplementation may be necessary to achieve optimal health. Personally, I think this hypothesis is one worth heeding.

She even features a chapter on exercise and movement that emphasizes the value of high-intensity, low-duration activities like sprinting and occasional lifting, coupled with plenty of rest and relaxation (sleeping) and low-intensity energy expenditure (walking outdoors) in between. The *spirit* of her approach to fitness and training, as I see it, is essentially a bricolage of what my friends Mark Sisson, Keith Norris, Robb Wolf, Art DeVany, Frank Forencich, and Erwan LeCorre have to say.

At the end of the day, Nora shares a kindred spirit with the rest of the ancestral health* community that has emerged recently (her book features notable quotes from Loren Cordain, S. Boyd Eaton, et al.), and she is playing an empowering leadership role in the movement.

So, take Nora's book as a field guide, as a map for your own evaluation and self-experimentation; hopefully, you'll stumble upon your own personal protocol along the way.

Get ready, it's *Primal Body, Primal Mind* time!

To good health.

BRENT POTTENGER holds a master of health administration degree from the University of Southern California and is earning his M.D. at The Johns Hopkins

---

*Special thanks to Navanit Arakeri for the term *ancestral health*.

University School of Medicine. He cofounded Ancestry, a nonprofit that organizes the Ancestral Health Symposium and the Ancestral Health Society. He also cofounded Game Plan Academy (GPA) to provide athletic and academic mentorship services to students who normally might not have access to these resources. He uses his blog at Healthcare Epistemocrat to build on the legacy of his ancestor Francis M. Pottenger Jr., M.D.

References

Bland, J. 1998. Foreword to *Biochemical Individuality: The Key to Understanding What Shapes Your Health,* by Roger J. Williams. New Canaan, Conn.: Keats Publishing.

Candela, M., et al. 2010. "Functional Intestinal Microbiome: New Frontiers in Prebiotic Design." *International Journal of Food Microbiolology* 140, no. 2–3: 93–101.

Hamilton, J. April 7, 2010. "How Gut Bacteria Evolved to Feast on Sushi." National Public Radio. www.npr.org/templates/story/story.php?storyId=125675700.

Peterson, J., et al.; NIH HMP Working Group. 2009. "The NIH Human Microbiome Project." *Genome Research* 19, no. 12: 2317–23.

Pollack, A. June 14, 2010. "Awaiting the Genome Payoff." *New York Times.* www.nytimes.com/2010/06/15/business/15genome.html?_r=1&src=busln.

Popper, K. 2002. *The Logic of Scientific Discovery.* London and New York: Routledge.

Qin, J., et al. 2010. "A Human Gut Microbial Gene Catalogue Established by Metagenomic Sequencing." *Nature* 464, no. 7285: 59–65.

Turnbaugh, P. J., et al. 2009. "The Effect of Diet on the Human Gut Microbiome: A Metagenomic Analysis in Humanized Gnotobiotic Mice." *Science Translational Medicine* 1, no. 6: 6ra14.

Preface

■ ■ ■ ■ ■ ■ ■ ■ ■ ■ ■ ■

As a clinical neurofeedback practitioner specializing in EEG biofeedback (also known as neurotherapy, neurobiofeedback, and brain training), I help individuals exercise or condition their brain in a way that allows for greater stability, enhanced cognitive functioning, and improved affect and ability to pay attention through what is largely a neurological modification of stress response. It is a means of impacting both the regulation and the functional dysregulation of a nervous system through a noninvasive and self-empowering process. Neurofeedback is best likened to highly specialized "brain exercise." At its best, neurofeedback seems to restore a neurological flexibility, a stress-coping capacity, and a certain improved homeostasis that should be everyone's birthright. It can free one from self-imposed obstacles and allow the full flowering of human potential.

Using neurofeedback, I myself was freed from over thirty years of intractable depression that had not responded to *anything else*. The concomitant anxiety and panic attacks I experienced almost daily, too, became part of the past. It provided a freedom and a liberation that has made me a devout practitioner of this miraculous form of brain training ever since. That was many years ago. The effect I have since witnessed in thousands of individuals has been so profound that I am convinced: neurofeedback is the most powerful means available to facilitate permanent and positive changes in neurological functioning. It is the most rewarding work I can possibly imagine.

However, I have found individuals repeatedly plateauing in their process, simply hitting walls they couldn't seem to hurdle. Some experience inexplicable backslides or have difficulty getting their brain to move at all. What such experience has revealed to me, over and over, is that typically there seems to be an issue with diet, food sensitivity, endocrine dysfunction, severe nutritional deficiencies, or a combination of conditions. Almost without exception, addressing these dietary issues allows the obstacles to be overcome, and healing improvements are then free to take place. Everything comes together far more efficiently. The brain and body simply have to have certain raw materials to work with in order to function properly. It is abundantly clear that all the brain training in the world (much less any other form of support or therapy) cannot create a nutrient where there is none or remove a problematic substance that does not belong.

My more than twenty-five years of background in the passionate, intricate study and application of nutritional science, and more recently, nutritional anthropology, served to beautifully cement and maintain my own neurotherapy results. Dietary intervention with clients has repeatedly provided a powerful solution to such dilemmas. Counseling my clients regarding diet, however, is something that proved to be time consuming and often overwhelming for all involved. As a believer in providing detailed education and not prescriptions, I found that there was simply too much information to convey and too little time to convey it. I was at a loss to recommend any single source of literature to provide answers to my clients, as no single source seemed adequate in its scope. I found myself spending untold time and money copying articles and pages from books and offering lengthy explanations. This arrangement was an enormous source of frustration for all involved.

As such, frustration became the mother of invention, and this book was born. In its infancy, this was little more than a five- or ten-page article, outlining basic principles and providing a few resources. With all the positive feedback, however, came more questions—lots of questions. I also realized that much of what I was providing as information was at times controversial and not voiced in the format of the mainstream health-oriented mantras. I needed to provide more clear references and illustrate the solid foundations of the framework I was gradually building in writing. More and more information seemed important to add, either as a clarification or as a pertinent adjunct to these principles. The modest five or ten pages began to grow. Increasingly positive feedback and excellent clinical results ensued, and there were still more questions. Eventually the whole thing grew and evolved. This newly revised, substantially expanded, and updated volume is the result.

Today, I use this book, nutritional counseling, and nutritional therapy with both my neurofeedback clients and those interested solely in dietary help. The results have been overwhelmingly positive.

Many, many individuals have benefited profoundly from the information presented here. Tremendously positive and inspiring results have been reported. I have seen weight loss when it was needed, restored digestive health when nothing else worked, substantially improved blood chemistry reports, and total liberation from food cravings and eating disorders—even addictions. I have also seen liberation from antidepressants, psychostimulants, and other types of medications; enhanced energy levels; improvements in mental clarity and affect; improved sustainability of attention; reduced anxieties and instabilities; and freedom from unnecessary dependence on gimmicks, gurus, and supplements. People are even reporting big savings on their grocery bills!

Most rewarding of all, I have come to see others become students of health themselves, no longer relying on controlling, confusing, or contradictory advice from diet pundits and "dictocrats," to borrow a creative term coined by Sally Fallon, president and founder of the Weston A. Price Foundation. Using sound, commonsense principles, not formulas, gives independence in the process of wellness and makes better educated consumers of us all.

It's been several years since I wrote the earlier versions of the manuscript for this book. So much new information and so many new clinical experiences, responses from readers,* and new realizations and scientific advances have driven me to present the information in a more expansive, comprehensive, better-illustrated, and more multidimensional way. This brand-new second edition has been updated and revised from the 2009 version and offers the reader clearer and more comprehensive information than ever before.

In addition, the birth of the Primal Body, Primal Mind website is an inspiration whose time has come (www.PrimalBody-PrimalMind .com). The field of nutritional science is now evolving exponentially and far faster than ever before. We live in exciting, if not perilous, times. The

---

*For more information relating to neurofeedback, visit my website, at www.northwest-neurofeedback.com, or go to www.eeginfo.com.

Primal Body, Primal Mind website is an up-to-date and evolving resource for ongoing, detailed, cutting-edge nutritional information and education. It is for all those seeking to expand their knowledge, radically improve their health, and maximize their mind's performance to the fullest extent. Also, look for the newly created website for the Nutritional Underground (www.nutritional-underground.com). The Nutritional Underground is a collective website devoted to a multifaceted approach to health and well-being as outlined by the paradigm presented in these pages. Multiple contributors from many facets of health and wellness provide you with a "one-stop shop" for support, resources, and ongoing education. Think of it as a community resource.

Addressing diet from an evolutionary perspective has been of immeasurable value in my practice and seems to speak in a commonsense way to even the most hardened skeptics; this includes even avowed junk-food junkies and devout vegetarians or vegans. A respectfully conveyed approach, combined with the hard science of basic human physiology, cuts through a lot. Newfound advances in the science of longevity research have added an entirely new dimension to these foundational concepts and promise to radically transform even the healthiest person into a manifestation of even greater potential. The implications are truly staggering.

We are boldly venturing here into extremely exciting frontiers never before imagined!

My interest is not to prescribe or dictate anyone's dietary habits. The information presented speaks for itself. Ample quality reference material is provided throughout to allow for further exploration. What readers choose to do with the information contained here remains entirely up to them. It has been wisely stated that it is abjectly impossible to actually teach anyone anything. The best one can do is inspire others to learn.

May you find this book inspiring.

Introduction

■ ■ ■ ■ ■ ■ ■ ■ ■ ■ ■ ■

Just what is it that genuinely constitutes a *healthy diet?*

Innumerable popular books, articles, and testimonials overwhelm and confound the average consumer in such a way as to render such a concept virtually meaningless. Misinformation driven by financial interests and emotional biases either sways the gullible to extremes or leads the skeptical-minded to cynicism. Either way, the truth is lost somewhere in the static and remains overwhelmingly clouded. It is my objective in writing this book to put forth an appeal to what can be readily defined as logic and sense, as well as to provide information that is sound and based on evolutionary, modern scientific and physiological perspectives. This book thinks outside the box of accepted dogma—away from corporate vested interests—and lays a clear foundation of *principles,* rather than *formulas,* that can serve as a guide. This is not just another "caveman" diet book or just another low-carb diet. Fasten your seat belt.

The optimal human diet is not something that should have to require overly careful formulation by calories or percentages, much less by blood type. A person should not need a calorie counter, a percentages guide, or any sort of manual in tow when going to the market to buy food. No one should need a blood test to determine blood type in order to know how to eat. Such tools, though they provide a seductive sense of structure and security, can be unnecessarily confusing and do not ultimately constitute a sound, principle-based, commonsense approach. Long term, these approaches tend to lack sustainability.

Fundamentally, as humans, we are much more alike physiologically

1

than not. Although it's true that we need to take into account something called *biochemical individuality,* the fact is that we are all subject to the same fundamental physiological laws. We all share a sophisticated endocrine system subject to certain interhormonal relationships; we all, of necessity, have a blood pH value ranging between 7.35 and 7.45; and we all have similar basic nutrient requirements. There are certain basic principles that apply to all of us that must be taken into account. To be fair, some of these truths are newly discovered and decidedly alter the landscape of dietary optimization. But there's much more to it than this—much more.

So where do we begin?

All of the structure and functions of the human body are built from and run on nutrients. All of them.

JANET LANG, B.A., D.C.

PART ONE

PRIMAL BODY

Science is in trouble whenever the will to believe overwhelms the duty to doubt.

SIEGFRIED OTHMER, PH.D.,
CHIEF SCIENTIST, THE EEG INSTITUTE

1

A Look at Where Our Dietary Requirements Originated

■■■■■■■■■■■■

All humans require similar ranges of both macro and micronutrients and all human groups have similar anatomical, physiological and endocrine functions in regard to diet and nutrition. We were all hunter-gatherers dependent upon wild plants and animals, and these selective pressures shaped our present-day nutritional requirements.

LOREN CORDAIN, PH.D., PROFESSOR OF EXERCISE AND SPORTS SCIENCE AT COLORADO STATE UNIVERSITY AND NOTED EVOLUTIONARY DIET RESEARCHER

99.99% of our genes were formed before the development of agriculture.

S. BOYD EATON, M.D., MEDICAL ANTHROPOLOGIST

As a species, we are essentially genetically identical with respect to genetic expression, regardless of blood type, to those humans living more than forty thousand years ago. Our physiology is fundamentally the same as that of people from the Paleolithic Era, which refers to the human evolutionary time period spanning from roughly 2.6 million to about ten thousand years ago—before the dawn of agriculture. We are the result of an optimal design, shaped and molded by nature over one hundred thousand or so generations. In other words, we are *all*—biologically, genetically, and physiologically—without exception—hunter-gatherers. And for much of our hominid evolution, we have been mostly hunters.

The hunter-gatherer diet can be described via at least two different perspectives: ice age Paleolithic and post–ice age, or neo-Paleolithic. The diet of neo-Paleolithic peoples, including modern-day hunter-gatherers with some regional variation, essentially consisted of high-quality animal-source protein, both cooked and uncooked (including organ meats of wild game, all clean), that was hormone-, antibiotic-, and pesticide-free, naturally organic, and entirely range-fed with no genetic alteration. This diet included some eggs, when available, insects (sorry to say), and seafood.

This diet was typically moderately high in fat, calorically, at a rate estimated to have been roughly ten times our modern intake (and fat was highly coveted). This included varieties of saturated, monounsaturated, and omega-3 fats, and balanced quantities of omega-6 fats, together with abundant fat-soluble nutrients. Neo-Paleolithic, primitive human diets, as well as diets during more temperate periods amid the ice age, generally included a significant variety of vegetable matter, some fresh raw nuts and seeds, and some very limited quantities of tart, wild fruit, as was seasonally available.

There was far more plant material in the diets of our more recent ancestors than our more ancient hominid ancestors, due to different factors. The current ice age (yes, "current"), known as the Pliocene-Quaternary glaciation, started about 2.58 million years ago, around the time the first hominids appeared, during the late Pliocene era, when the spread of ice sheets in the Northern Hemisphere began. Since then, the world has seen cycles of glaciation, with ice sheets advancing during extended time periods called *glacials* (glacial advance) and retreating during time periods called *interglacials* (glacial retreat). The earth is currently in an interglacial period, and the last glacial period ended close to 11,500 years ago.

In 1976, scientists at the Lamont-Doherty Earth Observatory spearheaded a project called Climate: Long-Range Investigation Mapping and Prediction (CLIMAP) to map the history of the oceans and climates. They exhaustively studied core samples and discovered that major cooling and glacial advances begin or end, almost like clockwork, every 11,500 years. Every one hundred thousand years or so, this transition to a major, especially brutal deep freeze occurs in a surprisingly abrupt manner, at times over no more than a few seasons. They refer to this regularly varying cycle of cooling periods as the Milankovitch cycle, also sometimes referred to as "the pacemaker of the ice ages."

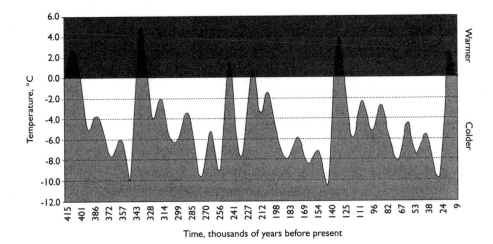

Fig. 1.1. Earth's average temperatures over the past 415,000 years. The dark peaks represent warm climatic periods. Human civilization emerged only during the last warming peak, which followed a 107,000 year-long ice age. We have spent most of our human history in ice age. From: J. R. Petit, J. Jouzel, D. Raynaud, et al. "Climate and Atmospheric History of the Past 420,000 Years from the Vostok Ice Core, Antarctica," *Nature* 399, no. 6735 (1999): 429–36.

There can be no question that our physiology is profoundly influenced by this climatologic history. We have spent highly significant time periods during our ancestral history locked in the grip of mostly ice and snow, with only the briefest periods of warmer reprieve when edible plant life could have grown over a significant portion of the Northern Hemisphere. Periodic swings in climatic conditions, from relatively brief periods of reasonably temperate conditions to prolonged, harsh, ice age conditions, are more recently understood by climatologists to have been relatively rapid.

Back in the late 1980s, a group of scientists known as the Greenland Ice Core Project (GRIP) drilled cores almost two miles deep into the ice, drilling deep enough to reach ice that had formed 250,000 years ago. By analyzing the data this provided, it was realized that each and every ice age during the last 250,000 years actually began quite abruptly, typically (ironically) following spikes in global temperature. Each time this change occurred, the climate descended into full-blown glacial severity within less than twenty years, sometimes well within ten years! Only those people adapted in their physiology and cunning would have survived such sudden onsets of frigid, and unforgiving conditions (Calvin 2002). Even while the Northern Hemisphere was gripped in snow and ice during these periods, Africa was being ripped apart by droughts and wildfires, with catastrophic areas of flooding elsewhere. During any ice age, the entire planet endures a relentless range of such extremes.

Studies of ancient human coprolites, or fossilized human feces, dating anywhere from three hundred thousand to as recent as fifty thousand years ago, have revealed essentially a complete lack of any plant material in the diets of the subjects studied (Bryant and Williams-Dean 1975). In other words, it is likely we subsisted for a very significant portion of our evolution largely on the meat and fat of animals we hunted. Fat was *the* prime commodity for its concentrated nutrient and energy value. This has even been true of neo-Paleolithic hunter-gatherers and traditional societies, as clearly shown by the exhaustive scientific work of Weston A. Price first published in 1939 (Price 1989). As omnivores and opportunists, we would always have certainly procured whatever might have been available to us for food. Permafrosts and droughts, however, left many of us limited options for long stretches of time. Fat, too, is our most efficient, dense, and prolonged-burning fuel. It is essential for an important multitude of bodily processes, not the least of which is the functioning of the human brain.

Another important limitation stems from the fact that we as a species have only relatively recently developed a universally controlled use of fire. By most accounts, this did not occur before fifty thousand to one hundred thousand years ago. Although scattered evidence of fire exists from as far back as three hundred thousand to four hundred thousand years ago, it is unlikely that the sophisticated development of cooking practices occurred much before the use of fire became more universal and commonplace—sometime after Cro-Magnon man migrated into Europe. (The oldest-known pottery dates only as far back as 6800 BCE, incidentally.)

What makes the use of cooking especially significant is the toxicity of most plant species. Wild plants contain any number of toxic compounds that would have made their use as food in any significant quantity perilous. Cooking is the only means by which many of these "antinutrients" can be neutralized.

Modern produce has been genetically modified to reduce the presence of harmful compounds to a significant extent. Most wild plants, on the other hand, require extremely careful selection and preparation. Most starchy roots, tubers, and legumes would have been prohibitively dangerous to consume without extensive cooking. Furthermore, the energy expended in the procurement of the remaining types of plant foods easily exceeds their potential caloric value, to say little of their meager, inferior available protein content, which is so critical to our needs. Mass die-offs of megafauna following the last ice age ten thousand years ago and overhunting by humans may have led to an increased dependence on plant foods and ultimately to the development of agriculture. Some people also hypothesize that it was an addiction to the exorphins (morphinelike compounds) in grains that sparked this widespread development.

A recent article published online by CNN revealed the "shocking" news that evidence had been discovered proving that our Neanderthal cousins cooked and ate veggies, and perhaps a few grains along the way (Said 2010). Well, *of course* as omnivorous hominids they would have eaten almost anything to stay alive. Presumably, we noshed on a grain or two (as certain wild species do exist) scraped up here and there when meat was scarce. Where else would we have gotten the idea to start using them more extensively later on? *Of course* we knew they were edible! This is a *far* cry away from Neanderthals getting behind a plow for eight hours a day in the field, baking bread, or eating Grape Nuts for breakfast. Setting aside the fact that Neanderthals are now known to have evolved down a very different hominid line from us, I am still comfortable assuming our Cro-Magnon forebears experimented with eating a variety of things, including the occasional handful of (nongenetically modified) grains—even enjoying a little salad-bar fare once in a while, as the environmental conditions allowed. Who wouldn't enjoy a bit of asparagus with her steak?

Nonetheless, it is widely accepted that it was, in fact, our extended dependence on the meat and fat of animals (rich in eicosapentaenoic acid, or EPA; and docosahexaenoic acid, or DHA) through these frozen winters of unimaginable duration that allowed for the rapid enlargement and development of the human brain. Meat and especially fat would have been the most coveted and important commodities of all. We *never* would have survived as a species without them.

Our increased dependence on hunting also likely helped facilitate and develop the very human qualities that we most intrinsically value—cunning, cooperation, altruism, sharing, advanced creativity, the power to foresee the future and to be able to call upon the past in terms of the future, the capacity to evaluate with complexity, and the ability to imagine solutions—qualities not particularly found in other primates (Ardrey 1976). Also, interestingly, the dominant form of fatty acids in the human brain is omega-3; in chimps and other primates, it is mostly omega-6. This is a very significant distinction and one that is the likely result of these evolutionary, ice age–induced dietary changes.

Many authors popularizing the notion of Paleolithic diets base their conclusive evidence on the diets of more-contemporary primitive peoples, forgetting that for most of our evolution, the world has been a very, very different place. Either way, it is evident from even the most recent analysis of primitive diets that animal-source foods and fat-soluble nutrients invariably play a critical, central role in such peoples' extraordinary physical and mental health and freedom from disease, as characterized in primitive peoples and more traditional groups. It is also quite evident that diets consisting of any significant quantity of carbohydrates are a strictly modern phenomenon, one that our ice age human physiology has evolved little adaptation to—or defense against.

Carbohydrates, other than the largely indigestible variety found in fibrous vegetables and greens, have generally played a minimal role at best through most of human evolution. Fruit was consumed only seasonally by our neo-Paleolithic ancestors in most places, and wild fruit is extremely fibrous and smaller in size, with less total sugar content. Many potatoes and tubers would have required extensive cooking to neutralize extremely toxic alkaloids. Wild varieties that would have been available to us through most of our history as a species can be especially toxic.

In other words, it isn't likely we were eating baked potatoes with our woolly mammoth steaks—or much starch at all.

In fact, of all the macronutrients (that is, protein, fats, and carbohydrates), the only ones for which there are no actual human dietary requirements are carbohydrates. This is a critical and very fundamental point to remember: **we don't ever have to eat any sugar or starch of any kind at all in order to be optimally healthy.**

Our bodies can manufacture glucose, as needed, from a combination of protein and fat in the diet. As a matter of fact, glucose is really needed only in an ongoing way mainly for fueling our red blood cells.

Most organs and tissues in the body, including the brain, actually prefer, if we let them, to use *ketones,* the energy-producing by-products from the metabolism of fats. This fact is very overlooked or misunderstood by the majority of medical and nutritional experts. There is abundant evidence that many modern disease processes, including those resulting in cardiovascular disease, elevated triglyceride levels, obesity, hypertension, diabetes, hypoglycemia, and cancer, to name a few, are the product *not* of excess natural fat in the diet, but of excess carbohydrates. Other contributing factors certainly include ultra-prevalent and unnatural trans fats; rancid fats; unnaturally high quantities of dietary omega-6 fatty acids from vegetable oils; heavy metals and other pollutants; artificial chemicals and additives; and the widespread use of xenoestrogens, the artificial estrogen-like compounds used in pesticides, lotions, shampoos, plastics, and many other common household items, cosmetics, and cleaning supplies.

Current marketing ploys and diet dictocrats unrelentingly cling to other notions, despite overwhelming and well-documented evidence to the contrary. More modern ills can be traced to chronic carbohydrate consumption than to any other single factor. Trans fats might come in at a close second. Note that trans fats are industrially produced, *artificially* saturated fats, which may also be identified on labels as "hydrogenated" or "partially hydrogenated." The method of this saturation produces an abnormal molecular configuration that is unrecognizable by the human body and therefore is inclined to be highly problematic in its effects.

Consider, for instance, that the first four cases of coronary thrombosis ever recorded were written up in *The Journal of the American Medical Association* in 1912. This disease was unknown by the medical profession before that time, and it was considered an unusual disorder. Dr. Paul Dudley White, personal physician to President Dwight D. Eisenhower and author of the very first medical textbook on coronary heart disease, had never heard the words *coronary thrombosis* when he graduated from medical school in 1911. When, as a physician, he decided to specialize in this newly emerging field of "coronary heart disease," his colleagues suggested he find an area of specialty that was more profitable. But by the 1950s, it was one of the leading causes of death among Americans. However, the consumption of animal proteins and saturated fat had been going on for one hundred thousand generations prior to that time. What had suddenly changed?

The quality, nutrient-laden dietary fats richly present in the organ meats, fatty fish, bone marrow, and tallows favored by humans throughout 2.6 million years of evolution constituted 60 percent or more of some primitive cultures' caloric intake—all without detriment to the heart. This consumption of naturally occurring dietary fat did not, all of a sudden, become problematic. It was, in fact, the advent of the food industry, leading to increased consumption of refined "Franken-foods," vegetable or hydrogenated trans fats, and sugar or carbohydrates, that more clearly and reasonably correlates to such a statistic.

And it was the combined egos of medical theoreticians and the designs of greedy, unscrupulous members of the vegetable oil industry that gave birth to and perpetuated the myth of the dietary heart disease hypothesis. The dietary heart disease hypothesis sought to vilify saturated fat and cholesterol as the culprits in heart disease. What started out as a plausible hypothesis has never, ever been proved, despite extensive efforts and millions of dollars spent. Today, there are billions upon billions of dollars—from government agencies, medical-establishment interests, the pharmaceutical industry, organizations such as the American Heart Association, and, let's not forget, the ever-popular food industry—all invested in the perpetuation of the antisaturated fat and anticholesterol agenda. This sordid history is well documented, though poorly publicized, as the media are beholden to their corporate advertisers.

Dr. George V. Mann, noted researcher in the Framingham Heart Study, stated, "On-going issues of pride, profit and prejudice cause outdated and never-proven notions of the saturated fat/cholesterol hypotheses to persist despite a lack of supportive evidence in the medical literature." In fact, the Framingham study—long considered the most important dietary-related heart study to date—presented data that can only be a secretly shattering disappointment to those keen on promoting the dietary heart disease hypothesis. Claims by biased investigators that the difference in cholesterol value from 182 to 244 led to an increase in heart disease by 240 percent were shown clearly by forty years of Framingham data to be in actuality a potential increase in risk of no more than **0.13 percent.** This is hardly damning evidence in favor of reducing saturated fat and cholesterol in the diet. In this range, there is virtually no difference among any individuals relative to their risk of coronary heart disease. Interestingly, in those people with cholesterol levels between 244 and 294, the rate of coronary heart disease *actually declined!*

Study after study (such as Framingham, the Minnesota State Hospital Trial, the Veterans Clinical Trial, the Puerto Rico Heart Health Study, and the Honolulu Heart Program) has shown a consistently distinct lack of correlation between dietary fat, dietary or serum cholesterol, and heart disease. Autopsy studies of vegetarians show the same degree of athero-sclerosis as nonvegetarians, despite a commonly lower level of serum cholesterol and fewer dietary sources of saturated fat and cholesterol. A group of scientists known as the International Atherosclerosis Project analyzed thirty-one thousand autopsies from fifteen countries and found **zero** correlation among animal fat intake, atherosclerotic disease, and serum cholesterol levels.

The fixation on cholesterol levels and recommendations toward eliminating dietary saturated fat and cholesterol bewilderingly persists to this day, despite an overwhelming degree of evidence to the contrary. Michael Gurr, Ph.D., a renowned lipid expert and coauthor of the textbook *Lipid Biochemistry,* said, "Whatever causes coronary heart disease it is not primarily from a high intake of saturated fat." He went on to refer to the steadfast preoccupation with the antisaturated fat and anticholesterol agenda as "the degree of self delusion in research workers wedded to a particular hypothesis despite the contrary evidence" (Fallon and Enig 1996). In the quest for answers with respect to the causative factors in coronary heart disease, there are many more viable contenders to more realistically blame: the increased consumption of dietary sugar and starch (and the development of AGEs and/or insulin resistance), certain vitamin and mineral deficiencies, elevated homocysteine levels, food sensitivities, damage from free radicals, inflammation (due to increased C-reactive protein levels; *H. pylori* overgrowth; intake of vegetable oils, omega-6 fats, trans-fats, or dietary sugars; or food sensitivity issues), stress, a lack of exercise, consumption of pasteurized milk products, and others.

United States Department of Agriculture (USDA) data from the early 1900s clearly show dramatic shifts away from animal fats and increases in the consumption of industrially produced vegetable oils, hydrogenated or trans fats like margarine and Crisco, refined flours, and, of course, sugar.

Note the following illustrations.

Enter: the food industry

It is increasingly clear from the current medical literature that many of the chronic, degenerative diseases and other uniquely modern disease processes are readily attributable not to natural saturated fats and cholesterol but to something increasingly known as *syndrome X,* more recently referred to as *metabolic syndrome.* Essentially, it is insulin resistance.

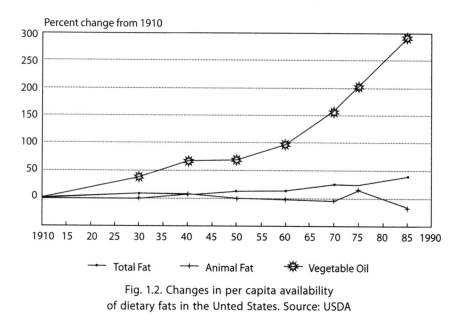

Fig. 1.2. Changes in per capita availability
of dietary fats in the Unted States. Source: USDA

Syndrome X, or metabolic syndrome, is both created and exacerbated primarily by chronic carbohydrate consumption in combination with dietary trans fats, unnaturally abundant omega-6 fats (vegetable oils), and, to some extent, potentially even excess omega-9 fats (oleic and olive oils).

Other contributors to insulin resistance include stress; food sensitivities; dieting; caffeine and other stimulants; sleep deprivation; alcohol; tobacco; steroids; lack of exercise; all prescription, over-the-counter, and recreational drugs; and excess or unnecessary thyroid replacement therapy. *Most important, insulin resistance is primarily a phenomenon associated with a diet deficient in protein and fats but overabundant in carbohydrates* (Schwarzbein and Deville 1999).

> It seems reasonable to suggest that resistance to insulin-mediated glucose disposal and the manner in which the organism responds to this defect play major roles in the pathogenesis and clinical course of what are often referred to as diseases of Western civilization.
>
> GERALD M. REAVEN, M.D., "PATHOPHYSIOLOGY OF
> INSULIN RESISTANCE IN HUMAN DISEASE," *PHYSIOLOGICAL REVIEWS*

It is clear that low-fat diets, promoted by numerous U.S. government agencies and even more numerous heavily funded health organizations, have

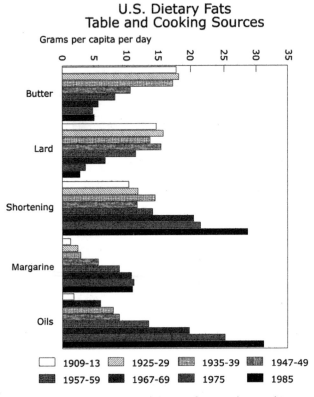

Fig. 1.3. Changes in consumption of dietary fats used in cooking in the Unted States. Source: Human Nutrition Information Survey—USDA

not prevented heart disease (which is still on the rise); obesity (now affecting more than an estimated 58 percent of the American public); diabetes (the most common result of insulin resistance, now recognized by the World Health Organization as epidemic and affecting as many as three out of five people and rapidly rising, even in children); cancer (now exceeding heart disease as the leading cause of death in the United States); or any of the other disease processes that the eating of low-fat diets—especially low-saturated-fat diets—is supposed to prevent. The numbers continue to climb.

Mood disorders, learning disabilities, attention deficit disorder (ADD), more commonly referred to as attention deficit hyperactivity disorder (ADHD), autism, Asperger's disorder, anxiety disorders, and immune- or autoimmune-related diseases are also equally unprecedented in our history and are rapidly on the rise. Although total dietary fat consumption has risen since 1900, fats coming from animal sources have substantially decreased in the American diet, while dietary vegetable fats, including trans fats, have risen almost exponentially. And many of these fats have entered the human diet within the past hundred years, for the first time in human evolution. In fact, the number one source of fat calories in America today is soybean oil, nearly all of which is partially hydrogenated and a prevalent source of dangerous trans fat.

Concomitantly, the percentage of the Western diet composed of carbohydrates, from all sources, is of a proportion equally unprecedented in all of human history. The overall, number one source of dietary calories at this time in the United States is actually *high fructose corn syrup,* an extremely toxic industrial sweetener found in almost all processed foods.

> The diet-heart hypothesis (that suggests that high intake of fat and cholesterol causes heart disease) has been repeatedly shown to be wrong, and yet, for complicated reasons of pride, profit and prejudice, the hypothesis continues to be exploited by scientists, fund-raising enterprises, food companies, and even governmental agencies. The public is being deceived by the greatest health scam of the century.
>
> GEORGE V. MANN, M.D.,
> RESEARCHER WITH THE FRAMINGHAM HEART STUDY,
> *CORONARY HEART DISEASE: THE DIETARY SENSE AND NONSENSE*

The agricultural revolution did not take place until roughly ten thousand years ago, probably as a result of necessity, with an increase in human populations and a decreased availability of wild game in certain regions of the world. This may have been due in part to extinctions of megafauna following the last ice age and possibly overhunting. The addictive nature of grains (due to their containing morphinelike compounds called *exorphins*) may have also played a significant role in their widespread adoption as a food source. The implementation of agriculture was far from an immediately universal phenomenon, however, and thousands of hunter-gatherer societies continued to thrive worldwide. Recent estimations assert that agriculture was not widely implemented in Europe until little more than two thousand years ago. By most accounts, it takes roughly forty thousand to one hundred thousand years for human genetic expression to adapt significantly to such a major change. We have yet to physiologically adapt to the agricultural revolution.

Consequently, it is logical to conclude and easy to demonstrate that modern agricultural foods such as grains and legumes, corn, wheat, soy, and so on are foods that are not especially compatible with optimal human health, particularly when consumed in any significant quantity. Grain consumption has been linked with allergies, food sensitivities, autoimmune disorders, colon cancer, pancreatic disorders, mineral deficiencies, celiac disease, epilepsy, cerebellar ataxias, dementia, degenerative diseases of the brain and central nervous system, peripheral neuropathies of axonal or demyelinating types, and myopathies as well as autism and schizophrenia, to name a few (Cordain 2002). Legumes are particularly rich in starch—roughly 60 percent of their composition—and contain numerous antinutrients that can cause mineral deficiencies and other problems.

There was, in fact, a marked decline in human stature, bone density, dental development, and overall health, including an increase in birth defects, malnutrition, and degenerative disease, following the early implementation of an agricultural lifestyle. Anthropologists and archaeologists know this well.

Our modern ability to transport fresh produce and broader varieties of fresh foods during all seasons throughout much of the industrialized world allows for greater varieties of foods in various regions and has helped improve health considerably. Such advances, unfortunately, are entirely dependent on the use of limited fossil fuels.

Even those cultures adopting the early agricultural lifestyle typically included as many animal-source foods as were available to them. No known primitive culture in the history of the human species has ever adopted vegetarianism by choice.

It is a popular misconception that prehistoric humans usually died when they were around twenty years old, so it didn't matter how much meat or fat or how few carbohydrates they ate because they didn't live long enough to develop heart disease or any of the other modern disorders that meat and fat consumption supposedly cause. This twenty- to forty-year figure that is commonly batted around as the average age of death for prehistoric humans is no more than exactly that: the average age of death. It incorporates infant mortality, as well. The figure, often misrepresented, states nothing about the rate of aging or maximum life span of our prehistoric ancestors. Authors and physicians Michael R. Eades and Mary Dan Eades wrote, "Other methods of determining true probable life span, as well as a look at modern hunter-gatherer societies, show it was probably about the same as ours" (Eades and Eades 2000).

It is important to note also that the above figures are frequently confused with postagricultural time period mortality statistics.

It is clear that postagricultural peoples became shorter in stature and had much higher rates of osteoporosis, rickets, and other bone-mineral disorders. They were also plagued with vitamin and mineral deficiencies not shared by their Stone Age ancestors: scurvy, beriberi, pellagra, and vitamin A and zinc deficiencies, together with iron deficiency anemia—all endemic to cereal-based diets. They had tooth decay, skeletal abnormalities, and maloccluded dental arches. They had infectious diseases in far greater numbers, more childhood mortality, and a decidedly shorter life span. Prehistoric or preagricultural humans had the capability to live as long as we do, without all our high-tech "health care"; they simply didn't have as comparatively controlled an environment and, as a result, were far more prone to accident and infection. In other words, "What we're actually comparing when we compare our average age of death to theirs is, in reality, the relative hostility of our two environments" (Eades and Eades 2000).

This is also misleading, however, since it is clear that primitive societies did not experience the same ranges of degenerative or chronic diseases shared by their early agricultural descendants or our modern-day populace. The primary causes of death in Stone Age societies were typically accident and infection. If one managed to get around those two primary causes of death as well as infant mortality, one stood a good chance of leading a long, healthful, and vibrant life, free of most of the chronic and degenerative diseases so prevalent in our aging population today.

It is also a popular misconception that people in primitive cultures were a great deal more physically active than modern humans are today and could therefore afford to eat a diet higher in fat and calories. The evidence from numerous anthropological studies of hunter-gatherer cultures suggests a typical "workday" of no more than about three hours, including procurement of food, housing, and clothing. And there were no jogging shoes or gym memberships. This is in sharp contrast to the lifestyle of postagricultural farmers, known to work eight or more hours a day performing often backbreaking labor in the field. Agriculture may have spawned civilization (not to mention overpopulation), but it clearly was not the fast track to easy living or radiant health. We paid a price for the change, as has our beleaguered planetary environment.

The bottom line is that we had access to most, if not all, of our dietary or physiological requirements long before the agricultural revolution, and *those requirements have not changed.*

Diets consistent with these principles and having a substantially higher nutrient content than our current diet, particularly of the fat-soluble nutrients, according to numerous anthropological studies, have, for hundreds of thousands of years, been consistent with superior health, strong and lean physical structure, and freedom from the chronic or degenerative illnesses so common today.

High carbohydrate consumption—sugary, starchy, and refined—and the vast tidal waves of insulin generated as a result are strictly modern phenomena that our primitive physiologies are ill suited for. One only need go and stand at a Safeway checkout line to see what the majority of people place on the checkout conveyer belt, and one can visibly see how that has affected their physical, and even mental, health. It certainly stands to reason that if something on the grocery store shelf would not have looked like food to someone walking around with a loincloth and a spear forty or fifty thousand years ago, it probably isn't food for us now, either (Eaton et al. 1997). (See the average contemporary hunter-gatherer nutrient intake table.)

AVERAGE CONTEMPORARY
HUNTER-GATHERER NUTRIENT INTAKE

NUTRIENT	PALEOLITHIC INTAKE	RDA	U.S. INTAKE
Vitamin C	604 mg	60 mg	77–109 mg
Vitamin E	33 mg	8–10 mg	7–10 mg
Calcium	1,956 mg	800–1200 mg	750 mg
Magnesium	700 mg	350 mg	250 mg
Potassium	10,500 mg	3,500 mg	2,500 mg
Zinc	43 mg	12–15 mg	5–14 mg
Fiber	50–104 grams	25–35 grams	10 grams

Source: Eaton, S. B., et al. 1997. "Paleolithic nutrition revisted: twelve year retrospective on its nature and implications." *European Journal of Clinical Nutrition* 51: 207–16.

Fig. 1.4. Nutrient intake of the average contemporary hunter-gatherer

The Prehistoric Food Pyramid the USDA
(and Other Vested Interests)
Didn't Want You to See

If one were to construct a food pyramid designed around a diet closely resembling that of our preagricultural ancestors, it would most easily appear as on page 20—mercifully leaving out insects and grubs for the sake of more-delicate modern-day culinary sensibilities.

This chart clearly contrasts with the largely scientifically unfounded USDA food pyramid so commonly promoted by registered dietitians and nutritionists, the same people who design hospital and school lunch menus. No human society in history has consumed a diet remotely resembling what the USDA pyramid suggests as optimal.

There are more than fifteen thousand papers on the subject of Paleolithic or primitive nutrition and innumerable books on the subject written by a variety of scholars and scientists in a variety of fields. No one owns this information, though many have borrowed from it. This is not a formulary approach to diet and health that requires a written

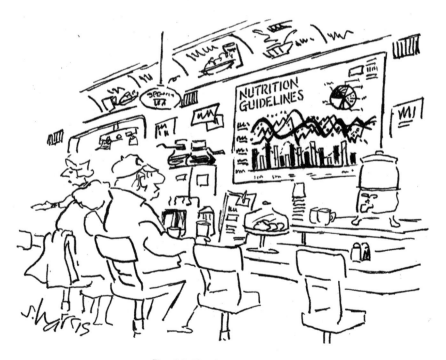

Fig. 1.5. Nutrition Guidelines?

guide. It is not a fad diet—or if it is, then it's the oldest fad diet known to humankind. Eating a diet as similar as possible to what our ancestors ate is purely common sense and is based entirely on how we have been genetically molded for the vast majority of human evolution. No gurus needed. Eat the way your body was designed for you to eat, and a lot takes care of itself.

The USDA Food Pyramid should be renamed "The Feedlot Pyramid." Its nutrient profile is the same as swine-fattening chow. And it is fattening the population in the same way.

MICHAEL R. EADES AND MARY DAN EADES,
*THE PROTEIN POWER LIFEPLAN: A NEW
COMPREHENSIVE BLUEPRINT FOR OPTIMAL HEALTH*

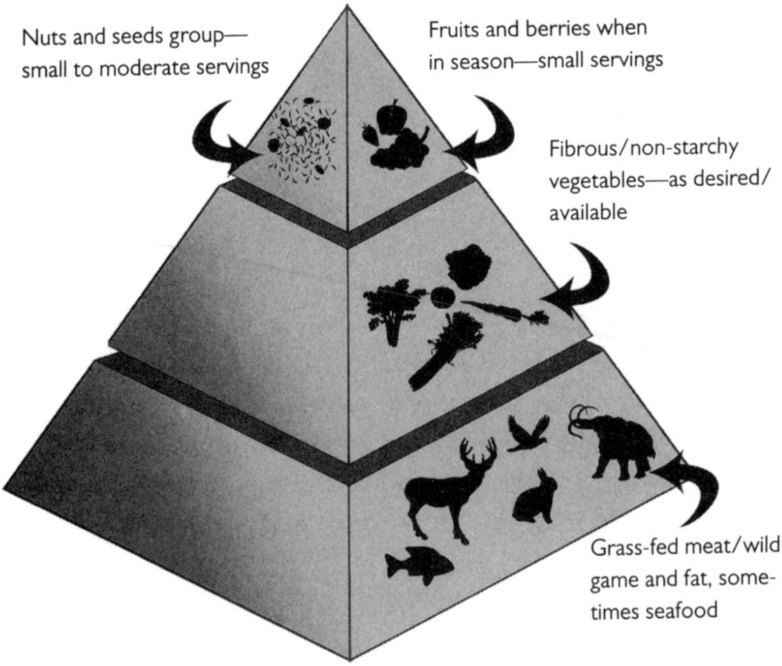

Nuts and seeds group— small to moderate servings

Fruits and berries when in season—small servings

Fibrous/non-starchy vegetables—as desired/ available

Grass-fed meat/wild game and fat, some-times seafood

Fig. 1.6. The prehistoric food pyramid the U.S. Department of Agriculture (and other vested interests) didn't want you to see

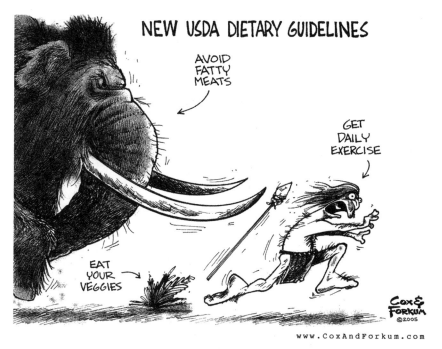

Fig. 1.7. "Caveman Diet"

Are Genes Really Everything
They're Cracked Up to Be?

Throughout your life the most profound influences on your health, vitality and function are not the doctors you have visited or the drugs, surgery or other therapies you have undertaken. The most profound influences are the cumulative effects of the decisions you make about your diet and lifestyle on the expression of your genes.

JEFFREY S. BLAND, PH.D., *GENETIC NUTRITIONEERING*

A great deal of press is being given today to the idea that we may have—through no fault of our own—a silent killer, or two or three, lurking in the entanglement of DNA deep within our cells. It's the ultimate boogeyman, a terrorist "sleeper cell" right inside our own bodies, lying in wait for just the right moment to unleash its deadliest intent. Everyone is running to get tested for his or her genetic profile in an effort to prepare for the unspeakable inevitability of any number of diseases. The medical establishment, not unlike homeland security, could not be more delighted to feed the rampant paranoia and offer, at a price, everything from pharmaceutical to surgical preventives to help save us from ourselves.

Although there is certainly some merit to the science of genetics, its revelations are more commonly abused, or blown entirely out of proportion, than related to any actual inherent threat. Our genes really aren't that special. We all have twenty-two thousand of them, far fewer than the Human Genome Project expected to find. We all have all sorts of genes for all sorts of things, good and bad. Not all are actively expressed—a decidedly good thing. Many remain dormant. Genes, however, do not lie in wait like some hungry, vicious predator waiting eagerly to pounce on you when you least expect it. *A gene will not express itself at all unless the environment surrounding it becomes favorable to that expression.* A cancer gene, for instance, needs certain environmental requirements to be met before it can activate. In other words, as Bruce Lipton wrote in his book *The Biology of Belief,* "It's the environment, stupid!"

The key isn't genetics; it's epigenetics.

Epigenetics can be described as the study of the heritable changes in gene expression that occur without a change in gene sequence, causing an organism's genes to behave (or "express themselves") differently. In an article published in the journal *Reproductive Toxicology,* the authors wrote, "If the genome is compared with the hardware in a computer, the epigenome is the software that directs the computer's operation. . . . A growing body of evidence suggests that epigenetic mechanisms of gene regulation, such as DNA methylation and chromatin modification, are also *influenced by the environment* and *play an important role* in the fetal basis of adult disease susceptibility. . . . Identifying epigenetic targets and defining how they are dysregulated in human disease by environmental exposures will allow for the development of innovative novel diagnostic, treatment, and prevention strategies that *target the epigenomic software* rather than the *genomic hardware*" (Dolinoy et al. 2007). In other words, it is not the genes themselves that predispose us to disease, but rather those things within our diet and environment that act upon our genes. **To a very great extent, we have control over this.**

The prefix *epi-* means "over," so the term *epigenetics* suggests those things that have influence *over* our genes. In another article, published in the peer-reviewed journal *Nutritional Perspectives,* the authors wrote, "The previous view that nutrients interact with human physiology only at the metabolic/post-transcriptional level must be updated in light of current research showing that nutrients can, in fact, modify human physiology and phenotype at the genetic/pre-transcriptional level" (Vasquez 2005). This influence of food and nutrients as the primary factor of importance in epigenetics is further narrowed in the field of nutrigenomics (the study of how different foods and their constituents can interact with specific genes to increase or lessen the risk of common chronic diseases).

Even by the most conservative standards in genetics, we actually control anywhere from a "low" of 80 percent to upward of 97 percent or more of our own genetic expression with respect to potential disease processes and even longevity. Genes are turned on and off by regulatory genes, and *regulatory genes are controlled mainly by nutrients.* Environmental chemical exposure also certainly plays a role.

Foods, however, fundamentally serve as our basic genetic instruction and guidance information. The thing to consider here is that our genes reside within the cells, and the nutrients that best protect them from mutation or undesirable influences are those that are best able to cross the cellular membrane into the matrix of the cell. For this, *fat-soluble* nutrients and antioxidants are critical as well as being long overlooked and underestimated in importance and value.

By keeping the public focused on the all-importance of genes themselves, the message conveyed to us is one of a basically predetermined helplessness, except through the possibilities afforded by modern medical technology (and its funding thereof). Poppycock. Those with vested interests in keeping you hostage to the illusion of your own inner "genetic threat" would rather you weren't aware of the fact that there is *no drug anywhere* that can regulate genetic expression better or more powerfully than your diet can.

2
So, What's for Dinner?

■■■■■■■■■■■

Although it is nearly impossible to replicate a truly Paleolithic diet in our modern everyday life (who has time to hunt and gather any more?), certain fundamental principles are easily derived and applied.

It is important to emphasize that once upon a time, literally everything we ate was free-range, fully grass-fed, and organic. It should be obvious that factory-farmed meat laden with chemicals, hormones, antibiotics, and pesticides that is further insulted by irradiation to extend shelf life is not quality food. Animals raised to provide such meat also lead tortured lives and are fed foods that are unnatural to them, including grain, which is used to fatten them up (take a hint). Grain-fattened animals yield a distinctly altered fatty-acid profile with unnaturally high omega-6 fatty acid levels and virtually no omega-3 fatty acids, which are otherwise found in highly significant quantities in wild game and exclusively pasture-fed animals. The same is true, unfortunately, of farm-raised seafood. (See the following illustration, borrowed with permission from Jo Robinson's book *Pasture Perfect*.) It is also logical to conclude that genetically engineered, pesticide-laden produce grown in mineral-depleted soil does not promote optimal health or longevity.

This being said, it can be a comfort to know that it is entirely possible to obtain clean, quality, humanely raised, grass-fed poultry and eggs, beef, lamb, and organ meats. These can come from easily available sources ranging from various co-ops and certain grocery markets to the farmers themselves. For the more adventuresome, venison, elk, buffalo, ostrich, and other more exotic varieties of game meat can be found via

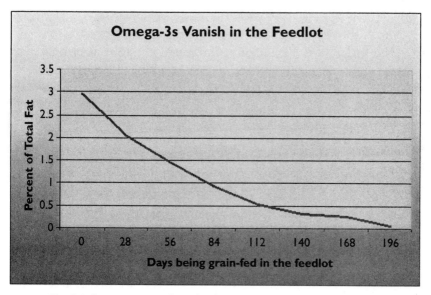

Fig. 2.1. Omega-3s vanish in the feedlot. Source: *Journal of Animal Science* (1993) 71(8): 2079–88

the Internet and at some of the better meat counters (although these can be expensive). Wild-caught seafood of all kinds and organic vegetables and greens, seeds, fresh nuts, berries, and some (just some) fruits are abundantly available.

Eating never has to be dull. Nor need it be too costly.

Some may argue that this seems like it would be an expensive way to eat. Putting aside the alternative specter of the ongoing and eventual health costs associated with the modern, conventional Western diet, one can save a tremendous amount of revenue merely by avoiding processed, prepackaged, refined, nutrient-devoid junk foods and beverages and putting the savings from that toward whole, unprocessed, organic vegetables and free-range meats with a minimum of financial difficulty. Nutrient-dense quality meats, fats, and vegetables are readily satisfying, and smaller amounts of food are far more filling. Naturally occurring fat, which our ancestors would have sought out as much as possible, is inherently satisfying to the appetite.

It is also a simple matter in many places either to grow a small vegetable garden of one's own in a backyard or community-garden plot or to shop seasonal farmers' markets, where produce is most affordable. Community-supported agriculture programs, also known as CSAs, are abundant and allow for considerable savings on a huge variety of organic, biodynamically grown produce—especially when orders are split with friends or neighbors. And organic, free-range, exclusively grass-fed meat, poultry, and eggs, even raw milk, can be readily purchased from family farms in your area. This is highly recommended as one can easily purchase meats in larger quantities to be stored in a chest freezer for convenience and considerable long-term savings.

This is also an advantage from the standpoint of having firsthand knowledge of where one's food is actually coming from—something conspicuously lacking in our modern-day world. Personally, I would much rather support the honest and ethical efforts of a small, local family farmer than the vast, faceless, and greed-driven food industry or the conglomerates of factory farms that care nothing for the nutritional content of what they produce, the health of their consumers, or the environment. For others, hunting or fishing for their food can be a viable option. This does not have to be expensive! Good-quality food can be within almost anyone's financial reach with a little resourcefulness and, initially at least, a little extra time.

Contacting a local chapter of the Weston A. Price Foundation (described in more detail in appendix E) can put one in touch with resources, recipes, cooking classes, and other families with which one can seek support and helpful ideas. Foundation members can pool resources to purchase membership in CSAs and can also be a wealth of information. See www.WestonAPrice.org for details. Additional resources for locating grass-fed meats and other such foods as well as other useful websites can be found in appendix G. A summary of general guidelines and suggestions for getting started on your road to health is in appendix A.

Things to Generally Avoid, Aside from the Obvious

Excess consumption of sugar, starch, and cereal-based carbohydrates *is easily the most destructive dietary tendency today.* It is a rampant problem, leading to heart disease, obesity, diabetes, cancer, and many other degenerative disorders as well as numerous mental health and cognitive problems.

As a whole, it is entirely preferable to avoid starch such as that found in rice and white or red potatoes, which contain easily one-quarter cup or more of very damaging high glycemic, glycating sugar, as well as anything containing gluten, including cereals, breads, pastas, and all the plethora of hidden sources.

Most conventionally produced dairy products are also best avoided. Milk, especially the "low-fat" variety, is very high in carbohydrates; heavy cream, however, has essentially none. Some traditional societies that raised grass-fed sheep, goats, and cattle were shown to have thrived on raw, whole-fat, unpasteurized, organic, grass-fed, hormone-free, antibiotic-free and pesticide-free, unhomogenized milk, cream, cheese, and nutrient-rich butter. Such dairy products are commercially unavailable at this time in most public markets, with the exception of some imported raw-milk cheeses (delicious!), but there are some online quality raw-dairy sources (see www.organicpastures.com). A list of states in which certified raw-milk products are legal can be found by contacting A Campaign for Real Milk (www.RealMilk.com) or at www.eatwild.com. (Nationwide sources of grass-fed meats can also be found on the latter website.)

Small amounts of raw, unprocessed dairy products *can* be healthful, if desired, *but only if they are well tolerated.* Butter and heavy cream can be used more liberally by all but those people who are casein sensitive. Butter oils and ghee are casein-free and therefore essentially safe for people otherwise sensitive to dairy products. **Do beware of sensitivity to casein (a milk protein);** it's a growing and increasingly common issue (very often accompanying gluten sensitivity), leading to numerous health problems that decidedly need to be taken seriously. Don't just assume you don't have a certain food sensitivity because you "haven't noticed any symptoms." Often, only careful testing using Cyrex Labs proprietary salivary arrays (www.cyrexlabs.com) or a stool antigen test (www.enterolab.com) can reveal this issue with reasonable accuracy. False-negative results (which show that a condition isn't present when it really is) when using standard blood tests are notoriously common. In fact, blood tests for food sensitivity issues that show "negative reactions" usually aren't more than 30 percent accurate, on average—hardly something to hang your hat on. Don't rely on them when they come up negative. Positive results are almost always accurate, however.

Don't expect to just know whether you happen to be casein sensitive or not. I didn't. Tests or elimination/provocation diets are the best available means of ascertaining whether it is an issue for you.

Pasteurized and especially ultrapasteurized milk products contain rancid fats and oxidized cholesterol and are especially likely to aggravate casein-related food-sensitivity issues. Low-fat (skim, 1 percent, and 2 percent) milks contain large amounts of oxidized cholesterol because powdered, denatured whole milk gets added in after the cream is removed in processing to add "body" to the texture. These milk products are highly processed and made up mainly of carbohydrates, and should be entirely avoided. They wouldn't even look like food to a baby cow.

Raw, organic, pasture-fed butter or ghee can be an especially rich source of commonly deficient but beneficial nutrients, including vitamin A, conjugated linolenic acid, and selenium as well as a beneficial substance known as *X-factor*, which is found only in butter from entirely pasture-fed animals. As such, butter or ghee can be included liberally in the diet. In addition, raw butter, milk, and cream contain the Wulzen factor, otherwise known as the "antistiffness" factor, which is potentially beneficial for healthy joints in non-casein-sensitive individuals.

Fast foods and processed snack foods such as chips, crackers, and rice cakes should always be avoided; they are laden with dangerous trans fats, processed or rancid fats, excess carbohydrates, chemical additives, and carcinogens. Save your hard-earned money for real food.

3
Grains

■ ■ ■ ■ ■ ■ ■ ■ ■ ■ ■

Are They Really a Health Food?

Grains and legumes typically contain very high levels of a substance known as *phytic acid*. Phytic acid actively binds minerals and eliminates them from the body, which results, with increased grain consumption, in widespread deficiencies of minerals, including calcium, iron, magnesium, and zinc. Legumes typically contain 60 percent starch and only relatively small amounts of *incomplete* protein, and they also contain potent protease inhibitors, which can damage one's ability to properly digest and use dietary protein and can also potentially damage the pancreas over time, when one is overly dependent on them as a source of calories.

Grains and legumes also contain *goitrogens,* or thyroid-inhibiting substances, as well as "foreign proteins" like gluten and gliadin, and they are an extremely common source of allergies and sensitivities that can lead to both physical and mental or emotional disorders, even when the best preparation methods are used. One additional hypothesis suggests that the lack of the essential amino acid L-tryptophan in grains, which are now an unnatural and primary food source for commercially raised beef and poultry (not to mention humans), may help account for rampant serotonin deficiencies, clinical depression, anxiety, and some forms of ADD/ADHD in our populations. Chronic carbohydrate consumption, in general, ultimately depletes serotonin stores and greatly depletes the B vitamins required to convert amino acids into many needed neurotransmitters.

Careful preparation by presoaking, sprouting, or fermenting these

29

foods can minimize or even eliminate phytic acid and certain other anti-nutrients. *Nonetheless, they remain a very-high-carbohydrate food source.* Many grains are also a source of an extremely damaging protein that has increasingly become a source of serious health problems for millions of people: gluten.

Since there is *no human dietary grain requirement* and since the consumption of grains causes so many known health problems due to their gluten content, antinutrient content, poor L-tryptophan profile, high omega-6 fat levels, and mainly starch-based content as well as their allergy and sensitivity potential, there is *little reason to include grains in the diet of anyone seeking optimal health.*

In fact, the fewer grains consumed, the better. Zero is by far the best.

The Weston A. Price Foundation, with whom I am proudly affiliated by membership, maintains that grains are okay since many more-traditional postagricultural societies were seemingly able to incorporate them healthfully as long as they were "properly prepared" (that is, presoaked, fermented, or sprouted). But rapid changes in the genetic robustness of our species (in our culture, particularly), especially as a result of poor prenatal diets over the last generation or two, have rendered many in today's world—particularly our children—much more vulnerable to and much more intolerant of grains, legumes, starch, milk, sugar especially, and other postagricultural and processed foods in any form. These are also very-high-carbohydrate foods.

Our genetic resilience has changed and is continuing to change for the worse at an alarming rate. Health in this country is declining rapidly; many degenerative processes and illnesses once thought to affect only our aging population are now afflicting the young—and sometimes the very young.

The money spent in the United States today on medical interventions for every imaginable type of illness is staggering. We are number one in the world in medical spending. By the year 2016, what Americans spend on so-called health care—already an astronomical two trillion dollars—is expected to *double* to more than *four trillion dollars,* according to economists with the National Health Statistics Group. Already, *sixteen cents out of every American dollar* is spent on health care. This is expected to rise to nearly twenty cents in ten years. Consequently, **out-of-pocket** consumer spending on health care alone is expected to rise to *440 billion dollars.* Things are going from bad to worse, fast. A culprit found in most grains may be a highly significant and little-appreciated contributor to these statistics.

Gluten: A "Cereal Killer"

Just What Is Gluten, Anyway?

Gluten (from the Latin word for "glue") is a substance found in numerous grains such as wheat (e.g., durum, semolina, graham, spelt, kamut, and triticale), rye, and barley. It is typically present in oats, too, due mainly to modern processing methods. Small amounts of gliadin and related compounds are also present in corn products and cornstarch. All foods with a high content of *prolamin* (a plant storage protein) should be considered suspect. This includes all cereal grains, such as wheat (which contains gliadin, see list of wheat types above), rye (which contains secalin), barley (which contains hordein), corn (which contains zein), and oats (which contain avenin). Gluten is actually made up of two proteins: gliadin (consisting of twelve different fractions) and glutenin, which make up at least 80 percent of the protein content in most grains. Used in baking, it gives bread dough its elasticity and baked goods their fluffiness and chewiness. It is also used as an additive and stabilizing agent in innumerable processed foods and personal-care products. Insanely, gluten is almost everywhere. Laws do not require its labeling on all products, so consumers are left to judge for themselves whether gluten may be an additive. I personally don't trust any product that isn't clearly labeled "gluten-free."

For us humans, who have spent nearly all of the past 2.6 million years as hunter-gatherers, gluten (and its closely related compounds) is a very new inclusion to the diet and is very difficult for us to digest. To say that gluten can add complications to your health is putting things mildly. Problems with gluten are becoming epidemic, and although public awareness about this issue is certainly growing, there is more that is poorly understood by most people (including those in the medical fields) than not. The weight of the scientific evidence supporting concerns associated with gluten is suffocating (with only the most minute smattering of scientific evidence actually presented here), while it is oddly and rather inexplicably ignored or even absurdly disputed by those in mainstream medicine. In light of the overwhelming evidence from innumerable solid studies, it is quite clear that the consequences of gluten sensitivity (diagnosed or undiagnosed) can be lethal. And, no, I am not being extreme when I say this. The consequences are far broader than most suspect and *very* real. Gluten can ruin your life.

Although it is commonly associated with celiac disease, many people do not appreciate gluten's potentially incredible and very broad impact on the health of countless individuals or the commonality with which people are afflicted with nonceliac "gluten sensitivity," which is every bit as lethal as celiac disease. In fact, celiac disease is in actuality only one form of gluten sensitivity. It can be said that all celiac disease is a form of gluten sensitivity but not all gluten sensitivity is celiac disease.

Celiac disease, incidentally, is diagnosable rather narrowly as a state of what is termed "total villous atrophy of the small intestine." *Villi* (and *microvilli*) may be likened to what looks like shag carpeting that lines the inside of your small intestinal wall. The "shags" add necessary surface area to facilitate proper absorption of nutrients from the diet. If the villi are only partially worn down, no diagnosis of celiac disease is given. One is "awarded" the actual diagnosis only if your villi are completely destroyed and your shag carpeting has been transformed to flat Berber carpeting. It's the equivalent of being told you can be diagnosed with heart disease only if you've actually suffered a heart attack. The diagnostic criteria, as well as the testing available to diagnose the condition, have been woefully lacking, to put it kindly.

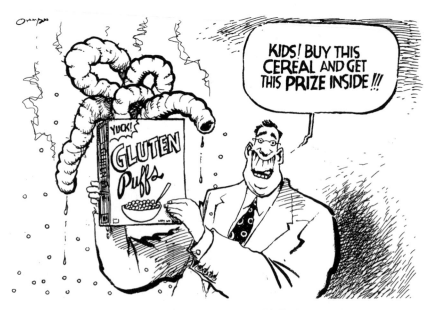

Fig. 3.1. Gluten, the "cereal killer"

The result of celiac disease is severe chronic malabsorption of nutrients, leading commonly to other disease states and degenerative processes. An article in the journal *Lancet Neurology* stated, "Coeliac disease, or gluten sensitive enteropathy, is only one aspect of a range of possible manifestations of gluten sensitivity" (Hadjivassiliou et al. 2010).

Gluten is undoubtedly the silent root of a great many of the health challenges that millions of people face today, both physical and mental. It is rarely suspected as the underlying culprit in most instances, however, even by supposed medical authorities. Furthermore, the inherent presence of the morphinelike compounds called *exorphins* in grains makes gluten-containing grains quite addictive and leaves many in frank denial of the havoc that gluten can wreak. Ignorance of gluten sensitivity and resistance to the awareness of what it is really all about are pervasive. The need for awareness and concern is very, very real. It is for this reason that the treatment of this particular subject here is so exhaustive. *You really need to get this.*

Allow me to elaborate.

Celiac disease (CD) and gluten sensitivity are generally defined as states of heightened immunologic responsiveness to ingested gluten proteins in genetically predisposed individuals. All celiac disease is a form of gluten sensitivity but not all gluten sensitivity is celiac disease. They are differentiated by their genetic markers—though the presence of genetic markers is not essential for gluten-induced enteropathy (intestinal damage) or "silent celiac disease" to occur, nor is the absence of these markers somehow "proof" that gluten isn't a problem. It was once believed the genetic markers were necessary. Current studies have refuted this assumption, however. Also, the primary form of damage in celiac disease has been recognized as villous atrophy within the small intestine, though additional forms of damage may be found elsewhere in the body and may affect *many* other systems, including the brain.

A study in the *Journal of the American Medical Association* shows that people with celiac disease or gluten sensitivity, whether diagnosed or undiagnosed, had a significantly higher risk of death, particularly from heart disease and cancer (Ludvigsson et al. 2009). It has been estimated (conservatively) that one in every two hundred people has full-blown celiac disease ("full-blown" being the only manner by which it is actually diagnosed), a devastating consequence of gluten consumption. Some researchers have recently hypothesized that this number may be closer to one in thirty—**or perhaps even a great deal more common.** In an article in the *Archives of Internal Medicine,* the authors wrote, "Celiac Disease is a much greater problem than has previously been appreciated" (Fasano et al. 2003). In an article in *The New England Journal of Medicine,* the author wrote, "Celiac Disease is one of the most common lifelong disrorders in both Europe and the US" (Fasano 2003). And in an article in *Pediatrics,* the authors stated, "In the past 7 years, *1 in 4 children was diagnosed as having celiac disease* [emphasis mine] in southern Alberta as a result of case-finding of associated conditions, consistent with data from the United Kingdom" (McGowan et al. 2009). Gluten sensitivity (as opposed to celiac disease, not included in these same statistics) is considerably more common than full-blown celiac disease and is currently almost epidemic, if not ubiquitous in its scope.

The effects of and the markedly increased mortality risks associated with both full-blown celiac disease and gluten sensitivity happen to be virtually identical. Both are autoimmune conditions that create inflammation and immune system effects throughout the body.

Gluten can affect all organ systems (including your brain, heart, and kidneys), your extended nervous system, your moods, your immunological functioning, your digestive system, and even your musculoskeletal system—truly almost all of you, from your hair follicles down to your toenails and everything in between.

When it comes to the effects of gluten in the brain, exposure to gluten in a sensitive individual essentially shuts down blood flow to the frontal and prefrontal cortex (a process called *cerebral frontal/prefrontal hypoperfusion*). This is the part of our brain that allows us to focus, to manage emotional states, to plan and organize, to consider the consequences of our actions, and to exercise our short-term memory. Over time, this can result in the generation of actual brain lesions, which in turn result in chronically impaired neurological functioning. In an article in *Pediatrics,* the authors stated, "The lesions in the brain may be the result of a decreased blood supply (hypoperfusion) caused by inflammation" (Kleslich et al. 2001). Note that hypoperfusion to the frontal and prefrontal cortex is additionally powerfully associated with cognitive impairment and conditions such as depression, anxiety, and ADHD. Know anyone with cognitive, emotional, psychiatric, or attentional issues? The frontal and prefrontal cortex is our brain's "executive function" control center and is the part of our brain that basically makes us the most human.

The inflammatory response invoked by gluten exposure additionally activates the brain's inflammatory microglial cells, which have no built-in inhibitory mechanisms and do not readily wind themselves down again. It can take many months for a brain-based inflammatory response to an antigen such as gluten to subside. The damage and neural degeneration this can cause over time, together with the effect of generating overarousal of the sympathetic nervous system (the "fight-or-flight" response), can be significant.

In routine blood tests, suspicion of gluten sensitivity should be raised when seeing chronic states of functionally to clinically depressed white blood cell counts (below $5.0 \times 10E3/\mu L$), subclinical anemia (serum iron levels below 85 µg/dL, ferritin levels below 10 ng/mL in women and below 33 in men and menopausal women, and hemoglobin levels below 13.5 µg/dL), functionally depressed or elevated serum protein levels (below 6.9 g/dL or above 7.4 g/dL), unusually depressed triglyceride levels (much below 75 mg/dL, especially where carbs play a significant dietary role) or alkaline phosphatase levels (significantly below 70 U/L), functionally depressed blood urea nitrogen levels (below 13 mg/dL), abnormally elevated high-density lipoprotein (HDL) levels (in excess of 75 mg/dL) or overly depressed HDL levels (below 55 mg/dL), excessively depressed or elevated total cholesterol levels, or chronically (even functionally) elevated transaminase or liver enzyme levels, especially when found in combination with the other above-mentioned markers. Other chronic inflammatory conditions and malabsorptive markers can also be causes for possible suspicion, but can't be used for diagnosis. One does not have to have all or most of these conditions to consider gluten sensitivity testing. Pay attention to other possible symptoms, as well. It takes further testing to be sure, though even some of the best testing methods can vary greatly in their accuracy.

Opening the Floodgates

Gluten can also be looked upon as a "gateway food sensitivity." It is known to increase the levels of an enzyme in the body known as *zonulin,* which controls intestinal permeability. Elevated zonulin levels in the presence of gluten can also serve to allow other types of undigested proteins to slip past what would otherwise be more selectively permeable barriers and cause additional immunological reactions to other foods. In an article in the medical journal *Diabetes,* the authors wrote, "We have recently reported a novel protein, zonulin, that modulates intestinal permeability by disassembling the intercellular tight junctions" (Sapone et al. 2006). They went on to say, "This protein, when upregulated, appears to play a key role in the pathogenesis of autoimmune disorders." It is gliadin that activates the zonulin signaling pathway. The authors of an article in the *Journal of Immunology* said, "Gliadin and its peptides interact with the intestinal epithelium increasing intestinal permeability through the release of zonulin that, in turn, enables paracellular translocation of gliadin and its subsequent interaction with macrophages within the intestinal submucosa" (Thomas et al. 2006). This is basically, in plain language, a total setup for autoimmune disorders.

Currently, as a collective whole, autoimmune disorders are the **number three killer,** behind heart disease and cancer, in the United States. Note that gluten is certainly not always the underlying cause of all autoimmune disorders. The most common causes are food sensitivities (particularly gluten sensitivity), environmental triggers, viruses, excess estrogen exposure, and heavy-metal toxicity. This said, even where gluten is not the primary cause of an autoimmune illness, it can almost always be suspected as an exacerbative factor. Let's just say it never helps. An article in the peer-reviewed journal *Cellular and Molecular Life Sciences* stated that "autoimmune disorders occur 10 times more commonly in celiac disease than in the general population" (Green et al. 2005). Of course, this is not even counting those people merely identified as gluten sensitive or those with less than full-blown celiac disease.

Despite the overwhelming association with autoimmune disorders, an article in the *Journal of the America Medical Association* stated, "Cardiovascular disease was the most common cause of death in celiac disease, followed by malignancy" (Ludvigsson et al. 2009). Is that piece of bread *really* worth the risk, especially considering the fact that **only 1 percent** of those people with celiac disease (or gluten sensitivity) have ever been properly diagnosed?

Healing the Gluten-Ravaged Gut

Even when gluten has been removed from the diet completely, this alone is not necessarily sufficient unto itself toward restoring intestinal integrity. Less than half of the patients with celiac disease on a gluten-free diet for an average of 9.7 years have complete normalization, as shown by intestinal biopsy test results (Duerksen et al. 2010). A systematic regimen of reducing inflammation and healing the existing damage *must* be implemented for long-term optimal results and true healing; this is a process that is likely to take at least one year of dedicated effort, although significant tangible benefits are typically seen much sooner—some within days of eliminating all exposure to gluten, in fact. The daily addition of omega-3 fat (EPA), the fatty acid GLA, vitamin D, glutathione-enhancing nutrients, and botanicals such as turmeric (curcumen) can help battle inflammation, while the use of other botanicals (marshmallow root extract, slippery elm bark extract, deglycyrrhizinated licorice extract, and aloe leaf extract can all be helpful) as well as additional substances such as L-glutamine and methylsulfonylmethane can help serve to support the healing of the existing damage. Proline-rich polypeptides from bovine colostrum and whole, minimally processed, grass-fed, organic bovine colostrum can also be of tremendous benefit in restoring healthy gastrointestinal integrity and immune function over time. There are more than nine thousand studies showing grass-fed bovine colostrum's potentially key role in restoring gastrointestinal integrity. Other food sensitivities must also be addressed.

The good news is that other food sensitivities often diminish over time once the aggravating factor of gluten (the granddaddy of them all) is finally out of the picture and intestinal integrity is restored. In an article in *Nature Reviews Gastroenterology and Hepatology,* the authors wrote, "This new paradigm subverts traditional theories underlying the development of autoimmunity, which are based on molecular mimicry and/or the bystander effect . . . and suggests that the autoimmune process can be *arrested* [emphasis mine] if the interplay between genes and environmental triggers is prevented by re-establishing intestinal barrier function" (Fasano and Shea-Donohue 2005). This is amazing news. The potential for healing is extraordinary once gluten is eliminated and the gut is repaired.

Also, a potent cross-reactivity to casein (the protein found in milk products) has additionally been demonstrated to be similar to an immunologic reactivity to gluten. In the journal *Clinical and Experimental Immunology,* the authors stated, "A mucosal inflammatory response similar to that elicited by gluten was produced by CM protein in about 50% of the patients with coeliac disease. Casein, in particular, seems to be involved in this reaction" (Kristjánsson et al. 2007). Casein is among the most common cosensitive agents with gluten, but the immune system can come to react to almost anything if gluten consumption persists. Cross-reactivity, which is the tendency to react to substances either genetically or structurally similar to gluten or that our immune system has merely learned to *associate* with gluten, is an added concern for many. This can be a very real and frustrating problem. Once multiple food sensitivities take over, they can cause a very vicious cycle that only worsens with time and becomes extremely difficult to correct. Living with this can be miserable at best. Autoimmune processes—often multiple ones—can be a very common result. Identifying cross-reactive substances (using Cyrex Labs Array 4 panel; www.cyrexlabs.com) may be necessary to identify other guilty culprits that are stalling or thwarting your healing process.

Among the most common *true* potentially cross-reactive compounds are:

- casein (milk protein and cheese included)
- oats (including the supposedly "gluten-free" kind)
- rye
- barley
- spelt
- kamut (also known as Polish wheat, Egyptian wheat, or camel's wheat)
- yeast
- coffee (so sorry!)
- milk chocolate (don't hit me)

Additional compounds tested for by Cyrex Labs (frequently substituted for gluten) that may cause problems and food sensitivity issues of their own include:

- corn (very common food sensitivity and almost always a GMO food)
- sesame
- buckwheat (note that most buckwheat and soy flour, apart from being potential sensitivities in and of themselves are most commonly contaminated with gluten due to processing methods)
- quinoa
- sorghum

- millet
- tapioca
- amaranth
- rice (yes, rice—increasingly, believe it or not)
- potato

Celiac Disease:
More Common Than Ever?

A study published in the peer-reviewed journal *Gastroenterology* compared ten thousand available blood samples taken from individuals fifty years ago to samples taken from ten thousand people today and found that there has been a **400 percent increase** in the incidence of full-blown celiac disease (Rubio-Tapia et al. 2009)! Changes made to American strains of wheat, giving them much higher gluten content, are likely a significant part of the problem. Increased genetic susceptibility due to a variety of causes is likely another. Additional reasons for this increased susceptibility also reasonably include modern gluten-processing methods (something called *deamidation* in processed foods); prolonged storage of gluten-containing grains, leading to enterotoxin contamination; chronic stress issues, leading to cortisol-related breakdown of immune barriers; digestive enzyme and hydrochloric acid insufficiency; and generally poor nutritional habits due to an increasingly processed and nutrient-depleted food supply. According to the same article, fully 30–50 percent of all people carry the gene for celiac disease (known as HLA-DQ8 or HLA-DQ2) and eight times more people with celiac disease have no gastrointestinal symptoms than do. Gluten-sensitivity genes are significantly more common (HLA-DQB1, alleles 1 and 2).

Fully **99 percent** of those people who have this entirely curable and potentially lethal condition are completely unaware of the dangerous vulnerability within themselves. Although a biopsy of the small intestine is commonly used to diagnose celiac disease, the actual diagnostic criteria are so restrictive as to be inherently untrustworthy as a final determinant. Gastrointestinal symptoms are, in fact, barely the tip of the iceberg. An article in the *British Medical Journal* stated, "The iceberg is a common model used to explain the epidemiology of celiac disease. The majority of patients have what is termed silent celiac disease, which may remain undiagnosed because the condition has no (gastrointestinal) symptoms" (Feighery

1999). In the journal *Gastroenterology,* an article stated, *"For every symptomatic patient with celiac disease there are 8 patients with celiac disease and no gastrointestinal symptoms"* [emphasis mine] (Fasano and Catassi 2001). In fact, an article in the journal *Neurology* stated, **"Gluten sensitivity can be primarily and at times exclusively a neurological disease, affecting not only the brain and nervous system directly, but also cognitive and psychiatric illness"** [emphasis mine]) (Hadjivassiliou 2001). In the *Journal of Neurology, Neurosurgery and Psychiatry,* an article stated, "Our finding . . . implies that immune response triggered by sensitivity to gluten may find expression in organs other than the gut; and the central and peripheral nervous systems are particularly susceptible" (Hadjivassiliou et al. 1997). In an article in *Cellular and Molecular Life Sciences,* the authors wrote, "Celiac Disease (CD) has also been termed Gluten Sensitive Enteropathy because the small intestine is the main target of injury; however, the clinical manifestations are extremely diverse, suggesting the disorder is in fact a multi-system disorder" (Green et al. 2005).

A review paper in *The New England Journal of Medicine* found that fully **fifty-five diseases** are known to be caused by gluten (Farrell and Kelly 2002). Among these are heart disease, cancer, nearly all autoimmune diseases, osteoporosis, irritable bowel syndrome and other gastrointestinal disorders, gallbladder disease, Hashimoto's disease (an autoimmune thyroid disorder responsible for up to 90 percent of all low-functioning thyroid issues), migraines, epilepsy, Parkinson's disease, amyotrophic lateral sclerosis (ALS, or Lou Gehrig's disease), neuropathies (having normal EMG readings), and most other degenerative neurological disorders as well as autism, which is technically an autoimmune brain disorder. Gluten can also cause many common psychiatric illnesses, including anxiety issues, ADD/ADHD, bipolar disorder, depression, dementia, and schizophrenia. In my opinion, it is always safest to simply *assume* the presence of gluten sensitivity in these populations, or, frankly, wherever significantly compromised health is an issue. Even where avoidance of gluten may not solve the problem, one has at least removed a potentially enormous obstacle from the path toward improvement.

Testing for Gluten Sensitivity

Although there are numerous methods for assessing the presence of gluten sensitivity and celiac disease, most are unfortunately somewhat unreliable in their accuracy (including the so-called gold standard approach of intestinal biopsy), which may be partly why so few people are properly diagnosed, even when testing is sought out. With respect to blood and saliva testing, out of twelve different subfractions of gliadin, for instance, typically only one—alpha-gliadin—is ever tested for. If you happen to have sensitivity to any of the eleven other forms of gliadin, it might not ever show. If a person happens to be sensitive or allergic to the glutenin fraction of gluten protein, it is not identifiable on tests. False-negative results are a notorious part of this type of testing, unfortunately. Accuracy (where negative results are concerned) is never 100 percent. Immunoglobulin testing for food sensitivities in people with autoimmune disorders and particularly Hashimoto's disease (autoimmune thyroid) is almost always skewed due to chronic imbalances of TH-1 (T cell) and TH-2 (B cell) immune response. **It's critical to look for multiple markers** (although the overwhelming association—almost 100 percent—between gluten sensitivity and Hashimoto's disease and most other autoimmune disorders makes the automatic assumption of gluten sensitivity a good idea).

Where blood testing is concerned, the most important tests to run are those for IgA (antigliadin antibodies and antientomysial antibodies), IgG (antigliadin antibodies), IgM (antigliadin antibodies), tissue transglutaminase antibodies (IgA and IgG, which are most associated with advanced small intestine villous atrophy), gluten antibodies, and total IgA antibodies, and if possible, always test for the presence of genes HLA-DQ2 and HLA-DQ8 as well as HLA-DQB1, alleles 1 and 2. I've seen individuals test negative for antibodies in blood and saliva, even when using the most accurate stool antigen tests (again, false-negative results are quite common), but they then test positive for both pairs of celiac disease or gluten-sensitivity genes, meaning that one can basically take the diagnosis of celiac disease or gluten sensitivity to the bank. *Note:* Positive results are almost always dependable. Negative results are not. I've found that a comparatively accurate assessment can be made by using an easily ordered proprietary stool antibody test from EnteroLab (www.enterolab.com). Its website also contains extremely helpful information on the subject, and the company offers fairly accurate testing methods for other major common food sensitivities as well. Getting the additional tests for genetic markers for gluten sensitivity and predisposition potential for celiac disease that they offer helps minimize false-negative results. Anyone can order this material without a physician referral.

As of January 2011, a new standard of excellence in testing for gluten sensitivity through affordable salivary panels covering not one but *all* fractions of gliadin—with an unprecedented accuracy rate—is available via Cyrex Labs (www.cyrexlabs.com). To quote the site itself, "Cyrex™ is an advanced clinical laboratory developing and offering cutting-edge tests based on the latest scientific advances in the field of immunology. These tests cover mucosal, cellular, and humoral immunology and specialize in antibody arrays for complex thyroid, gluten, and other food-associated autoimmunities and related neurodysregulation." Cyrex also offers testing arrays that address the often overlooked issue of what is termed *cross-reactivity* (defined as an immunologic state in which the body will react to some other substance *as if* it were gluten).

Cross-reactivity is a sticky conundrum that needs to be addressed whenever a gluten-free diet is insufficient to ameliorate the symptoms associated with it. Cross-reactive substances can comprise other, supposedly gluten-free grains, similar enough in molecular structure or genetics to cause reactivity in those particularly sensitive. Somewhat more mysteriously, they can also include entirely unrelated compounds that may have an immunologically associative relationship to gluten, such as casein (actually, surprisingly similar molecularly to gluten) *and even coffee* in some people. Coffee, in fact, according to the researchers at Cyrex Labs, may be the single most cross-reactive substance of them all. (How many people have done things like have coffee with their toast, cereal, croissant, danish, or doughnut for years on end?)

Cyrex Labs also makes available a testing array that can pinpoint the very areas in your body being most affected by gluten sensitivity. People often think that the symptoms to watch for when it comes to gluten issues are typically gastrointestinal, when gluten sensitivity can, in fact, profoundly impact your brain, nervous system, emotional states, endocrine functioning, neurotransmitters, immune system, bones, joints, skeletal system, and any possible aspect of your mental or physical physiological functioning. Make no mistake about it, Cyrex Labs *will* revolutionize the entire field of immunology. Note, however, that testing through Cyrex can be accomplished only through a licensed health care provider.

In time, there will likely be new and hopefully even more accurate diagnostic methods developed as studies demonstrating the devastating health impacts of gluten mount. EnteroLab's proprietary stool antigen test, which anyone can order online, is reasonable for accuracy, demonstrating a sixfold greater accuracy rate than available blood-antigen tests. The standard blood tests for gluten sensitivity have an accuracy rate of no more than about 30 percent (with false-negatives being the most common issue). Otherwise, elimination diets or testing for multiple markers using blood sampling are probably the next best bets.

Elimination diets can be an effective means of determining the potential for gluten sensitivity, but they must be strictly adhered to for at least six to eight months to make a genuinely clear determination. Avoidance of gluten must be **no less than 100 percent** from all (even hidden) sources, and not so much as even a single crumb of bread can be eaten. Beware, too, of many medications containing hidden gluten (crazy, but true; watch out for cornstarch). Also, beware of cross-contamination issues, where nongluten foods may come into contact with gluten-containing foods via cooking or preparation surfaces and utensils in restaurants or at home. (Yes, this matters.) The inflammatory effects in the brain especially and throughout the body from even trace gluten exposure can reverberate for fully six months in sensitive individuals. Any exposure of any kind (even seemingly innocuous and unintentional slipups) means you must basically start over on the elimination diet. Sorry to sound so fussy, but this is an issue that needs to be taken extremely seriously.

There are some helpful products on the market that can help curb excess inflammatory response to *trace* gluten exposure, but do not mistake these for being the equivalent of a gluten "morning-after pill" that can cancel out that birthday cake you wanted to indulge in.

An article in *Gastroenterology* stated, "During a 45 year follow up, undiagnosed celiac disease was associated with a nearly 4-fold increased risk of death. The prevalence of undiagnosed CD seems to have increased dramatically in the United States during the last 50 years" (Rubio-Tapia et al. 2009). In an individual with either full-blown celiac disease or gluten sensitivity, the risk of death from *all causes,* according to the journal *The Lancet,* was dramatically greater: "Death was most significantly affected by diagnostic delay, pattern of presentation, and adherence to the gluten free diet. . . . Non adherence to the gluten free diet, defined as eating gluten *once-per-month,* increased the relative risk of death *600%*" [emphasis mine] (Corrao et al. 2001). Next time you want to rationalize that one little cookie, slice of birthday cake, or piece of bread, think twice. Being "mostly gluten-free" or eating gluten-containing foods "only occasionally" just doesn't cut it. There are times where the saying (or perhaps rationalization) "all things in moderation" simply does not apply.

Brain and mood disorders, migraines, osteoporosis, diabetes, cardiovascular diseases, bowel diseases, autoimmune diseases, inflammatory disorders, and cancer are rampant. Grains are rarely suspected as the original culprit, though every one of these disorders, among many more, can potentially be traced to often insidious gluten intolerance. Gluten sensitivity is only rarely obvious to the afflicted, and many people are even entirely surprised to learn they have this sensitivity. I know I was.

> Only an estimated *1 percent* of all gluten sensitivity or celiac disease is ever diagnosed.

The Nitty-Gritty of Going Gluten-Free

The gluten-containing grains most associated with celiac disease are wheat (e.g., durum, graham, semolina, kamut, triticale, and spelt) as well as rye, barley, and most oats. Although oats technically are not part of the most problematic gliadin-containing family of grains, modern methods of processing nearly always ensure gluten contamination of oat products, and the presence of actual gluten should always be assumed unless a product is labeled "100-percent gluten-free." The prolamin (avenin) content of oats, however, still makes them at least potentially suspect for inherent cross-reactivity issues, even where they may be sold as gluten-free products. The very same can be said for many products containing corn and cornstarch. Buckwheat and soy flours are almost always contaminated with gluten due to processing and storage methods.

The good news is that the devastating symptoms of gluten sensitivity and celiac disease can often be entirely eliminated. The treatment solution? You *must* eliminate *100 percent*—not just most—of the gluten from your diet, and that means not just gluten-containing dietary grains, but all hidden sources as well, which can include (but are not limited to) commercial soups, broths, processed food mixes, soy sauce, teriyaki and other sauces, corn products and cornstarch, and salad dressings. Gluten can be listed as vegetable protein, seitan, hydrolyzed vegetable protein, modified food starch, and other names. Gluten is additionally hidden on food labels as other food starches, artificial food coloring, food stabilizers, malt extract (syrup or flavoring), dextrins, and food emulsifiers. Gluten is even an ingredient in many shampoos, cosmetics, and lipsticks (which can potentially be absorbed transdermally, which means through the skin), children's Play-Doh, medications, vitamins (unless specifically labeled "gluten-free"), and even non–self-adhesive stamps and envelopes.

Although I realize all this need for ultrastrict avoidance sounds rather tedious and inconvenient, an article in the *Journal of Neurology, Neurosurgery and Psychiatry* stated clearly, "Even minute traces of gliadin (gluten) are capable of triggering a state of heightened immunological activity in gluten sensitive people," meaning prolonged inflammation and other symptoms (Hadjivassiliou et al. 1997). Saying you've eliminated "most" of the gluten from your diet because you are gluten sensitive is a bit like saying you're just "a little bit pregnant." Either you are or you're not. There are *no* in-betweens. Avoidance must be strict and total.

I know you're thinking, "Wait just a minute, back up; did she just say 'personal-care products'? What?" It's crazy-sounding but true. You need to examine your shampoos, conditioners, and other hair-care and skin-care products for the presence of wheat protein, sometimes listed as hydrolyzed vegetable protein. Look for corn-related additives, also.

While you're at it, you might also want to consider avoiding toxic additives like parabens, pthalates, artificial fragrances, sodium laurel sulfate, methylisothiazolinone (MIT), and petroleum derivatives like mineral oil, toluene, petrolatum, and paraffin (slightly off-topic, but extremely noteworthy nonetheless). Note that the U.S. Food and Drug Administration (FDA) does nothing to ensure the safety of any chemical used in personal-care products, so you're left to trust the manufacturer. Even the FDA regulation (21 CFR Sec. 740.10) states, "Cosmetic products and ingredients are not subject to FDA premarket approval authority, with the exception of color additives. . . . Cosmetic firms are responsible for substantiating the safety of their products and ingredients before marketing." In 1978, congressional hearings presented evidence that the absorption of a known carcinogen, nitrosodiethanolamine (NDELA)—commonly found in shampoo products—was **shown to be more than one hundred times greater** when exposure came through the skin than through the mouth. Yes, you heard right; **one hundred times greater.**

Of the roughly 126 chemicals consumers regularly apply to their skin, 90 percent have never, ever been tested for their safety. Most people think nothing of the products they apply to their hair or skin, and the cosmetics industry readily capitalizes on this ignorance at tremendous potential cost to your health for considerable profit.

Why is this important? I mean, we're just talking about skin, right? It's not like you're drinking the stuff. . . .

In fact, it's probably worse.

Keep in mind that your skin is your largest organ and that it is *exceedingly* thin (less than one-tenth of an inch in thickness) *and* permeable. If you were to eat or drink these products, you'd have several things come into play to help protect you from direct bloodstream exposure, such as your gut lining, hydrochloric acid, and enzymes. In a hot shower, however, with your pores open wide, there is very little between you and the direct absorption of anything you are applying to your scalp and skin right into your bloodstream, where it is all free to travel throughout your body to your brain and all your other organs.

The concern here may seem trivial to some but it is very real. When you're reading a hair- or skin-care label, it's a good idea to ask yourself whether you would be willing to actually drink the contents of that product. If you are reading a list that includes a whole lot of difficult-to-pronounce chemicals or are seeing wheat protein or vegetable protein on the label, you'd do well to think twice about using that product. And don't let buzzwords like *organic* and *natural* fool you.

A partial listing of product sources can be found at www.celiac.com. Dr. Joseph Mercola, on his excellent health website (www.mercola.com), has additive-free shampoos and conditioners available. Another source for allergen-free hair- and skin-care products is Gluten-Free Savonnerie (www.gfsoap.com). Just do a Google search for "gluten and additive-free hair- and skin-care products" in your computer's browser. The potential selection is huge. If you happen to have a smart phone, there are also numerous "gluten-free" apps available to help you screen individual products, restaurants, grocery stores, and other shopping sources at your fingertips. The good news is that the awareness of these issues is rapidly spreading and resources are likely to grow exponentially in the very near time to come.

Many people will claim they have been adhering to a strict gluten-free diet when, in fact, they have been avoiding only the obvious sources and really haven't been paying enough attention to potentially hidden sources, including their personal-care products. They will eventually rationalize their lack of positive health results to the idea that they weren't gluten sensitive after all, and they will simply go back to eating whatever they want. This is a *huge* mistake! I have worked with clients who were gluten sensitive and were unable to make substantial progress until they addressed the issue of gluten in their personal-care products.

Even when adherence to a genuinely gluten-free diet doesn't seem to generate the expected turnaround in health and well-being, you have at least removed one very major hurdle to improvement. There can always be other hurdles yet to conquer. Gluten in personal-care products, medications, and even stamps and envelopes (the kind you have to lick) can be a problem. Cross-reactivity to other substances is another important possibility to consider when going gluten-free does not yield the expected improvements. Cyrex Labs has a testing array that can screen for this.

Gluten is, however, not the only modern substance challenging the health of the masses. Restoring health can be like peeling back the layers of an onion. It is a process. Often enough, by simply removing this one major dietary antigen, the turnaround in some people can seem nothing short of miraculous. It can also make a massive difference where seemingly more benign issues like resistance to weight loss are concerned.

So what about gluten-free substitutes?

Seeking out gluten-free substitutes is certainly an option, as there are scores of gluten-free products of all kinds available today. It's big business for food manufacturers these days, in fact. Clearly, gluten-free shampoos and cosmetics are a good and necessary idea. Unfortunately, even though other grains, such as quinoa, corn, millet, rice, and buckwheat (or soy), do not *technically* contain gluten, gluten contamination in many of these foods and cross-reactivity are extremely common. They are also more a source of starch than of protein, regardless, and the majority of gluten-free substitutes are highly, highly processed foods. Many are soy based as well (don't get me started on *that*). **Just because something is gluten-free does not mean it is actually healthy for you, anymore than the word *organic* does.** Beware of the plethora of junk food masquerading as a "healthy gluten-free option" or "substitute." Gluten intolerance *and* carbohydrate intolerance, in general, are far more the rule than the exception in today's world. It is logical to conclude that grain consumption of any kind, especially gluten-containing grains, just isn't worth the dietary risk, given our culture's innumerable health challenges and vulnerabilities. Why play Russian roulette? Why add to the unnecessary glycating, fattening, and neurotransmitter- and hormone-dysregulating carbohydrate load? In my view, it's better to take processed food off the radar screen entirely—period—and to stick to the foods that don't need a label you have to read every time. Truthfully, it's *far* less complicated and confusing to do so.

In short, there is no one alive for whom grains of any type are essential for health, and gluten, in particular, is a health food for no one.

It further stands to reason that the more symptoms a person has physically, cognitively, or psychologically, the more primitive a diet (in other words, preagricultural or "primal") he or she ought to consider adopting to reclaim rightful health. The commonality of degenerative diseases does not make these diseases a normal part of aging, or even remotely inevitable.

The choice is mostly ours.

For more information about gluten sensitivity and celiac disease, go to www.celiac.com. For the most accurate testing products and more information, go to www.cyrexlabs.com or www.enterolab.com. A good site for locating available gluten-sensitivity centers and public lectures is www.conquergluten.com.

4

So What about Soy?

■ ■ ■ ■ ■ ■ ■ ■ ■ ■ ■ ■

Contrary to popular belief, soy (particularly tofu, soy milk, and soy protein isolate) is among the newest additions to the human diet. Soy has been considered unfit for human consumption since ancient times, but chemical processing methods created by corporate interests have created an "all-new" soy, purported to be the cornerstone of health and longevity. The unsuspecting public has unfortunately succumbed to misleading claims and other marketing ploys to increasingly seek out meat substitutes, including texturized vegetable protein (also called TVP), tofu, soy milk, and soy protein powders. Many have been led to believe that these foods somehow prevent cancer and heart disease and provide improved-quality protein in their diets.

Nothing could be further from the truth.

Publicized studies attempting to show the health benefits of soy are largely funded and promoted to the media and the health-food industry by the multibillion-dollar, multinational soy industry in an effort to market its product. Innumerable independent studies, however, suggest considerable reason for concern.

The following points are cited from the Weston A. Price Foundation website (www.WestonAPrice.org):

- The high levels of phytic acid in soy reduce the assimilation of calcium, magnesium, copper, iron, and zinc. Phytic acid in soy is *not* neutralized by ordinary preparation methods such as soaking, sprouting, and long, slow cooking. High-phytate diets have caused

49

growth problems in children. (Also, soy contains the *highest levels* of phytic acid of any grain or legume.)

- Trypsin inhibitors in soy interfere with protein digestion and can cause pancreatic disorders. In test animals, soy containing trypsin inhibitors caused stunted growth.
- Soy phytoestrogens disrupt endocrine function and have the potential to cause infertility and to promote breast cancer in adult women.
- Soy phytoestrogens are potent antithyroid agents (goitrogens) that cause hypothyroidism and may cause thyroid cancer. In infants, consumption of soy formula has been linked to autoimmune thyroid disease.
- Vitamin B_{12} analogs in soy are not absorbed and actually increase the body's requirement for vitamin B_{12}.
- Soy foods increase the body's requirement for vitamin D.
- Fragile proteins are denatured during the high-temperature processing used to make soy protein isolate and texturized vegetable protein.
- The processing of soy protein results in the formation of toxic lysinoalanine and highly carcinogenic nitrosamines.
- Free glutamic acid (monosodium glutamate, or MSG), a potent neurotoxin, is formed during soy food processing, and additional amounts of it are added to many soy foods.
- Soy foods contain high levels of aluminum, which is toxic to the nervous system and kidneys.
- Recent studies suggest a link between soy consumption and kidney stones.

Additional Concerns
(As If All That Wasn't Bad Enough)

Soy has never been given the Generally Recognized as Safe status (GRAS) by the FDA. Soy is a phytoendocrine disrupter, inhibiting thyroid peroxidase, a thyroid enzyme that is necessary for the synthesis of the hormones T3 and T4. Effects include autoimmune thyroiditis (Divi and Doerge 1996; Divi et al. 1997) and hypothyroidism involving obesity, dry skin and hair, low blood pressure, slow pulse, depressed muscular activity, intolerance to cold, goiter, and sluggishness of all physiological functions.

Eating estrogenic foods may increase the risk for estrogen-dependent cancers. FDA scientists Daniel M. Sheehan and Daniel R. Doerge wrote a warning letter to the agency, stating, "A woman's own estrogens are a very significant risk factor for breast cancer" (Sheehan and Doerge 1998). In 1996, researchers found that women consuming soy protein isolate had increased incidences of epithelial hyperplasia, a precursor of malignancies (Petrakis et al. 1996). In 1997, a research study showed that consumption of genistein, a soy isoflavone, caused breast cells to enter into the malignant cell cycle (Dees et al. 1997). Soy also is known to alter menstrual cycle length (Cassidy et al. 1994).

Continued Still . . . Believe It or Not

Estrogens are known to be able to pass through the placenta. Sheehan and Doerge wrote, in their warning letter to the FDA, "Development is the most sensitive stage to estrogen toxicity because of the indisputable evidence of a wide variety of frank malformations and serious functional deficits in experimental animals and humans" (Sheehan and Doerge 1998).

Genistein causes alterations in leutinizing hormone regulation, which may cause abnormal brain and reproductive-tract development (Faber and Hughes 1991). When exposed to estrogen, 50 percent of human female offspring displayed one or more malformations in the reproductive tract (Sheehan and Doerge 1998). Babies on soy infant formula have estradiol levels thirteen thousand to twenty-two thousand times higher than babies on milk-based infant formula. C. H. Irvine and colleagues wrote, "Infants exclusively fed soy infant formula receive the estrogenic equivalent of at least five birth control pills a day" (Irvine et al. 1998).

In male infants, the estrogenic effects of soy interrupt the testosterone surge that occurs in the first few months, when testosterone levels can be as high as those of an adult male. Interruption may cause inhibition of male characteristics and sexual organs (Ross et al. 1983).

In female infants, the estrogenic effects of soy may speed the rate of maturation. Girls enter puberty earlier than normal: 1 percent show signs of maturation, including pubic hair and breast development, before the age of three; 14.7 percent of Caucasian girls and 50 percent of African American girls by age eight. Dietary estrogens have been linked as a possible cause of this early development (Herman-Giddens et al. 1997).

Soy consumption causes decreased testosterone levels in men. Buddhist monks ate tofu to reduce their libido. (Of course, there's always Viagra . . .) Soy consumption has been clearly linked to a higher risk of vascular dementia, or Alzheimer's disease, in men (White et al. 1996). The isoflavones of soy inhibit the enzyme conversion of testosterone to estradiol via the aromatase enzyme, which is necessary for male brain function and maintenance (Irvine et al. 1998).

Soy is not a complete protein. Like all legumes, it lacks the sulfur-containing amino acids cysteine and methionine. Lysine, which is essential for brain development and maintenance, is denatured during the processing of soy.

Still More Bad News

Soybeans contain hemagglutinin, a clot-promoting substance that causes red blood cells to clump.

Soy protein isolate, the main ingredient in most imitation meat and dairy products, goes through rigorous processing to remove inherent antinutrients. Soybeans are first mixed with an alkaline solution to eliminate fiber, then separated using an acid wash, and finally neutralized in an alkaline solution. The precipitated curd is spray-dried at high temperatures to produce a high-protein powder. To make texturized vegetable protein, this product is further extruded under high temperature and high pressure, creating carcinogenic nitrates from the denaturation of the original protein structure. Often, flavorings containing MSG, a powerful neurotoxin, are added under the guise of "natural flavors."

And here's the kicker: food manufacturers are using a gasoline additive known as hexane to process soy products (and some vegetable oils). Soybeans are soaked in large vats of hexane to assist in the extraction of substances such as protein and oils from them. An independent lab has found hexane residue in soy-based foods, but the FDA does not require any testing for hexane, even in baby foods. It is used by the food industry because it is cheap to do so and because the FDA lets them get away with it. The soy industry is incredibly powerful and influential. The U.S. Environmental Protection Agency lists hexane, incidentally, as a hazardous chemical.

Soy is also **the single most genetically modified crop there is**; it offers the most common examples of what are called "genetically modified organisms" (GMOs). These GMOs alone are enough of a health hazard to write an entire book about. In fact, anyone wanting to read something more horrifying than any Stephen King novel should read Jeffrey Smith's excellent book *Seeds of Deception* or watch the outstanding documentary *The Future of Food* (which can be accessed online for free viewing). Among the most common examples of GMO-containing foods are soy, corn, and wheat, but GMOs are insidiously infiltrating many, many unexpected areas of our food supply, and food manufacturers are fighting hard to even keep their presence in your food off the labels and hidden from consumer view. GMOs of all kinds may be the greatest danger to your health and the environment of anything ever created by the food and agricultural industry. To learn more, go visit the website for the Center for Food Safety, at www.centerforfoodsafety.org.

The only comparatively "safe" soy includes its fermented forms of miso, natto, and tempeh (only organic and non-GMO, please). Fermentation— and fermentation only—largely neutralizes trypsin inhibitors and phytic acid. Goitrogens or thyroid inhibitors, however, remain intact even following fermentation, so care must be taken not to overconsume even these soy foods.

For an extensive bibliography, visit the exhaustively referenced and informative SoyOnline Service website, at www.soyonlineservice.co.nz, in addition to www.Mercola.com and www.WestonAPrice.org.

5

Digestion and Nutrient Assimilation

■ ■ ■ ■ ■ ■ ■ ■ ■ ■ ■ ■

A North-to-South Journey

A person can consume the most-expensive, best-quality-source foods there are and still experience illness or marginal health. How can this be? One possible and critically important key is digestion. If you can't break down and appropriately assimilate what you eat, at best you are wasting your money on grocery bills. At worst, you are generating rancid, fermented, putrefied, and toxic compounds that can wreak havoc on every organ and system in your body. Quality digestion cannot be overrated, and it is a subject commonly overlooked when discussing a healthy diet. Every part of the body and mind depends to the extreme on proper digestion to supply it with nutrients necessary for functioning.

Poor digestion is an epidemic problem, as soaring sales of acid-blocking or neutralizing medications, gallbladder removals, and appendectomies neatly illustrate. Jonathon Wright, M.D., after using Heidelberg gastric telemetry equipment to examine the stomach pH values of thousands of his patients, estimated that approximately 90 percent of Americans produce too little hydrochloric acid. The implications of this are staggering.

A lack of adequate hydrochloric acid results in several rather major problems.

1. Poor digestion and absorption of the proteins or amino acids necessary for more than fifty thousand functions in the body, such as neurotransmitter production for regulation of mood; maintenance and repair of cells, organs, bone, and tissues; and many other indispensable functions.

2. Poor absorption of key minerals, including calcium, magnesium, phosphorus, boron, iron, and zinc. (The double jeopardy here is that it actually also *takes* zinc to make hydrochloric acid, leading to potentially severe deficiencies of these incredibly important minerals and all that this implies.)

3. Poor hydrochloric acid production by parietal cells in the stomach also impairs the proper vitamin B_{12} digestion essential for neurological health. This impairment can also lead to undersecretion of the intrinsic factor essential to vitamin B_{12}'s absorption in the gut. Vitamin B_{12} is a key methyl donor, which is necessary for cardiovascular and brain health. We also use it to make red blood cells. Prolonged deficiencies of vitamin B_{12} can result in irreversible neurological damage, severe mood dysregulation, impaired cognitive functioning, and dementia as well as macrocytic anemia and heart disease. Not pretty.

4. The poorly digested mass of rotting chyme in the stomach (sorry to be so graphic) goes on to wreak havoc elsewhere in the digestive tract, fermenting and being partially expelled as reflux symptoms, gas, and bloating. It generates irritation and inflammation in the small intestine. This can eventually lead to mucosal and microvillous erosion and what can be termed *leaky gut syndrome,* a hyperporosity of the otherwise selectively permeable membrane of the small intestine, where poorly digested proteins can then enter the bloodstream and be treated as antigens or foreign invaders by the immune system, initially resulting in allergies or food sensitivities and possibly leading to autoimmune disorders.

5. Enhanced vulnerability to parasites and other food-borne illness.

Going from Bad to Worse

There is one more unpleasant possibility here: If hydrochloric acid deficiency is allowed to become chronic, overgrowth of a normally benign denizen of our gastrointestinal tract, *Helicobacter pylori (H. pylori),* can occur. In an underacidic environment in the stomach, *H. pylori* can begin undesirably proliferating, leading to infiltration of the gut lining, suppression of parietal cells (making hydrochloric acid production even more difficult), and inflammation, thinning, or even ulceration of endothelial tissue. This can potentially generate gastritis and ulcers. Additionally, *H. pylori* can even spread to other endothelial tissue, infiltrating and inflaming arterial endothelium as a now known vector for vascular disease.

We do need some *H. pylori*, however. It plays a complex role in the regulation of leptin, so fully eradicating it with antibiotics is not the answer. Managing excess overgrowth with certain nutrients and restoring normal hydrochloric acid levels is the better alternative to total eradication.

The more difficult to digest a particular protein is, the more excessive the amount of food in a meal; the more overcooked and denatured the protein in that meal is, then the more ineffectual or strained hydrochloric acid production will be and the more likely it will be to cause problems. Gluten in wheat, rye, spelt, and oats; casein, especially in pasteurized milk and milk products; albumen in chicken eggs; heavily processed soy protein; and overly cooked, denatured proteins in general are all potentially problematic for many people and make hydrochloric acid's job much harder. Overeating is also a setup for inadequate digestion. Combining starches and protein in the same meal can also adversely impact hydrochloric acid secretion. Addressing these issues alone can often correct digestive problems and hydrochloric acid insufficiency.

So, Why Don't I Have Enough Hydrochloric Acid?

There are many possible reasons for hydrochloric acid insufficiency. Hydrochloric acid is produced only in the presence of proteins and is inhibited by the presence of sugars and starches. High-carbohydrate diets, particularly when combined with inadequate intake of dietary protein, such as in vegetarian and vegan diets, are an extremely common cause of hydrochloric acid insufficiency. Thyroid hypofunction (a low-functioning thyroid) suppresses the production of gastrin, a hormone necessary for signaling hydrochloric acid production. Certain nutrient deficiencies can also be culprits (vitamin B_1, zinc, and vitamin C are needed for hydrochloric acid production), as can overeating at meals; inappropriate food combination; excess alcohol consumption; and chronic stress, anxiety, and overarousal, particularly at mealtime.

Proper hydrochloric acid production is key to the rest of the digestive process, so it's an extremely important issue to address and among the most common deficiencies impacting health.

How It's All *Supposed* to Work: Digestion 101

Bear with me here; understanding how digestion naturally works is hugely important!

Remember that digestion begins in the brain and that it is a *parasympathetic* process, meaning that the body and mind must be in a relaxed, calm state for digestion to properly occur. Eating while rushed, otherwise preoccupied, or stressed paralyzes normal digestive function and inhibits necessary secretions. It's a great setup for reflux and indigestion.

Always wait to eat until you have time to relax and focus on the meal, take in the aroma of the food, and *take the time to chew.* In the mouth, the enzyme amylase begins the digestion of carbohydrates, and the food needs to be chewed thoroughly. Poorly chewed food creates far more work for the stomach and requires more hydrochloric acid to do the same job of breaking down the protein. Chew, chew, *chew!* (Sorry to say, your mother was right . . . about *that,* anyway.)

From there, the chewed food, or chyme, travels down the esophagus, enters the stomach (where it secretes self-protective mucus), and mixes with pepsin and hydrochloric acid to break down complex proteins into shorter chains, or peptides. The peptides are then further refined by pancreatic enzymes into dipeptide and tripeptide complexes and amino acids for absorption in the small intestine.

An extremely low pH value—roughly 0.8, almost pure acid—signals to the pyloric valve (the gateway to the stomach) that preliminary healthy digestion is complete, and like a key, the proper pH value opens the valve and allows the happily digested contents to empty into the duodenum. Improper pH signaling (i.e., inadequate hydrochloric acid pH values) can delay this gastric emptying, sometimes for hours, resulting in the fermentation of stomach contents and potentially generating reflux symptoms.

Try this experiment at home: Take a blender and throw some chopped meat in it, some mushy potatoes, some Pepsi (you might substitute a glass of wine), some ketchup, sour cream (for the potatoes), bread rolls and butter, and . . . what the heck, why not dessert. Now blend it all together, spit in it, then put it in a room that is 98.6° Fahrenheit for an hour or two (or more). I'll leave the results to your imagination. (With thanks to my colleague and friend Colleen Dunseth, M.A., N.T.P., for this very helpful and rather graphic analogy.)

Improperly digested chyme becomes rancid, putrefies, and ferments to become a mass of toxic compounds that the body, via the wise gatekeeper—the pyloric valve—is reluctant to allow through. When the pyloric valve (between the stomach and small intestine) is locked tight and won't let the food continue down, sometimes the contents will simply back up. Voilà—reflux!

The stomach is an acid organ. It thrives in the presence of extreme acid when healthy, and its contents *must be acidic enough!*

Even less than adequately acidic gastric pH values can feel extremely acidic to the delicate esophagus, which has zero protection from acid during reflux. But just think of what you're doing when you use an acid blocker or neutralizer to treat this symptom. Acid reflux is nearly always a consequence of *not enough* stomach acid, rather than too much! Short-term relief of symptoms by chronically using something that neutralizes stomach acid can lead to long-term disaster! These drugs were never meant to be used long term, yet many people today linger on them for years. Adequate hydrochloric acid is essential for the proper digestion of proteins, at least fourteen different minerals, vitamin B_{12}, and to some degree folic acid. It's also essential to the proper execution of the rest of the entire digestive process.

Having inadequate hydrochloric acid can be a real problem. Gas, bloating, belching, and a feeling of heaviness in the stomach after meals are all classic symptoms of inadequate hydrochloric acid production, as is reflux. Weak or brittle nails and, in some cases, excessive hair loss can also be common symptoms. These symptoms represent only the tip of the much bigger iceberg. This is also a wide-open gateway to developing multiple food-sensitivity issues.

Meanwhile, Farther South

At the same time that the appropriately acidic chyme enters the duodenum, the proper pH value signals the production of mucus to protect the vulnerable duodenum from stomach acids. The hormone secretin then signals the pancreas to release both bicarbonate to neutralize the stomach acid so the next phase of digestion can occur and pancreatic enzymes to further digest the food particles.

Another hormone, *cholecystokinin,* which senses the presence of fats, stimulates the gallbladder to release a sufficient bolus of bile into the bile duct, which then empties into the duodenum, where the bile can emulsify the fats there into smaller globules for easier assimilation. Bile function is also influenced by gastric pH signaling. In addition, gluten sensitivity can also markedly suppress cholecystokinin production and bile flow. The journal *Hepatology* stated, "Celiac Disease is associated with increased fasting gallbladder volume and reduced gallbladder emptying in response to meals" (Rubio-Tapia and Murray 2007). This, of course, can lead to biliary stagnation (sluggish bile) and the eventual precipitation of biliary calculi (gallstones). The article went on to say, "This is likely due to impaired meal-induced release of gut hormones (for example, cholecystokinin) secondary to the loss of enterocytes mass (villous atrophy) and increased somatostatin levels." Additionally, in an article in the journal *Gut,* the authors wrote, "Gall bladder emptying was measured on a minute-by-minute basis using ssniTc-HIDA scans. In the patients with celiac disease, gall bladder emptying was greatly decreased (34.6 ± 9.9 v 615 + 7 ± 5% at 60 minutes)" (Brown et al. 1987).

Poor bile function by any cause (including having no gallbladder at all) can seriously thwart the digestive process, leading to incomplete digestion of fats, poor fat-soluble-nutrient assimilation, and ultimately deficiencies of these vital nutrients. Trust me when I say this is a bad, bad thing.

Bile can become stagnant and unhealthy for many reasons, though among the most common culprits are poor hydrochloric acid production; gluten sensitivity; overconsumption of processed fats, rancid fats, or trans fats; an excess of estrogens; and an excessively low-fat diet. You see, bile is normally very watery in its consistency and is composed mainly of cholesterol (yes . . . *eeevil* cholesterol), bile salts, phospholipids, certain minerals, other nutrients, bile pigments, and taurine. Bad (i.e., processed, rancid, or artificial) fats or bile that is stagnating from disuse, as via low-fat diets, can alter bile's consistency, thickening it and making its expulsion from the gallbladder sluggish, painful, or almost impossible. Stagnant bile can then begin to precipitate out cholesterol, pigments, or calcium as small, or not-so-small, stones.

Heaven forbid one of these stones should attempt to traverse through or occlude the bile duct and then you eat a bucket of the Colonel's "Secret Recipe." This can trigger a nasty gallbladder attack and send you unceremoniously to the hospital, where doctors will be only too eager to surgically part you from your gallbladder forever. Sometimes doctors recommend removing a gallbladder preemptively or even (as insane as this is) "preventively," even when there is nothing wrong with it . . . *"yet."*

Don't be fooled into thinking you don't really need your gallbladder, though they may try to convince you that you don't. Living without a gallbladder can lead to lifelong issues with inadequate fat and fat-soluble-nutrient digestion, deficiencies of minerals and critical fat-soluble nutrients, fatigue, hormonal imbalances, and other problems. Carefully and systematically restoring biliary health should be a first choice whenever reasonably possible. Once you're in the middle of a full-blown gallbladder attack with a stone painfully lodged in your cystic duct, though, it's usually too late.

Taking bile salts (commonly sold as ox bile in health-food stores) with every fat-containing meal is a must in the absence of having a functional gallbladder. Additionally, care must be taken that one does not develop deficiencies of essential fatty acids and vitamins A, D, E, and K.

Inappropriate pH values in the stomach or biliary problems farther north along the digestive tract set the stage for irritable bowel syndrome, duodenal ulcers, yeast overgrowth, vulnerability to parasites and other food-borne illness, dysbiosis (imbalances of healthy gastrointestinal flora, or "healthy bacteria"), the "Big C" (constipation), and, ultimately, worse problems.

Suffice it to say, it is not a happy ending. (No pun intended.)

Yikes! What Do I Do?

So much can be accomplished toward optimizing proper digestion by following a few simple guidelines:

- Take time out and focus on being relaxed and calmly present at mealtime.
- Chew, chew, chew!
- Minimize fluid intake at meals. Stick to only small sips of water and avoid other beverages.
- Consume high-quality protein, not soy, cooked as minimally as possible (except, of course, chicken and pork) in small to moderate quantities at mealtime.

- Avoid combining proteins with starches and sugars, even fruit, at mealtime. Stick to fibrous, nonstarchy vegetables and greens.
- Test for gluten sensitivity if you know you have any digestive or gallbladder issues.
- Consider the incorporation of quality lacto-fermented foods and raw cultured vegetables with meals. These can help restore healthy bacteria and provide many enzymes that can assist in the digestive process. They are especially helpful when one is eating a lot of otherwise cooked and denatured foods. They are also delicious.
- Do not fear naturally occurring fat or get suckered into following a low-fat diet. Remember, we are designed to eat fat, and a significant amount of it. This is why we have a gallbladder in the first place. We're creatures of the ice age—remember? Use it or lose it.

  Important note: The one notable exception here is a person who may be experiencing gallbladder symptoms (gallbladder attacks, including aching pain under the right side of the rib cage, especially pain to the touch, or nausea at meals), in which case this should be dealt with cautiously, and a low-fat diet may be entirely appropriate until the issue is resolved. Consult with a qualified health care provider. Remember, don't be a hero and don't push it. *Listen to your body.*
- Avoid nonfermented soy (soy is a topic covered more exhaustively in chapter 4, So What about Soy?). Soy contains enzyme inhibitors that can, over time, ruin your ability to digest and absorb protein.
- Be sure to consume enough full-spectrum, unrefined sea salt (such as Celtic or Himalayan sea salt) as low-carbohydrate diets tend to result in sodium losses that can commonly contribute to constipation issues.

For some, taking hydrochloric acid as a supplement at mealtime may be appropriate and necessary for a time, until the stomach is able to resume its own production. If you experience gas, bloating, or excessive fullness after meals, the rule is start with one capsule of hydrochloric acid with a meal. If you do not experience a slight warming sensation with that, take two with your next meal and so on until a sensation of warming is achieved. Then back off by one capsule, and that is your dose. The amount of protein in the meal should be used as a gauge with dosing. (In other words, don't take a handful of hydrochloric acid capsules if all you're having is one or two lonely shrimp on your salad.) This process tends to be self-weaning, and your stomach will usually tell you when you need to start backing off.

Eventually, your stomach should be able to restore appropriate hydrochloric acid production on its own. If it doesn't, there may be some other underlying problem, such as *H. pylori* overgrowth, a poorly functioning thyroid, or some other issue. Seek out a natural, qualified, and knowledgeable health care provider for evaluation.

The exceptions to undertaking hydrochloric acid supplementation are people with ulcers, gastritis, or a current, acute reflux problem. The inflamed gastric and esophageal tissue needs to heal before people with these conditions should start taking hydrochloric acid supplements. This can be accomplished with supplements containing deglycyrrhizinated (DGL) licorice, vitamin U (or lots of very fresh raw cabbage juice, as long as you don't have a thyroid problem), vitamins A and D, high-strength and mucopolysaccharide-rich organic aloe vera, and L-glutamine.

Pancreatic enzymes, taken on an empty stomach, can further assist in digestion for people who lack adequate natural production. Consuming smaller, more easily digested meals, avoiding soy foods as well as other legumes and grains, and increasing the normalization of hydrochloric acid and gastric pH can also contribute to the normalization of pancreatic output.

Some individuals have a deficiency of an important pancreatic fat-digesting enzyme called *lipase*. Lipase deficiency may be more prevalent in people who are prone to diabetes and glucose dysregulation. Taking lipase as part of a pancreatic enzyme supplement on an empty stomach throughout the day can help restore healthy fat digestion for some and make eliminating the dependence on sugar as the primary source of fuel much easier.

Those people who are experiencing biliary stasis or who may have cholesterol-type gallstones often benefit from taking a couple of tablespoons of raw apple cider vinegar with their meals. The malic acid in the vinegar (also sold as a supplement) can help soften the stones and thin the bile over time. Other biliary support can be provided by beet juice (of mainly tops and stems), taurine, and phosphatidyl choline supplementation to help thin bile and restore better biliary function. Phosphoric acid supplements can be helpful with dissolving calcium-type gallstones. The use of bile salts may be necessary temporarily to help with digestion of fats until gallbladder function is more fully restored. *Note:* It is always recommended that a qualified and knowledgeable (preferably natural-oriented) health care provider be consulted before undertaking any regimen designed to address the issue of gallstones.

Remember, everything begins and ends with proper digestion. Improving this alone can result in what feels like a miraculous improvement in the way you feel and function!

6

Your Gut and the Immune Connection

■ ■ ■ ■ ■ ■ ■ ■ ■ ■ ■ ■

Few people are aware that up to 70 percent of our immune system resides in our gut. The mucosal layer, a mere single cell in thickness, serves as the superficial veil for the gut-associated lymphatic tissue (often referred to as GALT). It is the first line of defense in our immune system, and clusters of cells there, known as *Peyer's patches,* along with secretory IgA, which is located in the mucosa and protectively on the surface of lung tissue, are the sentinels that alert both T cells and B cells to possible invasion by unwanted antigens and microbes. Stress, excessively low or high cortisol levels, infection, and poor diet can strip secretory IgA from the gut and lungs, rendering them extremely vulnerable. The primary food for enterocytes (the cells of the small intestine) is the amino acid L-glutamine. Supplementation, along with maintaining the healthy dietary guidelines outlined in this book, can enhance and help facilitate more-rapid regeneration of eroded gastrointestinal mucosa and depleted secretory IgA levels, though this can still take time. Note that patients with celiac disease are ten to fifteen times more likely to have a secretory IgA deficiency (one reason why secretory IgA testing for gluten sensitivity is so unreliable).

There are more bacteria in our intestinal tract than cells in our body.

JEFFREY S. BLAND, PH.D.

Gastrointestinal flora, or healthy bacteria, are also an undeniably important part of this equation. Few individuals today maintain healthy populations of these vital gastrointestinal-system denizens, which outnumber all other cells in the human body combined! There are literally hundreds of probiotic species, most of which are, as yet, little researched or understood. The most common varieties are *Lactobacillus* (found primarily in the small intestine), *Bifidobacterium* (found primarily in the large intestine), *Bacteroides, Eubacterium, Peptococcaceae, Streptococcus, Ruminococcus,* and *Fusobacterium.* They can be either aerobic or anaerobic in nature.

These probiotic species are commonly established at birth via the birth canal and breast milk, and they colonize very quickly in infancy. In babies whose gastrointestinal probiotic colonization is poor, there is a greater tendency toward colic, gas, and diaper rash as well as the development of allergy, asthma, and eczema. Early problems with gastrointestinal integrity and healthy colonization are also exceedingly common in children with autism. Also, any child who is not breast-fed will likely never have normal gastrointestinal flora in the gut and will need to find a way to add probiotics or cultured foods to the diet on a daily and ongoing basis to have any real hope for optimal gastrointestinal health.

Our ancestors also obtained soil-based organisms through natural exposure to dirt on their food. This has recently been hypothesized to have been an important dietary source of beneficial flora that is lacking in today's more antiseptic food-preparation methods. (Note, however, that I do not advocate eating unwashed produce or mud pies today because of this.)

Most of us carry three to four pounds of bacteria in our gut at any given time. Ideally, at least 85 percent of that should be of the friendly variety; no more than 15 percent should be of the less favorable kind. These bacteria help convert fiber and other indigestible material into usable nutrients, facilitate the absorption of certain minerals, assist in detoxification, and maintain and protect the gastrointestinal mucosa. They can also help in the prevention of allergies, skin disorders, inflammatory bowel disease, ear infections, vaginitis, bladder infections, constipation, and diarrhea. Probiotics have more recently been demonstrated in studies to modulate immune responses via the gut's mucosal immune system. Certain exogenously derived soil-based organisms have also been hypothesized to be a more natural part of our ancient diets and may be uniquely beneficial in restoring gut health for some. They can be purchased in supplement form, as well.

Most probiotic supplements that are commercially sold tend to be of questionable viability, though there are exceptions. The brands available via health care practitioners may be somewhat more reliable in this regard because production for them tends to more rigorously adhere to certain standards. Probiotic supplementation is probably a good idea for most people. They are best taken on an empty stomach at least one-half hour prior to meals, though instructions may vary from brand to brand. Steer clear of budget brands. I recommend cycling through different quality brands, giving your gut a variety of strains and potencies. These tend to work synergistically.

The most effective and inexpensive solution to restore healthy gastrointestinal flora, by far, comprises the addition of raw cultured vegetables and, if tolerated, homemade, raw, milk-based or (tastier and healthier yet) dairy-free, coconut milk–based kefir and yogurt to the diet. This suggestion does *not* mean the conventional, commercial forms of kefir and yogurt sold in grocery stores, however. Pasteurized milk is a source of countless problems for many, if not most, people. Note, too, that lactobacillus cannot live in pasteurized milk products, rendering most commercial yogurts ineffective and unreliable as a significant probiotic source. Conventional, store-bought kefir and yogurt also tend to contain extremely high levels of carbohydrates and undesirable additives. Learning to make your own from quality raw cow, sheep, or goat's milk (assuming that you have no casein sensitivity) or even coconut milk (my personal favorite) is "easy-peasy." Raw cultured vegetables are also extremely easy and inexpensive to make at home. They are a wonderful addition to any diet. (See *Nourishing Traditions,* by Sally Fallon and Mary Enig.)

Perhaps the single most acutely damaging impact on the balance of gastrointestinal flora involves the use, particularly the extended use, of antibiotics. (There goes the intestinal neighborhood!) Reverberations can continue for many, many years beyond a single course of antibiotics, and reestablishing healthy gastrointestinal flora can be extremely difficult, particularly after the "bad guys" have moved in and taken hold. For this reason alone, antibiotics should be used only when absolutely and undeniably essential, which is rarely the case. If you absolutely cannot avoid the use of antibiotics, take care to supplement your diet with quality and abundant probiotics both during and after using antibiotics for up to several weeks or months, to help prevent long-term complications and common secondary infections.

A new, disturbingly common, and troubling phenomenon entering into the research literature in just the past two years involves something called small intestinal bacterial overgrowth (SIBO). The small intestine, unlike the large intestine, is not meant to be colonized by bacteria. These unwelcome bacteria interfere with our normal digestion and absorption of food and are associated with damage to the lining or membrane of the small intestine, resulting in what is termed "leaky gut syndrome." Bacterial growth here commonly (but not always) accompanies issues with gluten sensitivity and is strongly associated with IBS symptoms (particularly gas and bloating). In high enough amounts these bacteria can also generate acids that result in neurological and cognitive symptoms. According to Bures et al., "It is mandatory to consider SIBO in all cases of complex non-specific dyspeptic complaints (bloating, abdominal discomfort, diarrhoea, abdominal pain), in motility disorders, anatomical abnormalities of the small bowel and in all malassimilation syndromes (malabsorption, maldigestion)." In some (not all) cases—mainly a finding in those with celiac disease—bacterial colonies in the small intestine seem to involve rod-shaped strains *never before even found in humans.* One possible explanation could be the growing prevalence of genetically modified foods. For more information concerning SIBO go to www.SIBOinfo.com.

The Second Brain?

Although serotonin is a neurotransmitter widely associated with the brain and mood functioning, including the prevention of depression, anxiety, and insomnia, few people are aware that 95 percent of all serotonin production in the body lies not in the brain, but in the gut.

The gut, in fact, has even more neurons than the brain! The next time you find yourself struggling with mood issues, consider first the quality of your gastrointestinal health and digestion. The brain and gut are inextricably linked.

7
■ ■ ■ ■ ■ ■ ■ ■ ■ ■ ■ ■ ■

Dietary Fats

The Good, the Bad, and the Ugly

> *The commonly held belief that the best diet for prevention of coronary heart disease is a low saturated fat, low cholesterol diet is not supported by the available evidence from clinical trials.*
>
> L. A. CORR AND M. F. OLIVER,
> "THE LOW FAT/LOW CHOLESTEROL DIET IS
> INEFFECTIVE," *EUROPEAN HEART JOURNAL*

> *Even though the focus of dietary recommendations is usually a reduction of saturated fat intake, no relation between saturated fat intake and risk of coronary heart disease was observed in the most informative prospective study to date.*
>
> WALTER WILLETT, *NUTRITIONAL EPIDEMIOLOGY*

Dietary fat has a little-deserved and much maligned recent history in the popular press. Yet a diet moderately high in both saturated and monounsaturated fats and certain essential polyunsaturated fats such as omega-3 fats has been ongoing in our history, spanning nearly one hundred thousand generations.

What changed?

The multifold answer lies in the abundance of refined carbohydrates in the modern diet: highly polyunsaturated vegetable oils (these are new to the human diet and contain predominantly omega-6 fatty acids, which are essential but excessively present in modern diets and can cause serious imbalances), grain- or corn-fed meats, farmed seafoods (also rich in excess omega-6 fatty acids and having very little omega-3 fats), and hydrogenated and partially hydrogenated oils.

Cooking with such oils promotes carcinogenicity, inflammation, and unhealthy imbalances of fatty acids in the body. The excess omega-6, omega-9, and trans fats also exacerbates insulin resistance. Trans fats—hydrogenated or partially hydrogenated fats and oils found in margarine spreads, vegetable shortening, commercial vegetable oils (particularly soybean and canola oils), salad dressings, baked or packaged goods, and virtually all fast foods—are created in a laboratory, not in nature. They most certainly do not belong in our diet.

Care must also be taken to make sure that the animal fat consumed comes from clean, grass-fed-only, organic sources (i.e., pesticide-free, hormone-free). Many toxins are, in fact, fat soluble and readily stored in animal body fat. Meat from grain- or corn-fed animals should probably be as lean and trimmed of fat as possible or countered with extra omega-3 fat supplementation, and always organic. High, imbalanced levels of omega-6 fat in grain- and corn-fed meats tend to promote inflammatory processes, insulin resistance, and interference with omega-3 fat metabolism. *Exclusively* grass-fed meat is vastly preferable, though harder to come by, and the fat in such meat is rich in desirable omega-3 fat and conjugated linoleic acid—both highly beneficial fats.

We Are Creatures of the Ice Age

This is hugely important to remember. Fat, to all humans, means "survival" to our physiological functioning. Diets low in fat paradoxically cause the body to more easily synthesize fat from other sources, most notably carbohydrates, and to absorb and store this unwanted fat. Diets high in carbohydrates trigger our master hormone, leptin, to become severely dysregulated. Blood sugar surges lead to leptin surges, and ultimately to leptin resistance, in which leptin signaling is no longer effectively heard by the brain. This sends a message of "starvation" to the hypothalamus, which then reacts promptly with increases in appetite or cravings and inspires unhealthy binge eating.

For many people, low-fat diets, which are often replete with empty carbohydrates, have resulted in little more than accelerated weight gain, significant deficiencies in essential nutrients, general frustration, and feelings of deprivation, not to mention uninspiring menu selections. Nothing has contributed more to our obesity epidemic. So many taboos about dietary fat—particularly saturated fat—have likely arisen from the perception of "you are what you eat." Consider, instead, that *you are what your metabolism does with what you eat.* This helps change the perspective in a way that allows for the complexity of human biochemistry. The relationship between dietary fat and unwanted body fat or fat in your arteries is anything but linear. The controversy is fueled far more by the politics and related economic interests than by the actual science.

Moderate intake of natural dietary fat is only potentially problematic or "fattening" in the presence of dietary carbohydrates. Our more primitive ancestors sought out and ate plenty of quality fat, including saturated fat and cholesterol, containing ample amounts of critical fat-soluble nutrients—up to ten times our modern-day intake. They had none of our modern afflictions, including heart disease, diabetes, cancer, and obesity. It's no paradox.

All primitive and traditional cultures coveted and revered their sources of dietary fat. For the Plains and Northern Indians, it was pemmican (over which entire wars were fought); Canadian tribes relished bear and moose fat; the coastal Salish tribes revered oolichan grease (a marine lipid from a small, sardinelike fish, almost identical in its composition to human body fat, interestingly); the Inuit ate large amounts of seal, walrus, and whale fat; the northern Innus coveted caribou fat; and the Australian Aborigines depended on emu fat. The Masai consumed lots of high-fat whole raw milk.

> *In Framingham, Massachusetts, the more saturated fat one ate, the more cholesterol one ate, the more calories one ate, the lower people's serum cholesterol. We found that the people who ate the most cholesterol, ate the most saturated fat, ate the most calories weighed the least and were the most physically active.*
>
> DR. WILLIAM CASTILLI, DIRECTOR OF THE FRAMINGHAM HEART STUDY, "CONCERNING THE POSSIBILITY OF A NUT . . . ," *ARCHIVES OF INTERNAL MEDICINE*

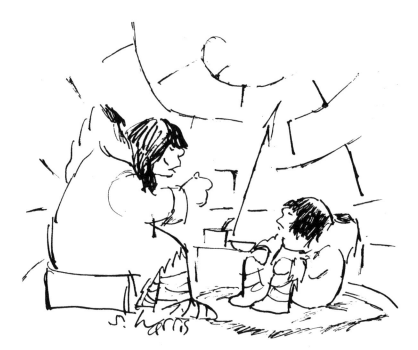

"EVERY DAY YOU SHOULD EAT SOMETHING FROM EACH OF THE FIVE BASIC FOOD GROUPS: FRIED BLUBBER, BOILED BLUBBER, STEWED BLUBBER, BAKED BLUBBER AND RAW BLUBBER."

Fig. 7.1. The Five Basic Food Groups

Reduced fat and caloric intake and frequent use of low caloric food products have been associated with a paradoxical increase in the prevalence of obesity.

A. F. HEINI AND R. L. WEINSIER, "DIVERGENT TRENDS IN OBESITY AND FAT INTAKE PATTERNS: THE AMERICAN PARADOX," *AMERICAN JOURNAL OF MEDICINE*

The idea that saturated fats cause heart disease is completely wrong, but the statement has been "published" so many times over the last three or more decades that it is very difficult to convince people otherwise unless they are willing to take the time to read and learn what produced the "anti-saturated fat agenda."

DR. MARY ENIG, CONSULTING EDITOR TO THE *JOURNAL OF THE AMERICAN COLLEGE OF NUTRITION*, PRESIDENT OF THE MARYLAND NUTRITIONISTS ASSOCIATION, AND WORLD-RENOWNED LIPIDS RESEARCHER, "THE OILING OF AMERICA," WWW.WESTONAPRICE.ORG

Consider the following:

- The French eat a richer diet and more saturated fats in the form of meat, liver pâté, butter, cream, and cheese than do people in almost any other Western nation, yet the heart-related death rate among middle-aged men in France is 145 per 100,000, compared with 315 per 100,000 in America. Heart-related deaths in France are actually at the lowest in Gascony, the region of France where people eat the most fat.
- Although it is a common perception that the Japanese eat a low-fat diet, this is a myth. The truth is that they get plenty of fat from eggs, chicken, beef, pork, organ meats, and shellfish. The amount of animal fat in their diet has gone up steadily since World War II, yet the rate of heart disease there is among the lowest in the world, and their average life span has actually increased.
- Scientists in India discovered that people in the northern part of the country ate seventeen times more animal fat than the people in the south, but their overall incidence of heart disease was **seven times lower.**

Elevated triglycerides, a known marker for increased cardiovascular risk, are generated not by dietary fats, but instead by dietary carbohydrates. Dietary fats (other than short- or medium-chain fats, which are used preferentially for immediate energy) are absorbed not into the bloodstream, but into the lymphatic system. In the textbook *Nutritional Biochemistry and Metabolism,* Maria Linder states, "The major portion of dietary fat (which has entered the lymphatic system) slowly enters into the bloodstream (as chylomicrons) through the thoracic duct, thus preventing large scale changes in the lipid content of peripheral blood" (Linder 1991). Excess carbohydrates in the diet are readily converted to triglycerides and enter the bloodstream soon after a meal (on their way to your "love handles"). When I see a blood chemistry report with elevated triglycerides, I know I am looking at the profile of a "carbovore." Always. And the closer that triglyceride number is to a person's total cholesterol number (it shouldn't be more than half), the closer that person is to full-blown *metabolic syndrome* (a common "parent" condition of heart disease, diabetes, and worse). A diet very low in carbohydrates not only results in low triglycerides but also substantially lowers saturated fat in the blood, even if the diet includes a substantial amount of saturated fat!

A remarkable, watershed study was published in January 2010 in *The American Journal of Clinical Nutrition* titled "Meta-analysis of Prospective Cohort Studies Evaluating the Association of Saturated Fat with Cardiovascular Disease." Catchy title, eh? The objective of the meta-analysis was to summarize the evidence related to the association of dietary saturated fat with the risk of coronary heart disease and cardiovascular disease, including stroke, that was noted in prospective epidemiologic studies involving 347,747 subjects—a sample well beyond "statistically significant" in number. The conclusions read as follows: "A meta analysis of prospective epidemiologic studies showed there is **no significant evidence** [emphasis mine] for concluding that dietary saturated fat is associated with an increased risk of [coronary heart disease] or [cardiovascular disease]" (Siri-Torino et al. 2010).

> *Whatever causes coronary heart disease, it is not primarily a high intake of saturated fatty acids*
> MICHAEL GURR, PH.D., *LIPID BIOCHEMISTRY: AN INTRODUCTION*

> In short: Saturated fat and cholesterol are not
> the culprits in heart disease! Hellllo!

The bottom line here is that your body *needs* saturated fat and cholesterol and is designed to make use of them.

Keep in mind, also, that all fats differ substantially from one another in their biochemical structure, in the way they are digested and absorbed, and in their specific physiological effects. They also may behave differently, even among individual types, depending on what other foods are consumed with them.

There are several different forms of saturated fat, in fact; short-, medium-, and long-chain varieties (and several different kinds of each) are used in the body in very different ways. Some are readily used for energy; others are more apt to be stored. You can never use just the term *fat* and encompass the myriad differences in their biological activity.

Perhaps the biggest misconception of all is that all fat is basically the same—or even that all saturated fat is the same. Natural dietary fats function with intricate complexity in the human body, and they are needed and used in varied ways under varied circumstances. For example, short- and medium-chain saturated fats have potent antimicrobial properties, bypass the gallbladder during digestion, and enter the portal blood to provide an immediate source of energy. Their structure makes them unlikely to be stored as body fat at all. Longer-chain dietary saturated fats (of which there are also a variety) fuel the muscles, including the heart, give structural integrity to our cellular membranes, assist in protein metabolism, assist in brain structure and function, are burned for energy via beta oxidation (at the same rate as all other natural fats), become lung surfactant (protecting our lungs from air pollutants and damage by oxidative processes), and protect the more delicate, polyunsaturated "essential" fats from damage and rancidity, improving their proper use. Some saturated fats even serve as substrates for conversion to the often overly revered monounsaturated fats (through the action of delta-9 desaturase)!

When the human body makes fat from carbohydrates, the vast majority are converted to palmitate (through the actions of acetyl CoA and insulin), which is the primary form of storage fat (the stuff you most want to get rid of) (Aarsland and Wolfe 1998). Only a very small amount is ever converted to palmitoleate, a monounsaturated fat—and usually only if the person is also using glucose to make a *lot* of saturated fat at the same time.

> Carbohydrates and unnatural fats—not healthy, natural fats in the diet—make you fat.

Only excess amounts of any dietary saturated fat are likely to be stored on your body, where you least want it. What's excess? Anything well over and above what you need to satisfy your appetite *in a low- or no-carbohydrate meal*. Once you add sugar or starch to a meal, you change everything. The less sugar and starch—*ever*—the better. Dietary fat, on its own, doesn't make you fat.

> *If you reduce saturated fat and replace it with high glycemic index carbohydrates, you may not only not get benefit you might actually produce harm.*
>
> DAVID LUDWIG, DIRECTOR OF THE OBESITY PROGRAM
> AT CHILDREN'S HOSPITAL, BOSTON

Saturated fats exist in the body because they are stable; they resist peroxidation (since we aren't refrigerated) in membranes exposed to free radicals. Saturated fats assist with our proper immune function, and their physical properties allow the body to regulate key membrane characteristics. Our body also regulates its own levels of saturated fat to a degree independent of dietary intake, especially when sugar and starch are most restricted from the diet. In short, our bodies *need* saturated fats!

I once heard Dr. Richard Feinman, professor of biochemistry at Downstate Medical Center in Brooklyn, New York, talk in a lecture about saturated fat this way: "The process of 'prosecuting' saturated fat is a lot like prosecuting in a courtroom. You can only be found 'not guilty.' You cannot be 'found innocent.' The problem in my view with saturated fat is that it should never have been indicted in the first place. It's like someone accused of being a child molester. They can be found 'not guilty' but still, no one wants to allow them to move into their neighborhood. Suspicion will forever persist."

The fact is that all natural fats have a role to play in our health, and what matters in the end is proper balance. Artificial, overly processed, or rancid fats, however, are the ones that need to be avoided altogether. Those are the real bad guys.

> *No diet will remove all the fat from your body because the brain is entirely fat. Without a brain, you might look good, but all you could do is run for public office.*
>
> GEORGE BERNARD SHAW

8
Dispelling the Cholesterol Myth

■ ■ ■ ■ ■ ■ ■ ■ ■ ■ ■ ■ ■

Besides real diseases we are subject to many that are only imaginary, for which the physicians have invented imaginary cures; these have then several names, and so have the drugs that are proper for them.

JONATHAN SWIFT, *GULLIVER'S TRAVELS*

As much as 90 percent of the published medical information that doctors rely on is flawed.

DAVID H. FREEDMAN, "LIES, DAMN LIES AND MEDICAL SCIENCE," *THE ATLANTIC*

Cholesterol is a vital substance in the human body. Using cholesterol, the body produces a series of stress-combating hormones and mediates the health and efficiency of the cell membranes. Cholesterol is found in the nerve sheaths, the white matter of the brain, and the adrenal glands. It also helps regulate the body's electrolyte balance. It is regarded by the body as such an important metabolic aid that every cell has a mechanism to manufacture its own supply (Erdmann and Jones 1995).

Cholesterol is also essential for brain function and development. It forms membranes inside cells, and keeps cell membranes permeable. It

76

keeps cells "waterproof," allowing there to be a different chemistry inside and outside the cell. It keeps moods level by stabilizing neurotransmitters and helps maintain a healthy immune system. No steroidal hormone can be manufactured without it, including estrogen, progesterone, testosterone, pregnenolone, adrenaline, cortisol, and dehydroepiandrosterone (DHEA)—or vitamin D.

Up to 2 g, or 2,000 mg, of cholesterol is produced by our bodies every day, several times the amount found in our diets. *Despite this ability to manufacture cholesterol, it is, in fact, critical to obtain cholesterol from dietary sources.* Although our cells technically have the means to manufacture cholesterol, it is quite difficult and inefficient to do so and involves a roughly thirty-step, complex biochemical process. Eating cholesterol actually gives the liver (the major internal source of cholesterol manufacture) a break, because it is so difficult to make. In fact, dietary cholesterol is so important that 90 percent of the cholesterol we consume is actually reabsorbed by the gut so it may be used again. The human diet has **always** contained significant amounts of it. Restricting or eliminating its intake basically indicates a crisis or famine to the body. The result is the production of a liver enzyme called *HMG-CoA reductase,* which, in effect, then overproduces cholesterol from carbohydrates in the diet to help make up for the dietary cholesterol deficit. Consuming excess carbohydrates while decreasing the cholesterol intake guarantees a steady and burdensome overproduction of cholesterol in the body. The only way to switch this overproduction off is to consume an adequate amount of dietary cholesterol and back off the carbs. In other words, the *dietary intake of cholesterol stops the internal production of cholesterol* (Schwarzbein and Deville 1999).

Most of the statin drugs used to lower cholesterol are designed to inhibit the action of HMG-CoA reductase artificially at the dangerous and costly expense of substantially depleting the body's own reserves of the coenzyme CoQ10 and overburdening the liver. *CoQ10 may be the single most important nutrient for the functioning of the heart.* Furthermore, statins have never even been proved to lessen the risk of a heart attack! Some studies promoting the supposed C-reactive protein–lowering effect of statins fail to mention that the reason this happens is due to liver damage by the drugs, disabling the liver's natural capacity to produce C-reactive protein, but in fact doing absolutely nothing to lower actual systemic inflammation!

A sobering aside: Political commentator Tim Russert was reportedly taking statin drugs at the time of his death. Tragically, he was prescribed these drugs even though his cholesterol was completely normal. His doctors had put him on statins "preventively." There is talk today of similarly prescribing statins "preventively" to children. A new report shows the number of kids taking statin drugs has sharply risen 68 percent in just five years. Pfizer has even introduced a new chewable, "kid-friendly" version of Lipitor, and there is a call among medical authorities to mandate a universal screening in schools to find children with high cholesterol and prescribe such drugs to those "in need of treatment." Cholesterol is a vital and utterly necessary nutrient in developing healthy brains and nervous systems. We simply cannot, in our right minds, allow this to happen!

Study after study has demonstrated the potentially debilitating effects of statin drugs. There are over *nine hundred* studies to date showing the adverse potential effects of statin drugs on everything from cognitive functioning to immune-system functioning. One recent study showed that the statin drug simvastatin (Zocor and Simvacor) actually hinders the ability of the body's immune system to kill pathogens! The same study showed that the use of these drugs also resulted in an increase in cytokine production, which increases damaging systemic inflammation (Hubbard 2010). Another review of nineteen large studies of more than sixty-eight thousand deaths by the Division of Epidemiology at the University of Minnesota found that low cholesterol levels predicted an *increased risk of dying* from gastrointestinal and respiratory diseases (Jacobs, Blackburn, Higgins, et al. 1992). Finally, the same University of Minnesota team did a study of more than one hundred thousand healthy individuals in the San Francisco area for fifteen years. At the end of the study, those who had low cholesterol levels at the start of the study had been admitted to the hospital more often because of an infectious disease. In other words, either low cholesterol made them more vulnerable to infection or high cholesterol protected those who did not become infected. The promotion of the low-cholesterol agenda and the use of statin drugs have been much more than wrong; they have been lethal.

Among numerous other things, the use of statin drugs can produce a confused state similar to that of Alzheimer's disease. They have additionally even been linked with Lou Gehrig's disease. A new study published in the *Journal of the American College of Cardiology* revealed that driving down cholesterol levels actually increases the risk of cancer (Alawi et al. 2007).

The many potential side effects of statin use include:

- Depression
- Confusion
- Memory problems
- Inability to concentrate
- Amnesia
- Disorientation
- Weakened immune system
- Increased risk of cancer
- Shortness of breath
- Liver damage
- Fatigue
- CoQ10 depletion or deficiency and weakening of the heart
- Lowered sex drive
- Impotence
- Kidney failure
- Nerve pain
- Muscle weakness
- Rhabdomyolysis (painful deterioration or destruction of muscle cells)
- Death

"Elevated" cholesterol in women of all ages and the elderly was demonstrated through data from studies to actually be a **positive longevity marker** (Hulley et al. 1992; Forette et al. 1989). Another, more recent study showed similar longevity benefits in elderly people who had higher levels of cholesterol and a mortality rate from heart attacks that was **two times greater in those individuals with low cholesterol!** (Krumholz et al. 1990) Many studies reveal the fact that low cholesterol levels are actually much worse to have than higher cholesterol levels.

By conveniently placing the blame on cholesterol-carrying low-density lipoprotein (LDL), nothing is done to address the underlying problems that actually cause heart disease. The deeply flawed focus on lowering cholesterol with medications also enables the various guilty corporate interests to keep or expand their considerable profits (big pharma, the corn industry and the rest of big agriculture, the sugar industry, and the entire unscrupulous processed-food industry). It's all about the money, folks. Your health and well-being have nothing to do with it. Fully 50–75 percent of people who have a heart attack have what doctors term normal cholesterol. (My own father, a prominent medical doctor and the man who wrote the medical textbook titled *Cardiovascular Radiology*, was one of them.)

The best basic dietary approach for anyone wanting to prevent heart disease is a normal, unrestricted dietary intake of cholesterol and healthy natural fat, total avoidance of highly processed or rancid vegetable oils and trans fats, and a reduced or eliminated intake of starch and sugar-based carbohydrates.

Dietary cholesterol can, in fact, be additionally beneficial to the gastrointestinal lining, where it improves cell-membrane integrity and can help prevent or reduce excessive permeability.

The bottom line is that we are fully designed, and well suited, for consuming and healthfully metabolizing naturally occurring cholesterol. Cholesterol is not our enemy.

No study to date has adequately shown any significant link between dietary and serum cholesterol levels *or any significant causative link between cholesterol and actual heart disease.* There are some uncommon cases of genetically based familial hypercholesterolemia in which natural mechanisms that regulate cholesterol production fail and the body cannot stop overproduction, and even in these cases, the proof of the problematic nature of cholesterol is dubious, at best (Sijbrands et al. 2001). Cholesterol is perhaps only potentially deleterious in and of itself in oxidized forms, occurring as a result of methods used in the processing of foods such as reduced-fat milks, powdered milk, and powdered eggs, and in high-heat cooking or frying. Statins, by the way, do absolutely nothing to reduce the already existing oxidized cholesterol.

Inflammatory processes can also cause healthy cholesterol to undesirably oxidize in the body, resulting in arterial plaques. The primary problem here is not cholesterol but the inflammation. Other than this, *all* cholesterol in the body is the same. Levels of HDL and LDL reflect only transport mechanisms for healthy cholesterol and are inherently meaningless measures of the risk of coronary heart disease risk (Ravnskov 1998).

Again, it is important to realize that HDL and LDL are not actual cholesterol at all, but merely the protein transport mechanisms for cholesterol.

All Cholesterol Is Exactly the Same

LDL takes cholesterol away from the liver to the extremities and other organs for various purposes, including the manufacture of important steroidal hormones and vitamin D. HDL merely returns the same spent cholesterol to the liver, where it can be recycled. LDL also serves as a transport mechanism for critical fat-soluble nutrients, including vitamin D and antioxidants as well as certain fats.

There is one undesirable variation of a certain LDL carrier molecule known as lipoprotein(a), which is smaller and denser than regular LDL. Within the arterial endothelium lie spaces between cells that serve as channels for the influx and outflow of nutrients. Lipoprotein(a) can actually lodge itself in the spaces between these vascular arterial cells and shut off those natural channels, resulting in poor nutrient flow to the endothelium and triggering a damaging inflammatory response. Lipoprotein(a) is the only lipoprotein of significant consequence. The drug companies, however, would rather you didn't know about it at all, as statin drugs do nothing to change the size of LDL particles or reduce lipoprotein(a); *only diet can do this.* It is high-carbohydrate diets and the presence of excess insulin that are responsible for the production of this undesirable lipoprotein. Diets rich in natural fats and moderate protein with low carbohydrates result in normal LDL. Actual levels of regular LDL and HDL are of little actual consequence, though they can serve as a relative marker for illuminating certain dietary tendencies. High fructose diets, for instance, are known to greatly increase the production of LDL. They can also in part reflect other disorders and can be useful to look at in that regard. Note that HDL levels in excess of 70 to 75 mg/dL, in people for whom there is no inherent genetic predisposition toward very high HDL, can often imply the presence of undesirable inflammatory processes and potential autoimmune issues. This is because what is termed the *inflammatory peroxidase system,* when activated, can actually raise HDL in excess of normally positive indication ranges, as they are formed through related pathways. Higher HDL is *not* necessarily better. Excessively high HDL on your lab report may not be the "bee's knees," but it is **still only an indicator, a clue toward other things**—and not a *cause* of anything.

Furthermore, cholesterol is the human body's version of duct tape. It travels to areas where there has been arterial damage and patches up lesions. Higher serum levels of cholesterol can serve as a message that "something is going on" for which it is needed. Serum cholesterol is simply an indicator, *not* a diagnosis. Allegedly high cholesterol is in no way a form of a pathologic condition, in and of itself. But it may be telling you something, much like the engine warning light illuminating the dashboard of your car. Unscrewing the bulb (i.e., taking statin drugs) isn't going to fix the engine. You need to dig deeper. What has been deemed high cholesterol by some, however (i.e., anything over 200 mg/dL) is an entirely **arbitrary** and unscientifically derived number fabricated solely by pharmaceutical interests. Levels approaching 250 to 300 mg/dL might be an indication to look under the hood to see why serum cholesterol seems to be going up. Rest assured, however, that cholesterol isn't being sent there like an evil villain to cause you trouble; it's simply trying to do its job. In my view, it is important to simply let it, while pursuing the trail of evidence to its more meaningful source.

Going in with statin drugs to stamp out cholesterol is the equivalent of preventing the firemen who arrive to put out a fire from doing their job—and blaming them for the fire. Elevated glucose or insulin levels, for instance, damage arterial walls and lead to an increased need for cholesterol to repair them.

Roughly 80 percent of what actually clogs arteries is not even composed of cholesterol or saturated fat but is composed of oxidized or rancid *unsaturated* fats (Enig 2001). Statistically, individuals whose blood cholesterol levels are low develop just as many plaques in their blood vessels as individuals whose cholesterol is high (Ravnskov 1998).

Cholesterol is no more a cause of heart disease than gray hair is the cause of old age.

Many people are unaware that cholesterol is also an antioxidant or that levels that are too low (below 150 mg/dL) actually *increase* your risk

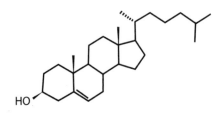

Fig. 8.1. Molecular structure of cholesterol

Cholesterol

Cholesterol mg/dl	205–234	235–265
MEN	**DEATHS/1000**	
Age 35–44	3	6
45–54	11	11
55–64	20	21
65–74	22	23
35–64 (age adjusted)	13	14
WOMEN		
Age 35–44	1	1
45–54	4	2
55–64	8	7
65–74	11	13
35–64 (age adjusted)	5	4

Fig. 8.2. Framingham Heart Study data, thirty-year observation

for cancer, hormonal imbalances, depression, sexual dysfunction, memory loss, Parkinson's disease, stroke (yes, stroke), suicide, and violent behavior. I personally worry far more about someone with cholesterol levels that are too low than someone whose levels are supposedly too high. In addition, normal hormonal production and balance are utterly dependent on the availability of cholesterol in the body. Cholesterol is the primary building block of many hormones. It is also essential for normal cognitive functioning and brain development. *We cannot live or function optimally without it.*

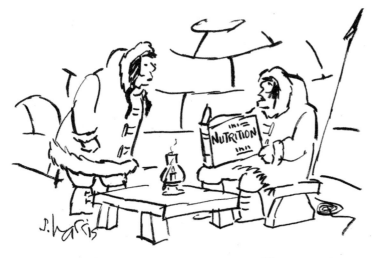

"IT APPEARS THAT OUR DIET IS ALMOST ONE HUNDRED PERCENT CHOLESTEROL. THAT APPEARS TO BE VERY, VERY, VERY BAD."

Fig. 8.3. The Cholesterol Problem

CHOLESTEROL EATEN PER DAY, IN MG

		PATIENTS WITH CHD	HEALTHY SUBJECTS
Male Chicago workers		721	757
Framingham citizens	men	708	716
	women	520	477
Puerto Rican men	urban	449	442
	rural	335	358
Puerto Ricans		419	417
Honolulu citizens		549	555
Men from Zutphen, The Netherlands		446	429
Irish men from Ireland and the US		854	832
Citizens from Rancho Bernardo, California	men	470	409
	women	226	309
Participants in the LRC study	age 30–59	427	416
	age 60–79	423	355
Hawaiian citizens	Hawaiian men	510	680
	Japanese men	466	587

Fig. 8.4. Comparison in ten study groupings of the amount of cholesterol eaten per day by patients with coronary heart disease (CHD) and by healthy age- and sex-matched control individuals.

> *Perhaps the biggest obstacle to a more rational debate about cholesterol, heart disease, or any other health problem is the simple fact that too many of the people we turn to for advice on such matters—our doctors—are tied to the makers of drugs. Sometimes those ties involve several hundred thousand dollars a year, sometimes just a few warm doughnuts.*
>
> RAY MOYNIHAN AND ALAN CASSELS,
> *SELLING SICKNESS*

Furthermore, it is an interesting irony that many of the most vital, protective, and supportive nutrients promoted for cardiovascular health in their most usable forms are those found (richly, predominantly, or exclusively) in animal-source foods and/or are best absorbed from these foods, which are typically rich in fat, cholesterol, and complete proteins. These nutrients include CoQ10, taurine, EPA and DHA, conjugated linolenic acid, the key glutathione precursor L-cysteine, L-carnitine, vitamins A (retinoic acid), D₃, and K₂, the antihomocysteine vitamins B₆ and B₁₂, folic acid (richly abundant in the liver), R-lipoic acid, magnesium, zinc, and sulfur, to name a few.

Saturated fat, particularly 18-carbon stearic acid, is the preferred fuel for the human heart, liver, and kidneys (Enig 2001).

> **Children should never, ever be put on a low-fat or low-cholesterol diet.**

Studies have overwhelmingly shown that the younger the child, the more critical fat and cholesterol are to the brain and nervous system's development. In fact, excessively low cholesterol levels in the brains of autistic children are increasingly recognized as a concern and a detriment to normal brain development and function in these populations, and increasing the dietary cholesterol has been shown to have a benefit in many cases. Breast milk is especially rich in omega-3 fats, saturated fat, and medium-chain triglycerides, an important component of some saturated fats, such as coconut oil. Fats are also essential for the absorption of many solely fat-soluble nutrients, such as vitamins A, E, D, and K, as are the many minerals that rely on such vitamins as cofactors and are necessary for their proper absorption.

The presence of dietary fat is critical for the proper use of dietary protein. We need quality natural fat in significant quantities, if not in abundance, for the optimal functioning of our body and our brain.

The human body and brain's primary source of fuel is designed to be fat in the form of ketones and free fatty acids—not glucose!

Amounts of critical fat-soluble nutrients, particularly true vitamin A (retinoic acid, found only in animal sources, as opposed to inefficiently converted "provitamin A," such as in carotenoids) and bioactive vitamin D₃, were especially high in primitive and traditional diets—often ten times higher than in modern diets (Price 1939). Beta-carotene, a fat-soluble nutrient, by the way, is not, contrary to the popular press, the equivalent of vitamin A, nor is its conversion to vitamin A a simple matter. Children under the age of five and individuals with liver or thyroid impairment cannot make this conversion at all.

The conversion also requires the presence of dietary fat. Furthermore, it takes no less than six units of beta-carotene to biochemically form a single unit of vitamin A (Enig 2001). One should never rely solely on vegetable sources for this incredibly vital nutrient. Remember, vitamin A (retinol) is not the same thing as beta-carotene (see figure 8.5). Cod-liver oil, which is high in vitamins, can be an excellent supplemental source of true vitamins A and some D (mostly A) as well as some omega-3 fats, and it may be additionally helpful in the reversal of mineral deficiencies.

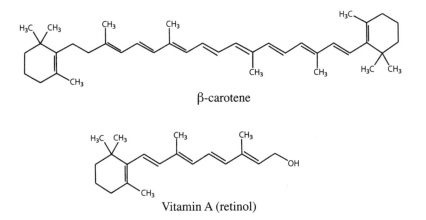

β-carotene

Vitamin A (retinol)

Fig. 8.5. Molecular structure of beta-carotene and vitamin A (retinol)

9
Vitamin D

■ ■ ■ ■ ■ ■ ■ ■ ■ ■ ■ ■

What All da Buzz Is About

> *[Vitamin D] may be the single most important organic nutrient for your overall health. In fact, if this were a drug, it would be considered the discovery of the century.*
>
> AL SEARS, M.D., *YOUR BEST HEALTH UNDER THE SUN*

Vitamin D has gotten quite a bit of press in recent years—and deservedly so. Innumerable studies are touting it as the single greatest preventive nutrient against cancer. Recent studies in Canada, in fact, showed that vitamin D lowered the risk of all forms of cancer in women by a remarkable 77 percent. In men, this figure was closer to 60 percent.

Vitamin D has also been shown to:

- Greatly reduce inflammation
- Help prevent most forms of cancer, including skin cancers
- Help prevent autoimmune diseases like multiple sclerosis and rheumatoid arthritis
- Support healthy immune function
- Help prevent cardiovascular disease
- Help prevent Parkinson's disease
- Help maintain healthy musculoskeletal structure
- Help prevent both type 1 and type 2 diabetes
- Support a healthy mood and prevent seasonal affective disorders

- Support brain health
- Be critical for the absorption and use of calcium and phosphorus

Plus, this news flash: *Vitamin D is also arguably the most potent antioxidant in the body, hands down.*

As much as vitamin E is the primary protective nutrient for omega-6 fats in nature, vitamin D is similarly the primary antioxidant and protective nutrient for omega-3 fats in nature (Sullivan 2006). Vitamin D (known specifically as a secosteroid) is also much more an actual steroid hormone than a vitamin.

What is seen as a nutrient's action is not always the same result gotten with supplementation, however, and more research is needed to determine not just the effects of vitamin D levels in the body but the effects of supplementation as well.

The Unfortunate Flaw in Nutrient Research

All this renewed attention paid to such a clearly important and previously undervalued and even irrationally feared nutrient is, of course, wonderful.

The problem lies in one simple fact: All nutrients operate in a complex system of interrelationships in the body, and requirements will vary greatly from person to person. Furthermore, modern-day research simply fails to take all these variables into account, instead studying nutrients in relative isolation, compartmentalizing what is never compartmentalized in nature.

The role of certain nutrients in relation to others and the need for certain cofactors in order to optimize a nutrient's function or prevent imbalances aren't normally discussed at all.

This, of course, leads to problems. For instance—and perhaps critically—for each and every receptor for vitamin D, there are two receptors for vitamin A on every cell. Because of the compartmentalized approach to vitamin D research, this sort of thing does not get recognized or discussed. A relative balance of these two nutrients is vital to their healthy functioning in the body. An excess of one can create a relative deficiency of the other. For instance, if you take large amounts of vitamin D without vitamin A, you are potentially more likely to develop symptoms of vitamin A deficiency and experience an actual immunosuppressive effect. Conversely, taking certain commercial cod-liver oil supplements that are rich in vitamin A but poor in vitamin D can lead to more severe vitamin D deficiencies. (It's important to read labels. The amount of vitamin D in a serving of high-vitamin cod-liver oil is around 1,000 IU. Most commercial brands don't exceed between 20 and 400 IU). Recent research from Spain indicates that vitamin A is necessary for both vitamin D binding and vitamin D release to receptor sites. The two vitamins are synergistic and should always be balanced in the diet or in supplementation. Individual needs for both may vary considerably.

A Possible Dark Side to the Sunshine Vitamin

There is some recent evidence and an "alternative vitamin D hypothesis" put forward by the Autoimmunity Research Foundation, a nonprofit organization, suggesting that excess supplemental vitamin D may actually be immunosuppressive in effect and may actually interfere with healthy immune function and recovery rather than protect against disease. Offering a conflicting perspective to the more common favorable view of vitamin D supplementation held by the Vitamin D Council, the head of the foundation, Professor Trevor Marshall, Ph.D., of Australia's Murdoch University School of Biological Medicine and Biotechnology, suggests that low vitamin D levels in some people may actually be the *result* of a disease process or immune compromise and not the actual underlying cause—and that supplementation may not always be desirable.

Marshall says, "Our disease model has shown us why low levels of vitamin D are observed in association with major and chronic illness. . . . Vitamin D is a secosteroid hormone, and the body regulates the production of all it needs. In fact, the use of supplements can be harmful, because they suppress the immune system so that the body cannot fight disease and infection effectively" (Marshall 2008).

It's clear that further research is needed to clarify the roles of vitamin D in human health before everyone goes off half-cocked and starts popping vitamin D pills in willy-nilly fashion. What is referred to broadly as vitamin D is also found in the body in different forms. Vitamin D_2, or ergocalciferol, which is sometimes found in plant foods, is largely inactive and requires the action of sunlight and 7-dehydrocholesterol (there goes that eeeevil cholesterol again!) to be usable. Also, 1,25-dihydroxyvitamin D_3, a metabolite of vitamin D metabolism (converted endogenously), seems to be most directly responsible for immune activation through the activation of what is known as the *vitamin D nuclear receptor*, which essentially mediates the way vitamin D in the body is used. 25-hydroxyvitamin D$_3$, the form most commonly measured in serum blood tests to determine vitamin D levels and the form most commonly sold as supplements, may actually serve to *inactivate* the vitamin D nuclear receptor, suppressing immune function either when necessary or when oversupplemented. Marshall also says, "Vitamin D affects the expression of over 1,000 genes, so we should not expect a simplistic cause and effect between vitamin D supplementation and disease" (Marshall 2008). Not meaning to confuse everyone, but it seems that much more needs to be understood here. People should not be running out to their health-food stores and popping vitamin D pills like candy. Testing is essential in ascertaining healthy vitamin D levels. Vitamin D gotten from sun exposure is much more naturally regulated in the body and probably the safest way to get vitamin D, though it isn't always practical, but the doses we get from sun exposure are far from predictable.

A growing, very real problem, too, is the excessive "fortification" of processed foods with vitamin D as a means of marketing and selling more of certain food products in an effort to capitalize on all the media hype about vitamin D's benefits. This is a potentially great cause for concern and could lead to toxic and even immunosuppressive effects in people who consume vitamin D in excess, particularly where preformed vitamin A deficiency might also be an issue.

What is certain is that both vitamin D and vitamin A have important roles to play in the human body, but they do not exist or function in isolation. Vitamin E helps recycle vitamin A, vitamin A needs zinc in order to be properly used, zinc and copper need to be in an 8:1 to 12:1 ratio in order to function properly, and on and on. Inadequate levels of either vitamin A or vitamin D, coupled with a significantly higher level of one or the other, can also result in a relative toxicity at much lower levels than if the two were properly balanced. This complex web of interrelationships is rarely discussed in the articles promoting vitamin D, or any other nutrient, as the answer to all ills. This is deeply problematic.

Furthermore, often no mention is made of all the varying requirements for vitamin D relative to individual needs or time of year. Taking any solitary nutrient (or hormone) doesn't just affect one thing; it affects many, *many* things. This needs to be intelligently considered. Plus, people with impaired biliary function or who no longer have a gallbladder may find it particularly difficult to absorb and use even supplemental fat-soluble nutrients.

Complex systems models, functional medicine, and functionally, foundationally based nutritional therapy must be the next evolution of research and practice across the spectrum of health care. Science and medicine can no longer be compartmentalized in their thinking or sell their souls to pharmaceutical and corporate greed if we are to genuinely uncover useful truths toward our enhanced well-being.

With all that in mind, back to vitamin D . . .

According to the Vitamin D Council, the amount of vitamin D most of us should have—measured as the amount of 25-hydroxyvitamin D_3 in the blood—in order to prevent cancer is about 60 ng/dL. The recommended range of serum 25-hydroxyvitamin D_3 according to a wide variety of experts lies somewhere between 40 and 80 ng/dL. The optimal amount, in light of the Vitamin D Council's findings, is probably closer to 60 to 80 ng/dL. If you happen to have an autoimmune illness, your ability to effectively use vitamin D is potentially impaired and your requirements are said to be generally higher. The guideline there is to shoot for between 80 and 100 ng/dL. Vitamin D can also help to mitigate the balance between TH-1 and TH-2 immune responses—a critical issue for people with an autoimmune condition. Currently, it is advised that no one exceed 100 to 150 ng/dL because of toxicity concerns.

Deficiencies of vitamin A, however, can make vitamin D toxic at much lower levels. Excesses of vitamin A can also result in greater vitamin D

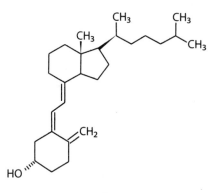

Vitamin D_3

Fig. 9.1. Molecular structure of vitamin D_3

deficiencies. Again, proper balance is needed. **Getting most of our nutrients from quality, nutrient-dense food sources is what seems to make the most sense, wherever possible.** That helps take the guesswork out of it.

When vitamin D supplementation is determined to be necessary, care, in my opinion, must be taken to use a supplement with a vitamin D complex containing the vitamin's numerous cofactors in relative balance, or rather, with vitamin A in its *true* state, as found in beef liver, grass-fed butter and ghee, and what is called "high-vitamin" cod-liver oil (rich in both vitamins A and D)—not simply beta-carotene. Taking a "vitamin D pill" may not necessarily be the best option. Emulsified, liquid forms of supplemental vitamin D may be a better choice for some people, as they are far better absorbed by most people and are much safer. Emulsification improves the vitamin's water solubility, so excesses can be more readily excreted. Far and away the safest means of obtaining vitamin D is through exposure to sunlight (which contains ultraviolet B, or UVB, light). This allows the body to make what it needs as it needs it. It is possible now to buy UVB-based vitamin D–enhancing light systems for home use.

It is very difficult to ascertain just how much vitamin D to recommend for any given individual, supplementally, to adequately and safely meet his or her needs. Recommended supplemental amounts of vitamin D may vary from as low as 1,000 IU for relative maintenance in an otherwise vitamin D–sufficient individual to upward of 10,000 IU per day for someone with an autoimmune condition. The woefully outdated government guideline established as the recommended daily allowance (RDA) for Americans is a meager 400 IU. Available data from modern-day, primitive hunter-gatherer societies generally estimate that the daily dietary intake was probably close to 4,000 IU of dietary vitamin D per day (Price 1939). This does not include vitamin D synthesized in the body from sun exposure, another highly variable and unpredictable process, depending on geographic location, time of year, and one's own inherent density of vitamin D receptors (and metabolic functioning). Higher amounts may be needed for a time to remediate deficiency states, however, or for specific conditions.

Your need for D depends on much more than (your geographic location); your skin color, your age, your sunning habits, your diet, your genes, your weather (clouds, fog and some urban pollution,

aka urban ozone, block UV-B). The only way to know how much D you have and how much D or sun you need and if the supplemental D or sun, or tanning bed you are using is working is TESTING. TEST and RETEST, don't guess.
KRISPIN SULLIVAN, NOTED VITAMIN D RESEARCHER,
NAKED AT NOON: UNDERSTANDING SUNLIGHT AND VITAMIN D

Active, usable dietary vitamin D_3 is found almost exclusively in animal and fish body fats and is not stored in any one organ.

The dogmas promoting low-fat diets, ultraviolet sunlight fear-mongering hysteria, and sun protection factor (SPF) sunscreen lotions have been responsible for rampant deficiencies of this potentially lifesaving nutrient (vitamin D_3) and its important cofactors. The body is able to manufacture vitamin D from a combination of its precursor ergocalciferol, vitamin D_2, which is found in some plant foods, and a form of cholesterol in the skin when exposed to UVB sunlight. Of course, this presupposes adequate levels of UVB sunlight (which is markedly insufficient in the more northern latitudes), adequate sun exposure (which almost no one gets, even in sunny locations), and an absence of any sunscreens worn. SPF sunscreen lotions stop natural vitamin D production dead in its tracks and may actually make you more susceptible—not less—to various skin cancers (including deadly melanoma) and many other cancers.

Living in the Pacific Northwest, where there are above-average rates of cancer and seasonal affective disorders, I have yet to measure vitamin D levels in a person (other than yours truly) that showed actual blood levels even approaching optimal sufficiency (according to Vitamin D Council guidelines).

If you have a need or interest in taking vitamin D, first take the time to get your blood tested. Anyone can order the test for 25-hydroxyvitamin D_3 online via www.directlabs.com without a prescription or a doctor's visit (blood can be drawn at any LabCorp location; see www.labcorp .com). It's relatively inexpensive. Keep in mind that the standard lab test result ranges offered for comparison to your results are ridiculously low, outdated, and relative only to everyone else who went into that particular lab system for blood work. Try, instead, to generally meet the requirements as laid out by the Vitamin D Council. It may well be (in light of evidence provided by the Autoimmunity Research Foundation) that measuring 1,25 dihydroxyvitamin D_3 levels also makes sense and that both should be monitored. Be warned, however, that testing for 1,25 dihydroxyvitamin D_3 can be expensive.

General blood-chemistry caveat: Reference or lab-range values in *all* conventional blood chemistry reports are *not* standardized, or scientifically agreed upon, by anyone. This lack of standardization is also true, by the way, of *every single blood marker* measured in standard blood tests, not just vitamin D.

As the population gets less and less healthy and everything gets averaged out (with the useless exception of lipid panels, which are the only markers actually standardized, although arbitrarily and for the purpose of selling statin drugs), many lab ranges have become too broad to be meaningful to a major portion of the population. They don't tell you in the least how you compare with "normal and healthy." The lab ranges are exclusively meant to reveal pathologic conditions, which may or may not be accurately represented. As such, many functional or subclinical dysregulations of, for instance, thyroid markers and other markers commonly go unnoticed by your doctor. The American Endocrine Society and the American Association of Clinical Chemists both agree this is a significant problem. Scientifically standardized normal-and-healthy functional ranges *are* available, but they are typically used only by certain enlightened natural health care providers specially schooled in *functional* blood chemistry analysis and some Certified Nutritional Therapists (CNTs), also referred to as Nutritional Therapy Practitioners.

Far and away the safest manner of obtaining adequate vitamin D is exposure to natural sunlight. In many areas of the country and during much of the year, however, this can be an impractical, if not impossible, proposition. Tanning beds using UVB bulbs can be another surprisingly viable option. Vitamin D obtained via natural sunlight has no potential vitamin D toxicity, though it *will increase your requirement for vitamin A*. Note that only UVB light, from the sun or tanning bulbs, will convert to vitamin D in combination with nutrient precursors and cholesterol in your skin. If you are inclined to use a tanning bed, always ask for one with the highest percentage of UVB bulbs for this purpose and patronize only reputable and sanitary tanning establishments. Take care not to overdo it; a sunburn is never a good thing!

Make sure to take quality cod-liver oil, too, to get adequate vitamin A, especially after being out in the sun, as sunlight exposure depletes vitamin A levels (Sullivan 2006). Beta-carotene and other carotenoids found in many vegetables and other food sources can be additionally helpful to your skin as singlet-oxygen free-radical scavengers and protective nutrients in their own right, other than as limited vitamin-A precursors.

Those people with a diet excessively high in omega-6 fats (from soybean oil, sunflower oil, canola oil, safflower oil, corn oil, and cottonseed oil), trans fats, and other processed fats and excessively low in both saturated fat and cholesterol are far and away the most vulnerable to skin cancers as well as numerous other cancers. These diets are also much more likely to wrinkle your skin. Damaged, rancid, artificial, or overly processed fats are known to damage DNA and generate particularly dangerous free-radical activity. The problem is not natural sunlight or some "SPF lotion deficiency" or some deficiency of any other magic potion marketed for your skin, but rather, it's what you put *inside* your body that most determines your susceptibility to skin cancer and wrinkles.

Malignant melanoma, the deadliest form of skin cancer, has been widely associated with vitamin D deficiency. *And what is everyone rushing to do?* They lavishly apply sunscreen to supposedly prevent the very thing for which they're actually increasing their risk. It's crazy! People almost seem to suffer from sunlight-avoidant hysteria. *The only people genuinely benefiting from sunscreens in this world are the ones who sell them.* Most SPF sunscreens use a base made of omega-6 oil (likely rancid), and they tend to be formulated with many toxic and carcinogenic chemicals for the ultimate effect of blocking not only sunlight but vitamin D production as well.

Remember: The best protection against unwanted ultraviolet light is a good tan or a hat. We evolved in fresh air and sunshine and have an actual nutrient requirement for sunlight, including ultraviolet light. Don't deny yourself your day in the sun!

> We are designed, cell by cell, as creatures of the sun. Virtually every organ system in your body is dependent on sunshine for optimal performance.
>
> AL SEARS, M.D., *YOUR BEST HEALTH UNDER THE SUN*

10

Making the Omega-3 Fatty Acids Connection

■■■■■■■■■■■■

Few people are aware that omega-3 fatty acids, which include ALA, EPA, and DHA, are easily the most deficient nutrients in the modern Western diet. Insufficient intake of these vital and essential dietary components is linked with virtually every modern disease process, weight problem, affective disorder, and learning disability.

Just What Is Omega-3 Fatty Acid, and What Makes It So Important?

Deep within the cellular structure (chloroplasts) of plankton, green and leafy plants such as grass, and other sources such as walnuts and flaxseeds lies ALA, the "parent" form of a class of essential fatty acids known as *omega-3 fatty acids*. The term *essential* here means that something cannot be manufactured by the body and *must* be supplied by the diet. When a grass-eating animal or plankton-eating fish comes along and consumes this substance in plant foods, a series of enzymatic and metabolic conversions take place to transform the ALA into its derivative forms: EPA and DHA. Herbivores make these conversions quite readily, though they are able to make only limited amounts of DHA. Humans make these conversions much less efficiently, and numerous factors may complicate this process.

To initiate this important metabolic conversion, a critical enzyme, known as *delta-6 desaturase,* must be present. It is essential to the process of elongation and desaturation into the active derivative forms of omega-3 fatty acids (EPA and DHA) from ALA. Once the body has either consumed or manufactured EPA, it can manufacture from this a series of eicosenoids such as series-3 prostaglandins, thromboxanes, and leukotrines. All are essential to the functioning of the human body as complex hormones that work on the tissue or cellular level.

DHA, another derivative, makes up the highest percentage of the fatty acids in the human brain, facilitating visual and cognitive function, forming neuroreceptors for neurotransmitters such as serotonin and dopamine, and serving as a storage molecule that the body can reconvert to EPA if needed later on. Omega-3 fatty acids also make up a significant portion of all cellular membranes, giving them fluidity and helping facilitate all metabolic and bioelectrical processes. No one can function optimally without them.

Although they are indispensable for the healthy functioning of the human brain and body, insufficient intake of omega-3 fatty acids is a nearly unavoidable problem that is endemic to modern diets and that can result in a complex array of symptoms, which are readily contributing to our current national health care crisis.

Omega-3 fatty acid (EPA/DHA) deficiency may be a contributing or causative factor in the following disorders:

- ADD/ADHD
- dyslexia
- depression
- weight gain
- heart disease
- allergies
- arthritis
- violent tendencies
- memory problems
- cancer
- eczema
- inflammatory diseases
- diabetes
- dry skin
- dandruff

- postpartum depression
- alcoholism
- Crohn's disease
- irritable bowel syndrome
- cirrhosis of the liver
- premenstrual syndrome (PMS)
- hypoglycemia
- cravings for carbohydrates and sweets cravings
- noncancerous breast disease
- ulcerative colitis
- scleroderma
- Sjögren's syndrome
- hypertension
- bipolar disorder
- irritability
- soft or brittle nails
- lowered immunity or frequent infections
- frequent urination
- fatigue
- dry, unmanageable hair
- hyperactivity
- excessive thirst
- dry eyes
- poor wound healing
- learning problems
- alligator skin
- patches of pale skin on cheeks
- cracked skin on heels or fingertips

If We Used to Get So Much Omega-3 Fatty Acid, Where Did It All Go?

Traditional and primitive sources of EPA and DHA in the diet have included such things as the meat and organs of wild game and other exclusively grass-fed meats and wild-caught cold-water seafood. At one time in our evolution, these essential fats were so prevalent in our diet that it is hypothesized that they alone were responsible for the threefold increase in the size of the human brain (Aiello et al. 1995). As much as 10 percent of human brain size has been lost in just the last century alone, likely due to the decreased amounts of available dietary EPA and DHA and the increased consumption of processed foods (Leonard et al. 2003).

Increased consumption of grains and legumes—as well as nuts, particularly, seeds, and, more recently, vegetable oils—added excessive levels of another essential fatty acid: omega-6. Although omega-6 fatty acids are needed in balanced quantity with omega-3 fatty acids for optimal health, recent trends in agriculture, food processing, and animal husbandry practices have resulted in dangerous dietary imbalances. Because *delta-6* and *delta-5 desaturase enzymes* are also needed for metabolism of omega-6 fatty acids, the resulting competition more often than not squeezes omega-3 fatty acids out of the picture. The result is that omega-6 fatty acids, along with trans fats and others, dominate the composition of membrane phospholipids and of fatty acids found in the brain and nervous system in the absence of the much needed omega-3 fatty acids. Excess omega-6 fatty acids—particularly in the presence of insulin—also results in excess production of *series-2 prostaglandins,* many of which promote or exacerbate inflammatory processes.

In today's world, however, excess omega-6 fatty acids are not the only culprit interfering with delta-6 desaturase activity and the use of omega-3 fatty acids. Among the most insidious sources of interference with this vital nutrient are the man-made trans fats, found in margarine, vegetable shortening, most commercial baked goods, nearly all fast foods, most processed foods, and commercial salad dressings and vegetable oils, including all commercial canola and soybean oils. They may appear on labels as "hydrogenated" or "partially hydrogenated" substances.

Labeling laws do not require full disclosure of processing methods, however, due to certain loopholes in them, and the presence of trans fats in most commercial vegetable oils remains largely hidden. Once they are consumed, it can take at least *two full years* for the body to get rid of dietary trans fats, causing untold metabolic chaos in the meantime (Enig 2001).

Trans fats should always be avoided 100 percent *at all* costs.

Read all labels very carefully and avoid commercial canola and soybean oils as well as all foods prepared with them (e.g., tortillas, potato chips, fries, boxed cookies, microwave popcorn, commercial breads, fast foods).

Deficiencies of biotin, vitamin E, protein, zinc, magnesium, and vitamins B_{12} and B_6 all interfere with the action of delta-6 desaturase and other enzymes involved in healthy prostaglandin production. Consumption of sugar and starch also interferes with the desaturating enzymes, and the concomitant production of excess insulin can readily divert omega-6 fatty acid elongation toward proinflammatory prostaglandin pathways (Enig 2001). As if all this weren't dismal enough, diabetes, poor pituitary function, and low thyroid function are also synonymous with altered and inhibited delta-6 desaturase function.

Individuals of northern European, coastal Irish, Scandinavian, Inuit, and Native American descent may not produce this enzyme at all and may actually have an increased requirement for EPA and DHA due to genetic adaptation to the abundance of these substances in their ancestral diets. Deficiencies of omega-3 fatty acids and insulin resistance (metabolic disorders) are exceedingly common among these populations.

Sources

Modern dietary sources of omega-3 fatty acids, particularly preformed EPA and DHA, include wild-caught seafood from particularly cold waters, such as salmon, halibut, cod, herring, mackerel, and sardines. Albacore tuna may contain small amounts. Farm-raised fish such as Atlantic salmon and other varieties are usually devoid of significant omega-3 fatty acid content. (Important: If it doesn't specifically say "wild caught," it isn't.) Wild game is another excellent and reliable source, though not everyone has access to this.

Exclusively grass-fed and finished beef, lamb, venison, and buffalo meat are also superb sources. Unfortunately, virtually all beef sold, even beef labeled as organic in natural foods–type markets, *unless otherwise specifically labeled,* is feedlot-finished on grains, corn, and soybeans, eliminating virtually all omega-3 fatty acid content and containing highly imbalanced quantities of omega-6 fatty acids. Be warned, too, that all beef-source animals—even feedlot beef animals—spend at least part of their lives out in the pasture and may be misleadingly labeled as grass fed. Be sure to inquire whether *any* grain feeding took place prior to the animal going to market.

Websites such as www.eatwild.com and www.grasslandbeef.com offer either regional or local sources or mail-order sources for high-quality, fully grass-fed and finished meat. Also, your local chapter of the Weston A. Price Foundation can provide you with a wealth of local resources as well (see www.WestonAPrice.org).

Regardless of whether one makes these healthy dietary changes, it is likely that, for a time, some period of additional supplementation of the omega-3 fatty acids EPA and DHA from either fish oil or Antarctic krill oil may be necessary for remediation of deficiency states.

Supplements of flaxseed and hemp oils are commonly promoted as rich sources of vegetarian omega-3 fatty acids. Although this is true, flaxseed and hemp oils contain omega-3 fatty acid exclusively in its parent form, ALA, and they contain zero EPA or DHA. ALA requires the action of delta-6 desaturase and highly involved metabolic processes in order to be fully elongated and used by the body and brain in its most abundantly needed forms (see the detailed prostaglandin pathway illustration on page 102).

These conversions occur very inefficiently, if at all. Under optimal conditions and with certain individuals, one might expect a maximum of about 6 percent of the ALA in flaxseed oil to convert to EPA and about 4 percent to DHA—assuming none of the aforementioned limitations is present. Should excess omega-6 fatty acid or dietary trans fats be present, this reduces to an average of only about 2.7 percent proper conversion overall, at best (Enig 2001).

Clearly, flaxseed oil is not the most preferable source of omega-3 fatty acids—particularly in a deficient individual—though there may be other benefits to flaxseed oil supplementation, and small amounts are okay. Walnuts also contain some ALA. Cod-liver oil is an excellent source of omega-3 fatty acids, rich in the EPA and DHA forms (also containing a little ALA, as well), but it is mainly a supplement for vitamin A and—to a lesser extent—vitamin D.

Regular fish oil or Antarctic krill oil supplements for omega-3 fatty acids, combined with small amounts of cod-liver oil, are far and away the best supplemental sources. Many companies molecularly distill their fish oil to remove any impurities or contaminants. Keep in mind that mercury is generally concentrated in protein and not very fat soluble, so it's usually not considered a significant contaminant risk where fish oil is concerned. Also, sufficient tissue zinc and dietary selenium levels can help mitigate the potential for mercury toxicity and retention.

Other potentially very important adjuncts to omega-3 fatty acid supplementation include vitamin E, CoQ10 (when affordable), and selenium, which, in addition to vitamin D, protect these highly polyunsaturated oils from breaking down and going rancid. At the very least,

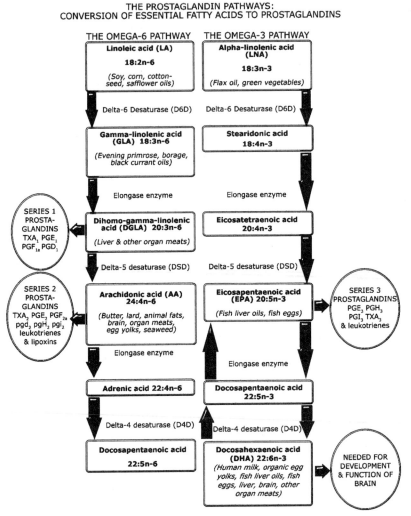

THE PROSTAGLANDIN PATHWAYS:
CONVERSION OF ESSENTIAL FATTY ACIDS TO PROSTAGLANDINS

Adapted from source: Mary G. Enig, Ph.D., adapted from R.R.Brenner, Ph.D. *The Role of Fats in Human Nutrition* 1989

Fig. 10.1. The metabolic pathways and conversions involved in the body's use of omega-6 and omega-3 fatty acids.

some vitamin D and vitamin E should be added to any regimen using supplemental levels of these highly polyunsaturated and delicate oils. The trace mineral selenium is required for vitamin E-complex (composed of natural mixed tocopherols, rich in gamma tocopherol, and preferably also containing tocotrienols) to work properly and is inexpensive to add to one's regimen. (*Note:* If you're buying vitamin E as a supplement, be sure to get it in a mixed tocopherol form rich in gamma tocopherol and only in a glycerin base, and not a soybean or canola-oil base). Selenomethionine is a highly bioavailable form of selenium and usually comes in 200 mcg doses. Selenium can also be readily derived from foods such as Brazil nuts, garlic, and grass-fed butter.

Added fat-soluble antioxidant supplementation is critical with an elevated polyunsaturated fat intake (such as omega-3 or omega-6 fatty acids). Also, dietary saturated fats, which are inherently resistant to oxidation, play an important role in the protection and use of both omega-3 and omega-6 fatty acids. Unlike trans fats, they do not interfere with but actually help your body safely make the best use of these important and delicate nutrients (Enig 2001). It's **never** a good idea to eliminate dietary saturated fats entirely.

Dosages

Standard fish oil capsules contain roughly 180 mg of EPA and 120 mg of DHA. At these concentrations, one therapeutic recommendation offered by Dr. Joseph Mercola (www.mercola.com) for remediating marked deficiency states of these nutrients involves taking one capsule for every ten pounds of body weight, preferably in two divided doses. This translates to approximately 1 teaspoon of liquid-form omega-3 fish oil for every forty pounds of body weight (much easier). Another recommendation, offered by Andrew Stoll, M.D., director of the Psychopharmacology Research Laboratory and a McLean Hospital faculty member at Harvard Medical School, is if you are using omega-3 fatty acids for health, mood, or cognitive enhancement, roughly 2,000 mg per day is probably adequate.

Current research in the area of human longevity and life extension puts this closer to 3,000 mg. Much is going to depend on how deficient or symptomatic you are. If needed for mood elevation or stabilization in more-serious mood disorders or bipolar disorder, 10,000 mg of omega-3 fatty acids or more may be appropriate in some individuals. In these instances, capsules become far less practical, and using a liquid form makes more sense. The traditional Greenland Eskimo diet included at least 14,000 mg per day of omega-3 fatty acids. Where deficiencies are likely an issue, as with ADD/ADHD and depression, it is probably better to err on the higher side, as far as dosage is concerned, for at least a period of time. If by some chance a worsening of symptoms is experienced with increased omega-3 supplementation, you may want to screen for a condition known as pyroluria (see appendix F). In these individuals there is a much greater need for omega-6s, and the condition may worsen by too much omega-3.

Always remember the increased need for fat-soluble antioxidant protection with high-dose omega-3 fatty acids supplementation. Supplementation of any essential fatty acid should, at the very least, contain added vitamins D and E with selenium, and CoQ10 and R-lipoic acid may serve some additional protection, if affordable. (*Note:* People taking warfarin [brand name Coumadin], high doses of aspirin, or any other related anticlotting or blood-thinning medication should be under close supervision by their health care provider when combining these medications with high doses of omega-3 fatty acids or vitamin E.)

If using cod-liver oil, start with one to two teaspoons a day for children and one to two tablespoons or more for adults. Remember, our adult primitive ancestors probably received ten times the current RDAs for vitamins A and D, and current research increasingly points to a greater need for vitamin D in the treatment or prevention of inflammatory disorders and cancer than ever previously suspected. Cod-liver oil, a source of omega-3 fatty acids in addition to vitamins A and D, is best used as an adjunct to other fish oil supplementation, particularly when therapeutic doses of omega-3 fatty acids are needed.

A little flaxseed oil added to salad dressings is okay; just don't try to use it as an exclusive omega-3 fatty acid source, *and never, ever cook with it!* Efforts, particularly by vegans, to compensate for low EPA or DHA conversion rates by increasing flaxseed oil consumption proportionally can lead to a dangerously increased risk of stroke and cancer. Remember always to supplement with some preformed EPA and DHA and to include some saturated fat and cholesterol in the diet for healthier, stronger membrane and vascular integrity.

Polyunsaturated vegetable oils have a weakening effect on cellular membranes when consumed in excess. Also, keep in mind that it is mostly rancid unsaturated and polyunsaturated oils lining clogged arteries rather than saturated fat or cholesterol. (Another myth bites the dust.)

A newer source of EPA and DHA, Antarctic krill oil, may be a superb alternative for people who want to avoid any fishy aftertaste (sometimes present with conventional fish oils) and is also a source of an extremely potent, naturally occurring protective antioxidant and anti-inflammatory agent, a carotenoid known as *astaxanthin*. This, along with naturally occurring phospholipids, can actually improve the use and protection of EPA and DHA in the body and brain better than conventional fish oil. Be prepared to pay big bucks for this alternative to fish oil, though; on the plus side, with krill oil "less does more."

Other Important Essential Fatty Acid Considerations

Given the difficulty in relying on the activity—even the very presence— of the delta-6-desaturase enzyme in the metabolic conversions of parent and vegetable forms of omega-3 *and* omega-6 fatty acids to their active derivative forms, it is important to consider the plight of certain forms of omega-6 fatty acid as well. Delta-6-desaturase is also responsible for the conversion of alpha-linoleic acid (ALA, the parent form of omega-6 fatty acid) to gamma-linolenic acid (GLA), an important precursor to dihomo-gamma-linolenic acid (DGLA), which is naturally abundant in liver and other organ meats. In turn, DGLA gives rise to series-1 prostaglandins, which are necessary for certain anti-inflammatory actions as well as mood regulation, cognitive function, hormonal balance, and prevention and treatment of skin disorders, and they may be conditionally essential.

It is probably advisable for most people to consider supplementation with small amounts (the recommended dosages on labels are probably sufficient for most people) of either black currant seed oil or evening primrose oil to cover this base and prevent imbalances from occurring. Borage seed oil, although arguably the richest natural source of GLA, contains pyrrolizidine alkaloids that are known to be hepatotoxic. I'd avoid making this my sole source of GLA. Also, be certain these delicate seed oils are labeled as hexane and solvent-free.

There are essentially three classes of prostaglandins. Prostaglandins are hormonelike substances made from essential fatty acids that operate on a cellular level to mitigate inflammation and various bodily processes. (*Note:* The process that gives rise to these substances, known as the *prostaglandin pathway,* is outlined in the detailed prostaglandin pathway illustration on page 102.)

Series-1 prostaglandins arise from GLA, a unique form of omega-6 fatty acid found in evening primrose oil, borage seed oil, and black currant seed oil, and from DGLA, which is found in organ meats. Both **have an anti-inflammatory effect.**

Series-2 prostaglandins are manufactured from arachidonic acid (AA), also an omega-6 fatty acid, which is commonly found in organ meats, animal fat (especially pork), eggs, butter, and seaweed. They are typically associated with proinflammatory processes (though this is a little overly simplistic). Both inflammatory and anti-inflammatory compounds can result from AA, and this is partly mitigated by the presence of insulin.

Series-3 prostaglandins are manufactured from omega-3 fatty acids, more specifically EPA, and are found abundantly in exclusively grass-fed meats, wild-caught cold-water fish (such as salmon and sardines), fish oil, and krill oil supplements.

Worthy of comment here is the widespread controversy and vilification of arachidonic acid (AA), an important form of omega-6 fatty acids, by the popular writer Barry Sears, author of *The Zone Diet,* who insists that this omega-6 fatty acid is to be avoided at all costs due to its proinflammatory properties.

Commonly found in liver, butter, and eggs, AA comprises 11 percent of the fatty acids found in the brain, and it is *absolutely required* for healthy cognitive functioning as well as being necessary for healthy inflammatory response following injury. There is also more recent evidence that the interaction of AA with vitamins A and D is absolutely essential for healthy neurotransmitter functioning. It is additionally the precursor to what are known as series-2 prostaglandins, some of which are inflammatory and some of which are anti-inflammatory.

There are no bad prostaglandins, only imbalances. Lipids researcher Dr. Mary Enig writes:

> Sears also asserts that perfect balance of the various prostaglandin series can be achieved by following a diet in which protein, carbohydrate and fat are maintained in certain strict proportions. This is a highly simplistic view of the complex interactions on the prostaglandin pathway, one which does not take into account individual requirements for macro and micro nutrients, nor of imbalances that may be caused by nutritional deficiencies, environmental stress or genetic defects. Like all systems in the body, the many eicosenoids work together in an array of loops and feedback mechanisms of

infinite complexity. Furthermore, liver and eggs are both highly nutritious foods. Liver supplies DGLA, a precursor of the Series-1 prostaglandins, and both liver and eggs supply DHA, an important nutrient for the brain and nervous system. Arachadonic acid found in butter and eggs is also an important constituent of cell membranes. (Enig 2001)

Up to 20 percent of the population may actually be deficient in AA. Individuals with the genetic metabolic disorder pyroluria actually have a much higher requirement for AA and much less need for omega-3 fatty acids. Furthermore, not all AA derivatives are necessarily proinflammatory. Excess insulin because of high-carbohydrate diets, however, strongly influences the prostaglandin pathway toward inflammation and is ultimately the biggest culprit in chronic inflammatory disorders, especially when coupled with excess vegetable oil consumption. American diets are clearly slanted toward excess proinflammatory series-2 prostaglandin production in an unhealthy way. All prostaglandins, however, do have their rightful place in human physiology.

The optimal ratio of omega-3 to omega-6 fatty acids seems to be about 1:1 and no more than 1:4. Modern diets are supplying as much as twenty parts of omega-6 to every part of omega-3 fatty acids. This invariably leads to undesirable consequences.

What is critical here is balance, not absolute amounts of any one type of fatty acid. Balance is achieved by observing three important things:

Ensure the adequate intake of viable omega-3 fatty acid sources or supplements.

Minimize or, better yet, eliminate dietary grains, legumes, feedlot meats, and vegetable oils (a little olive oil is okay) as well as other sources of sugary and starchy carbohydrates.

Completely avoid trans fat sources, including margarine, vegetable shortening, commercially processed foods and baked goods, commercial canola and soybean oils, commercial salad dressings, and fast food.

In the end, research seems to indicate that additional omega-3 fatty acid supplementation over and above that needed to remediate deficiency states can be additionally beneficial to cognitive functioning. Inuit diets that were studied were shown to contain anywhere from 14 to 20 g or more, that's 14,000 to 20,000 mg per day, of omega-3 fatty acids in combination with protective saturated fat, to no apparent detriment.

The bottom line here seems to be, if in doubt, it can't hurt to supplement!

> *Your foods shall be your remedies, and your remedies shall be your foods.*
>
> HIPPOCRATES

11

The Tyranny of Trans Fats

Just what are trans fats, and why should we need to go out of our way to avoid them, anyway?

Trans fats are a form of artificially saturated, hydrogenated, or partially hydrogenated fat typically made from vegetable oil (canola and soy oils are commonly used, though commercial lard is also usually hydrogenated). Making them is an involved, complex, and exceedingly unnatural chemical process that takes largely polyunsaturated oil and combines nickel and hydrogen ions, along with a little bleach, coloring, and steam cleaning along the way, in an effort to change the chemical configuration into something resembling saturated fat.

The commercial value of this process lies in its ability to extend product shelf life. By altering the natural molecular structure, an "imposter," a "Franken-fat" is produced that in no way behaves biochemically as its natural counterpart does. Metabolic chaos is the result of trans fat consumption, and the consequences range from neurological problems to cancer.

The following list—taken from a lecture by Mary Enig, Ph.D., at the National College of Naturopathic Medicine in October 2001—includes some of the known adverse effects of trans fats in the human diet:

- Raises levels of the atherogenic lipoprotein(a) in humans.
- Increases blood insulin levels in humans in response to glucose load, increasing the risk for diabetes.
- Decreases the response of red blood cells to insulin.
- Increases the risk of type 2 diabetes.

- Lowers the volume of cream in milk from lactating women, thus lowering the overall quality available to the infant.
- Increases trans fat levels in human milk, resulting in dose-response decreased visual acuity in breast-fed infants.
- Correlates to lower birth weights in human infants.
- Decreases the levels of testosterone and increases the number of abnormal sperm in men and interferes with gestation in women.
- Adversely interacts with the conversion of plant omega-3 fatty acids to elongated omega-3 fatty acids in human tissues.
- Escalates the adverse effects of essential fatty acid deficiency.
- Inhibits the functioning of membrane-related enzymes such as the delta-6 desaturase, resulting in decreased conversion of linoleic acid to AA and decreased conversion of ALA to EPA and DHA.
- Causes alterations in the activities of the important enzyme system that metabolizes chemical carcinogens and drugs or medications, (i.e., the mixed function oxidase cytochromes P-448–450).
- Affects immune response by lowering the efficiency of B-cell response and increasing the proliferation of T cells.
- Causes alterations in the physiological properties of biological membranes, including membrane transport and membrane fluidity.
- Causes alterations in adipose cell size, cell number, lipid class, and fatty composition.
- Increases peroxisomal activity (potentiates free-radical formation).
- A January 2001 paper in a peer-reviewed journal reported that margarine consumption is related to allergies in children, especially in boys.
- Research reported in 1997 and 1999 showed trans fatty acid intake related to asthma.
- Dutch researchers reported in March 2001 in *The Lancet* that trans fatty acids were again shown to be responsible for an increase in heart disease and calculated that a 2 percent energy intake of trans fatty acids is associated with an increased risk of heart disease of 25 percent (Aro 2001).

Because trans-fatty acids have no known health benefits and strong presumptive evidence suggests that they contribute markedly to the risk of developing [coronary heart disease], the

results published to date suggest that it would be prudent to lower the intake of trans-fatty acids in the American diet.
G. J. NELSON, "DIETARY FAT, TRANS FATTY ACIDS, AND RISK OF CORONARY HEART DISEASE," *NUTRITION REVIEWS*

The Danish Nutrition Council recommends that the addition of industrially produced trans-fatty acids to food stuffs ceases before 2005 and until then that the declaration of the content in foodstuffs becomes mandatory.
S. STENDER AND J. DYERBERG, "THE IMPORTANCE OF TRANS-FATTY ACIDS FOR HEALTH," *UGESKR LAEGER*

Clearly, hydrogenated and partially hydrogenated fats and oils have no place in the human diet. Obvious sources such as margarine, "spreads," vegetable shortening, and products clearly labeled as containing hydrogenated or partially hydrogenated oils are easy enough to identify and avoid. Few people realize, however, that current labeling laws in the United States do not always require manufacturers to list the presence of hydrogenated or partially hydrogenated fats in foods and that their presence is far more ubiquitous than suspected. Virtually all prepackaged snack foods, chips, cookies, and baked goods contain hydrogenated or partially hydrogenated oils, often even when they claim to be trans fat–free. They are able to get away from this because a certain amount of trans fat per serving is allowed before the manufacturer is required to disclose it on the label. All microwave popping corn, for instance, contains partially hydrogenated oils, yet many claim to be trans fat–free.

It's a simple, unscrupulous loophole—and far from harmless. Nearly all fast-food restaurants use these oils, and all commercial canola and soybean oils contain some level of trans fats as a by-product of their deodorization process. Clearly, in this instance, reading labels carefully may not be enough.

Figure 11.1 lists the content of trans fats by weight percentage in several commercial bakery and snack-food brands and some typical trans fat levels in U.S. foods back in 1990. Companies continue to regularly utilize trans fats, despite the more recent laws passed requiring disclosure on labels and improved public consciousness about the issue. Let's just say that old habits die hard, and laws today are better at protecting the

BRAND	# OF PRODUCTS	TRANS (WT%)
Bravo	1	49.7
Duncan Hines	1	36
Dunkin Donuts	2	35.1
Entenmann	1	31.7
Frito Lay	6	25.8–47.4
Gerber	1	42.2
Giant	3	27.1–45.5
GNC	5	24.1–37.8
Keebler	4	29.4–46.9
Murray	4	33.1–35.2
Nabisco	14	12.6–53.9
Pepperidge Farm	14	10.4–28.0
Safeway	3	8.8–27.7
Sunshine	2	34.5–42.7
Thomas	2	30.4–32.5
Wise	2	15.4–36.8

Presented at the 1990 American Oil Chemists Society Meeting, Baltimore, Md. Data from Mary G. Enig, Ph.D., Enig Associates, Inc.

Fig. 11.1. Content of trans fats in several commercial bakery and snack foods and some typical trans fat levels in U.S. foods in 1990

interests of the food industry, through convenient legal loopholes, than the health interests of you and me.

Here is a quick comparison of the biological effects of saturated fatty acids compared with trans fatty acids, just for the heck of it, compiled from a lecture given by Mary Enig, Ph.D., at the National College of Naturopathic Medicine in October 2001.

1. Saturated fatty acids raise the levels of HDL cholesterol, the so-called good cholesterol, whereas trans fatty acids lower the levels of HDL cholesterol.
2. Saturated fatty acids lower the blood levels of the atherogenic lipoprotein(a), whereas trans fatty acids raise the blood levels of lipoprotein(a).
3. Saturated fatty acids conserve the good omega-3 fatty acids, whereas trans fatty acids cause the tissues to lose these omega-3 fatty acids.

4. Saturated fatty acids do not inhibit insulin binding, whereas trans fatty acids do inhibit insulin binding.

5. Saturated fatty acids are the normal fatty acids made by the body that do not interfere with enzyme functions, such as those of delta-6 desaturase, whereas trans fatty acids are not made by the body and interfere with many enzyme functions, such as those of delta-6 desaturase.

6. Some saturated fatty acids are used by the body to fight viruses, bacteria, and protozoans, and they support the immune system, whereas trans fatty acids interfere with the function of the immune system.

For countless years, scientists studying the effects of dietary fat lumped together saturated and trans fats as being the same thing, making absolutely no delineation between the two. Nearly all research vilifying the biological effects of saturated fat has been greatly tainted by this and has been misleading consumers and health care experts alike for decades.

Don't Get Greased by Vegetable Oils

Vegetable oils, particularly commercial soybean, safflower, sunflower, corn, cottonseed, and canola oils, are an unnatural, very recent addition to the human diet. They are extremely prone to rancidity and cause mutagenic and atherogenic changes in the human body. Mutagenic changes result in damage to DNA that can lead to various cancers and atherogenic changes result in the building of arterial plaques associated with cardiovascular disease. High levels of consumption of these oils contribute to premature aging, wrinkles, cancers, and many inflammatory processes. They should never, ever be used in cooking.

Canola oil, by the way, touted by many as a "heart-healthy" oil, has been shown to produce heart lesions in animal studies, even after the suspected culprit, erucic acid, was bred out of the seed. Also, canola seeds contain abnormally low levels of vitamin E, which is needed for the prevention of oil rancidity; this increases the requirement for vitamin E of anyone consuming this oil and depletes the vitamin E in people who consume it as well. Additionally, all commercial canola and soybean oil is always partially hydrogenated as part of its deodorization process. As such, any claims by some authors that canola or soybean oil has "omega-3 content" are inaccurate since this is the very thing hydrogenated out of commercial oils due to their poor shelf life and proneness to rancidity. The only exceptions here would be canola or soybean oil labeled "organic and expeller-pressed," but then you're looking at a product quite prone to dangerous rancidity.

Moderate amounts of extra-virgin olive oil in salads and a dash or two of sesame oil, which contains a potent heat-protective antioxidant, sesamin, for flavoring in medium-heat cooking are fine. Excessive amounts of olive oil, however, along with other vegetable oils, have been shown to interfere with the use of omega-3 fats in the diet and have also been shown to potentially enhance insulin resistance (Enig 2001). In contrast, omega-3 fats (in the form of EPA and DHA)—abundant in wild-caught fish, wild game, and exclusively pasture-fed meats—are known to significantly improve insulin sensitivity. Saturated fats like coconut oil, palm oil, butter, lard, and tallow are essentially neutral and benign in moderate quantities, some having numerous beneficial antimicrobial properties. They are also important for the proper use of both essential fats (omega-3 and omega-6 fats) and protein in the body.

Margarine, hydrogenated or partially hydrogenated vegetable oils, and vegetable shortenings should be avoided at all costs. These artificial, "plastic" trans fats have no place in human health! Period.

Use a little olive oil on your salads; accent stir-fries with sesame oil; and use raw, organic butter or ghee (if you are casein sensitive) liberally on steamed veggies, as they assist in the absorption of oil-soluble nutrients in the vegetables. Use organic coconut oil, palm oil, organic lard, or quality tallow for higher-heat cooking or sautéing. These fats are highly stable and will not easily go rancid, and rancid fats are extremely damaging to your body and DNA. Short- and medium-chain saturated fats that are found in butter and coconut oil are far more likely to be used as energy by your body, including the heart and other organs, rather than be stored as body fat.

12

So, How Much Natural Fat Do I Need, Anyway?

■ ■ ■ ■ ■ ■ ■ ■ ■ ■ ■ ■

Recent advances in leptin and life-extension research point to a potentially important value in consuming a relatively higher *percentage* of fat in our diets (to be elaborated on later in this book). The implications of this research are quite exciting and show how the very thing we thought was our worst enemy may well, in fact, be our best friend after all. Eating a diet containing higher percentages of dietary natural fat—using an optimized macronutrient ratio and eating only as much as you really need to satisfy hunger—can actually help reverse disease and support a radically increased healthy life span, but we'll get to that.

Keep in mind that all natural fats have a role to play in our health and that overemphasizing one or another isn't particularly advisable. What is important, certainly, is making sure we get our necessary essential fatty acids (EPA, DHA, and GLA). The rest should simply be fat from a variety of natural and healthy sources: grass-fed meat (beef, buffalo, lamb, elk, pork, yak, venison), pastured poultry (chicken, pheasant, duck, goose—all with skin on), wild-caught seafood, coconut (milk, cream, and oil), avocado, grass-fed butter or ghee, heavy cream (preferably raw), olive oil, sesame oil (in small amounts), tallow, organic lard, nuts, and seeds.

Where omega-3 and omega-6 fatty acid intake is concerned, current recommendations by the most knowledgeable lipid researchers and biochemists suggest an intake of *no more than* three to four parts of omega-6 fatty acids to one part of omega-3 fatty acids. Omega-3 fatty acids should make up at least 0.5–1.5 percent of the total daily caloric intake. Omega-6 fatty acids should make up no more than 2–3 percent of the total daily caloric intake. One-to-one ratios are probably more optimal. Higher intake of omega-3 fatty acids may be desirable or necessary for a time (several months) to reverse a deficiency state.

Among the best sources of omega-3 fatty acids are grass-fed or wild game meats and organ meats and cold-water, wild-caught fish such as salmon, herring, sardines, and mackerel. The best supplemental sources are high-quality fish and krill oils. Quality matters.

Please be aware: Cod-liver oil contains some omega-3 fatty acids but is mainly a source of vitamin A and some D. Raw, preferably soaked and dried, nuts and seeds are a rich source of the parent form of the omega-6 oils and a less rich source of the parent form of omega-3 oils. We do need some of the parent form ALA, found readily in fresh walnuts, in flaxseed oil, and even in small amounts in fish oil supplements. Balanced levels of omega-3 and omega-6 fatty acids are also found abundantly in grass-fed meat and wild-caught fish, along with needed protective saturated fats. Black currant seed oil and evening primrose oil are the best sources of supplemental GLA, an important omega-6 fatty acid derivative. Our ancestors got a lot of this, in the form of DGLA, eating organ meats. Periodic supplementation with these oils or increased dietary consumption of organ meats may be desirable in cases of GLA deficiency due to impaired delta-6 desaturase activity, which manifests as eczema, skin disorders, hormonal imbalances, mood disorders, and some forms of cognitive dysfunction. Most people with deficient levels of omega-3 fatty acids are also deficient in this very important anti-inflammatory omega-6 fatty acid derivative.

What about Ketosis?

Ketones are a perfectly normal constituent of human metabolism. They are the energy-producing by-products of the metabolism of fats. They are used safely and effectively for energy in all tissues in the body, including the brain. In fact, ketones are *the* preferred fuel for every organ and tissue, and current research shows that they are a far less damaging source of energy than glucose, far more stabilizing, less excitatory, and may, in fact, even help extend your life span!

One particularly interesting study showed a marked benefit for a ketogenic diet for children with epilepsy. They went on ketosis-inducing diets, and their seizures were either greatly brought under control or stopped altogether (Prasad 1996). In fact, what we refer to today as "a ketogenic diet" was the number one treatment for epilepsy until the drug Dilantin was discovered in 1938. Recently rediscovered, a ketogenic diet is returning to mainstream acceptance and is again recognized as a highly effective therapy for seizure and neurologically related disorders. In fact, there are studies to show the strong benefits of ketogenic diets on virtually every manner of neurological disorder. Some examples of neurologic uses of a ketogenic diet other than epilepsy are migraines, Alzheimer's disease, Parkinson's disease, Lou Gehrig's disease (ALS), autism, brain tumors, depression, sleep disorders, schizophrenia, post-anoxic brain injury, posthypoxic myoclonus glycogenosis type V, and narcolepsy, to name a few.

All other vital organs are also able to thrive on ketones. The human heart prefers ketones, in fact, to any other fuel. Some evidence also shows that a state of healthy ketosis can help starve cancerous tumors, as they are unable to use ketones for fuel and must rely on glucose.

The vilification of ketosis was popularized by Jane Brody, of the *New York Times* (a major proponent of low-fat, high-carbohydrate diets), who ridiculously warned of ketones as "toxic compounds." Dr. Luber Stryer, professor of biochemistry at Stanford University and the author of the biochemistry textbook used in most medical schools, says ketones are "normal fuels of respiration and are quantitatively important as sources of energy. Indeed, heart muscle and the renal cortex use ketones in preference to glucose." Drs. Donald and Judith Voet, authors of another popular medical biochemistry textbook, say that ketones "serve as important metabolic fuels for many peripheral tissues, particularly heart and skeletal muscle." Far from poison. In fact, both mitochondrial function and energy levels actually improve on ketogenic diets. Dr. Richard Veech, a researcher at the U.S. National Institutes of Health, calls ketones "magic" and has shown that both the heart and the brain run 25 percent more efficiently on ketones than on blood sugar. He said, "Doctors are scared of ketosis. They're always worried about ketoacidosis. But ketosis is the normal physiological state. I would argue that it is the normal state of man" (Taubes 2002).

In the textbook *Nutritional Biochemistry and Metabolism,* the mobilization of fat for energy and production of ketones is described in detail:

> As the body enters the postabsorptive period when glucose is no longer entering the blood from the intestine (so insulin is no longer released), the pattern of fat flow (and glucose) into storage is gradually reversed. **As breakdown of glycogen begins in the liver to maintain blood glucose, the liver switches to fat as an energy source, and the same transition is increasingly made by other tissues** [emphasis mine]. Free fatty acids released into the blood travel on albumen to organs, where they diffuse across cell membranes and are carried into mitochondria for oxidation (burning for fuel). Transport across the mitochondrial membrane is accomplished with the help of carnitine (notably found most abundantly in the diet in red meat).
>
> Increasingly, as fasting continues, larger proportions of the free fatty acid in the circulation are converted to ketone bodies, principally in the liver. **Ketone bodies are a form of fuel** [emphasis mine; note that the term used is *fuel* and not *toxic waste product*] much more water soluble than fatty acids. The pathway for their synthesis is via acetyl-CoA. These ketones are used as fuel by the muscles and other tissues and, as fasting continues, eventually also by the central nervous system and brain. . . . Ketone production increases gradually . . . reaching its maximum by about 10 days. **The same occurs in individuals consuming little or no carbohydrate** [emphasis mine]. (Linder 1991)

Humans and hominids have been on ketogenic diets for close to the last three million years. Were ketones dangerous, it is unlikely we as a species would have survived to this day. In fact, both the body and the brain actually prefer ketones as a fuel to glucose, as they are nonglycating and therefore nondamaging on a cellular level. Ketones are a steady, long-burning, efficient fuel that we were designed to use as our ongoing primary source of fuel for most things (except in an emergency, which is when glucose gets released as a turbocharged supplemental source of energy). Fat is our safest, most natural, most fundamental aerobic energy source. We *always* pay a price for the use of glucose as an energy source, even in low amounts. Our red blood cells do need a certain amount of glucose—it is unavoidable—but the less of it we use or depend on, the better. Note that dietary protein in significant excess of what is needed for essential maintenance and repair will convert to glucose and can slow or stop the process of ketosis.

Having said this, it is important to note that there are four possible types of people for whom a state of ketosis is potentially questionable: (1) people with **uncontrolled** type 1 diabetes (ketoacidosis—a very different, more serious condition of particular concern under certain conditions—is often confused with ketosis), (2) people with renal disease (maybe, depending), (3) people who are pregnant (if they are unaccustomed to being in a state of ketosis), and (4) *people who sell diet drugs.* Ketoacidosis, by contrast, is an extreme, abnormal, uncontrolled, and pathological condition in which the body is unable to normally regulate ketone production and accumulates keto acids that plunge the pH levels into a dangerously acidic state. This condition is rare and typically occurs in people with untreated type 1 diabetes. Normal ketosis resulting from low-carbohydrate diets or fasting, conversely, is completely benign—and entirely desirable. Note, however, that overwhelmingly, even people with type 1 diabetes who apply the principles outlined in this book commonly—and enthusiastically—report nearly miraculous improvement in their conditions. So much for ketone fearmongering. If you have type 1 diabetes and are interested in applying these principles to your diet, I still suggest (to be on on the safe side) consulting a qualified and informed health care provider first.

Ketosis (simply put) is essentially the state in which the body is burning fat for energy instead of carbohydrates. This is the state we all want to be in. Many ancient hunter-gatherers would have lived in a functionally ketogenic state most of the time. There is no evidence that it is a harmful state for normal, healthy individuals to be in at all. To the contrary, the newest longevity and leptin research readily concludes that the more you use ketones for energy in your lifetime as opposed to glucose, the longer and healthier you will live—*by far.*

For people who are especially overweight and undertaking a more ketogenic diet, the initial excretion of ketones will be greater. During the initial stages of weight loss in an individual who is insulin resistant, the body can be used to using glucose as a more primary and inefficient energy source and may not yet be adept at using ketones or burning fat efficiently. Ketones may initially be excreted as more of a waste product. It takes time for the body to adapt to this change, as little as three weeks in younger individuals and longer in older individuals, but about a month to six weeks for most, on average. Certain individuals who have candida yeast overgrowth, are extremely addicted to carbohydrates, or have undiagnosed or unmanaged food sensitivities may take longer and may need additional supplementation and special attention to help facilitate the necessary metabolic changes.

Care must be taken to drink a good deal of water so that more ketones can be lost through the urine than the breath or skin (which may impart a mildly undesirable odor in the beginning). Adding a squeeze of fresh lemon juice can be additionally alkalinizing and can help somewhat with yeast issues. Sufficient water can also help dilute any toxic material commonly stored in adipose tissue so that it can get released in the bloodstream during ketotic states. (*Note:* Excess ketones in the urine may be associated with diabetes and marked insulin resistance. This means that they are excreted rather than burned for fuel and that sugar is being burned, preferentially, instead. Some excess ketones are additionally passed in feces.) Eventually, when dietary consistency is maintained, the body adapts to the primary use of fat for fuel, and not sugar. People often report that this is the day they feel truly liberated from their need for frequent meals and finally free from uncontrollable cravings.

Using additional herbal and antioxidant detoxification measures and supplements, which support improved insulin sensitivity, can be beneficial in this process. Focusing on healthy and clean sources of fat in the diet is also important for these and many other reasons. If a person is not particularly overweight and is metabolically geared for burning fat instead of sugar, ketosis is a natural state and easily and effortlessly managed.

Supplementing the diet with high doses of L-carnitine (2–5 g per day) can also help minimize any discomfort, maximize energy levels during the initial stages of weight loss, and facilitate the transition to using fat as a primary source of fuel. L-carnitine, which is not an amino acid but a quaternary ammonium compound that is a derivative of amino acid metabolism, assists in transporting fat into the mitochondria, where it can be burned for energy. Supplemental doses of pancreatic lipase can also help better facilitate the proper digestion and use of dietary fats. It's also important not to overconsume dietary protein because protein in significant excess of the RDA (roughly 0.8 g/kg of ideal body weight per day, 25–30 g of pure protein, or 2–3 ounces of meat, fish, eggs, etc., per meal) can convert to sugar and be used in the same way, slowing or reversing the state of ketosis for many people.

In short, ketones are a natural product of fat burning. When body fat is mobilized for oxidation, ketones are produced. Unless you want to keep all the excess body fat you have, you can't and shouldn't prevent the generation of ketones. Period.

13

Carbohydrate Metabolism 101

■ ■ ■ ■ ■ ■ ■ ■ ■ ■ ■ ■

Annual refined sugar consumption in the United States:

1750: 4 pounds per person, per year
1850: 20 pounds per person, per year
1994: 120 pounds per person, per year
1996: 160 pounds per person, per year

According to the USDA's Economic Research Service (www.ers
.usda.gov/Data/FoodConsumption), global sugar consumption continues to increase by about 2 percent per annum, and in 2006 and 2007
was expected to reach almost 154 million tons. *Note:* This does not
include the use of other industrial sweeteners such as high fructose
corn syrup!

High fructose corn syrup is now estimated to be the *number-one
source of calories in the American diet*! Increases in obesity, heart disease,
cancer, and diabetes correlate almost perfectly with the introduction of
HFCS nearly thirty years ago. The average person is consuming ⅓ **of a
pound of sugar each and every day,** which is 5 ounces or 150 grams—
half of which is fructose (sucrose is made up half and half of glucose and
fructose). This is roughly 300 percent more than the amount that can
trigger biochemical chaos. Our physiology has no defense against this sort
of onslaught. Fully 90 cents out of every US food dollar is spent on pro-

cessed food, and HFCS (the most glycating sugar of them all) is in *nearly every single processed food product*. Remember, too, that these sugar consumption amounts are considered **average** and that many consume more than twice this amount. Based on the most updated 2011 USDA estimates, the average American consumes roughly 12 teaspoons of sugar a day, which is the equivalent of about **3,550 pounds of sugar in a lifetime** (**close to *two tons***—picture an overflowing dumpster or a large pickup truck load filled with granulated sugar). If you want to get a mental picture of the average annual consumption of sugar picture a large, overflowing wheelbarrow (Toney 2011, Taubes 2011, and Lustig 2011).

None of these statistics begins to include the amount of sugar in our diets from *other* sources of dietary carbohydrate—starches such as cereals, bread, pasta, grains, potatoes, rice, or so-called natural sweeteners such as honey, maple syrup, agave, or others—or from *excess* protein consumption (which significantly converts to sugar). When you truly add it all up it is literally astonishing that the obesity, diabetes, cancer, and heart disease (to name a few sugar-related diseases and conditions) epidemics aren't far worse than they are. Our ancestors wouldn't even know how to *begin* to comprehend this sort of insanity.

All nonfibrous forms of carbohydrates (from grains, rice, potatoes, and other starch-based foods) in addition to refined sugar and natural and industrial sweeteners (such as high fructose corn syrup) **are sugar once they are metabolized by the body.** The dietary carbohydrate load in the human diet has grown unnaturally, exponentially, and grotesquely from what our Paleolithic ancestors once knew. This includes starchy or complex forms, with the exception of indigestible forms such as fiber, as well as simple carbohydrates found in fruit. Wild fruit was a very different food from the modern cultivated varieties (often more tart than sweet, usually much smaller, lower in sugar, and very fibrous) and was only seasonally available, at best.

All nonfibrous carbohydrates stimulate the secretion of insulin, which is the fat storage hormone, or damage the body and brain via a process known as *glycation* (in which sugars in the bloodstream react with proteins and fats and cause them to deteriorate). Among examples of carbohydrate foods in this context are bread, pasta, cereal, rice, potatoes, granola, dried fruit, juices, candy, chocolate, desserts, alcoholic beverages, and even most fresh fruit (an exception being something like avocados).

Added Sugar Consumption, 1970–2005

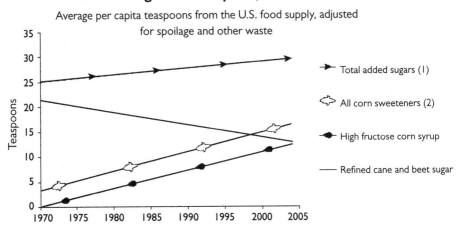

Average per capita teaspoons from the U.S. food supply, adjusted for spoilage and other waste

Total added sugars (1)

All corn sweeteners (2)

High fructose corn syrup

Refined cane and beet sugar

Fig. 13.1. Average daily added sugar consumption over a 25-year period.
Source: USDA/Economic Research Service, 2006

Fructose, the simple sugar in fruit, may not impact insulin much (except when it's in high fructose corn syrup), but it is *extremely* glycating and damaging. It is also more likely to raise uric acid levels (such as with metabolic syndrome and gout). In this context, the carbohydrates we are talking about here don't include fibrous vegetables and greens, which are very beneficial and have negligible sugar or starch content.

The body is obsessed with maintaining glucose levels within a minimally necessary range, which can differ from person to person in relative terms, varying on how dependent they have become on glucose for energy and how insulin resistant they are.

There are actually several hormones designed to raise glucose levels and only one that actually lowers them. This is because carbohydrates tended to be an extremely limited commodity in primitive diets, and as such, our ancestors very rarely had an "emergency" need to lower blood glucose levels, as is so common today. The ability to hormonally raise blood glucose levels in an emergency situation, however, is essential to survival.

It is fairly optimal for healthy, insulin- and leptin-sensitive humans to have a blood glucose value of no more than roughly 70 to 85 mg/dL at any given time (without any symptoms of hypoglycemia). The available scientific evidence from studies of human longevity and caloric restriction points to this range as optimal. Some current functionally healthy ranges are established as being more typically between 85 and 100 mg/dL, which is considered more the norm, though lower ranges are by far more desirable for people who normally maintain low insulin levels, even if the higher range is more common in many individuals. Fasting blood sugar, from a functional standpoint, in excess of 100 mg/dL, is already reflective of dysregulation. The most current human longevity studies indicate that the ability to maintain a fasting blood glucose level between 70 and 85 mg/dL—without accompanying symptoms of hypoglycemia—and not allowing glucose to spike higher than 40 mg/dL over your fasting value following meals has a favorable effect in activating *sirtuins* (our longevity genes).

A study of nearly two thousand men over a period of twenty-two years showed the startling results that men with fasting glucose levels **over 85 mg/dL** had a **40 percent** increase in risk of death from cardiovascular disease! The researchers conducting this study stated that "fasting blood glucose values in the upper normal range appear to be an important independent predictor of cardiovascular death in non-diabetic apparently healthy middle aged men" (Bjornholt et al. 1999).

What is referred to as hypoglycemia or even reactive hypoglycemia becomes a relative thing, depending on the context. A fasting glucose level of 90 or 100 may feel like marked hypoglycemia and may even induce seizures in someone who is used to levels of 400 mg/dL, as with some diabetics. Someone used to functioning between 85 and 100 mg/dL may feel reactively hypoglycemic (foggy, emotionally volatile, shaky, fatigued, or irritable) at 70 mg/dL. A healthy person maintaining consistently low glucose and insulin levels may not exceed 90 or 100 mg/dL, even following a meal, and may feel absolutely comfortable and symptom-free with fasting blood glucose levels at 70 mg/dL. Again, it is relative and contextual.

The rule of thumb is the lower you can maintain your blood glucose levels in a healthy and functional way (that is, without experiencing low-blood-sugar symptoms), the better off you are.

Those people who are more optimally healthy should maintain a range between 70 and 85 mg/dL or lower; this is equivalent to no more than 1 teaspoon of sugar, or about 5 g or 20 kcal, total. Keep in mind that the body is adamant about maintaining the minimal necessary levels of glucose at any given time because glucose is inherently damaging to vessels, organs, and tissues in the body. **The less glucose that is absolutely necessary, the better.**

Two slices of bread or a single small bagel contain about 6 teaspoons of glucose—*six times* the amount normally allowed in the bloodstream! Dietary carbohydrates, with the exception of fiber, are *all* absorbed by the liver and converted to the simple monosaccharide glucose, which is then released into the bloodstream. Cereals and potatoes can raise blood sugar levels even faster than a candy bar!

Glucose (and other sugars) in the bloodstream auto-oxidizes, which, in excess, produces potent free-radical activity that damages arterial walls and forms cross-links with proteins called *advanced glycosylation* (also known as *glycation) end products* (AGEs). AGEs are known to accelerate the age-associated declines in the functioning of cells and tissues and to cause mutations in DNA. Also, AGEs bind with certain receptors in the bloodstream, appropriately called RAGEs, and induce widespread inflammation, leading to more advanced cardiovascular disease. A simple, inexpensive blood test that can measure up to a three-month window of glycation of red blood cells is called a hemoglobin-A1c test, and it can be used to more accurately monitor these glycation tendencies over time. Fasting blood sugar as a marker is not sufficiently accurate for this.

Glucose is what ages (or AGEs) us. It is an irony that a thing we all need to stay alive, to feed our red blood cells, and to fuel anaerobic processes is what science has discovered is ultimately what degenerates and kills us. We have to have *some* sugar to fuel our red blood cells, but not so much for our brains, as many people think. Remember, our brain can run beautifully—in fact, better—with mostly ketones, which are the energy units of fat.

Ketones are a much more steady, reliable, and abundant source of fuel for our brain and organs to depend on. Our red blood cells, however, *need* to burn sugar (glucose) for fuel anaerobically to preserve their precious cargo, which is oxygen, so they burn sugar instead of fats.

Unfortunately, in the end, we pay a price for what is somewhat inevitable. Aging is now being understood by people researching longevity as essentially a gradual process of glycation of all tissues, including the brain. Chronic diseases associated with aging and certain forms of mental decline may be directly associated with these processes. The lower we maintain our blood sugar levels, the slower this process occurs and the longer and healthier we live—and the more gracefully we age.

A more pronounced and advanced state of the consequences of glycation effects can be seen in people with full-blown diabetes. The irony is that, given our most current understanding of how aging (which is now being viewed as a disease process) actually occurs, we can all be technically viewed as having diabetes—only to varying degrees. And the current evidence that even modestly elevated "normal" glucose levels significantly increase disease risk cannot be ignored.

Looking at it this way can really shift your perspective and hopefully your dietary habits. In a study of 33,230 men, high glucose levels were independently associated with a **38 percent increase** in deaths from digestive tract cancers (Matthews et al. 2010). Other studies certainly show that diabetics have even greater increases in cancer risks! What is clear and irrefutable from the current understanding of antiaging medicine and how degenerative processes and DNA mutation (leading to cancer) develop is that the lower the levels of blood sugar we are able to maintain and the less insulin we produce, the longer and healthier we live and the "kinder" and slower the aging process will be. (*Note:* Glycation and its damage is ultimately a cumulative process, so every bit of sugar or starch we eat eventually counts. Every piece of candy, cookie, bread, or potato, every spoonful of honey, and every drop of soda effectively shortens your life—something to think about. Though some glycation and its effects can be reversed, some cannot. It's all a matter of what you choose to prioritize.)

Another consequence of chronic dietary carbohydrate consumption is candida yeast overgrowth. Yeast overgrowth is extremely common in those people in the U.S. population eating a high-carbohydrate diet. It is especially common in diabetics and is created by an imbalance of organisms in the gastrointestinal tract as well as antibiotic use, poor diet, and certain exogenous hormone use. Most people with candida overgrowth have an allergy to yeast, as well. Both can provoke symptoms. Symptoms of yeast overgrowth can include postnasal drip, rectal itching, chronic sinus infections, sinus headaches, congestion, gas, bloating and heartburn, brain fog or spaciness, white tongue, vaginal yeast symptoms, frequent urination, constipation or diarrhea, skin eruptions, water retention, and cravings for sweet, starchy, or "yeasty" foods like breads, alcohol, and pizza. Complete avoidance of sugar- and starch-based foods in addition to most cheeses and sour cream, pickled or fermented foods (including soy sauce), and vinegars is often necessary to get candida under control.

The Relationship between
Insulin and Blood Sugar

Following a meal, significant levels of blood sugar generated above homeostasis stimulate the release of insulin, which works rapidly to remove glucose from the blood. Whatever glucose is not needed immediately—for outrunning, say, a hungry lion via anaerobic energy (i.e., peak, turbocharged energy output or exertion)—converts rapidly either to glycogen, which is stored in very limited amounts in the liver and muscle tissue for times of extreme anaerobic exertion, or to triglycerides through the activation of an enzyme called *glycerol-3-phosphate dehydrogenase,* which converts blood sugar into fat, which is then moved into storage via *lipoprotein lipase* as adipose tissue (body fat).

We need to understand a certain rather major point: **our ancient ancestors never really had an emergency need to lower their blood sugar levels.** It's critical you understand this. And here's a news flash: Something even many doctors do not understand is that insulin's actual biological function and purpose is ***not,*** in fact, to regulate blood sugar. We have several other hormones actually designed for blood-sugar regulation: glucagon, epinephrine, norepinephrine, cortisone, and growth hormone. The regulation of blood sugar by these hormones is designed to *increase* blood glucose when we need it.

Insulin, by default, does lower blood sugar (very crudely), but insulin's primary purposes are actually to simply store away excess nutrients in case of a famine and to *regulate the coordination of energy stores with life span and reproduction* (Rosedale 1999). Blood sugar lowering is a trivial sideline for insulin, a key hormone that has much bigger fish to fry. This is hugely important to understand and a key factor in new understandings by scientists in the quest for advancing human longevity, which we'll discuss later.

The Need for Steady Fuel

Where fueling the fire of our brain and body's metabolism is concerned, carbohydrates can best be described as kindling. Whole grains and legumes are somewhat like twigs; starch, such as in cereals and potatoes, and simple sugars are like paper on the fire; and alcohol might best be described as gasoline on the fire. If you're relying on carbohydrates as your primary source of fuel, you need to feed that fire often, regularly, and consistently. You will be craving that fuel. Unfortunately, most people today have forcibly adapted their bodies to this sort of an unnatural dependence by overconsuming carbohydrates in their diet.

Most, if not all, alcoholics (for instance) have severe issues with dysglycemia and sugar addiction. Alcoholics are utterly dependent on and regularly seek fast sources of sugar—alcohol being the fastest. This is one reason why they say "once an alcoholic, always an alcoholic." This is because the problem in alcoholism, in fact, isn't really alcohol, per se, but severe carbohydrate addiction. By merely giving up alcohol, one is **still** left with the real underlying problem: sugar addiction. The typical Alcoholics Anonymous meeting is replete with doughnuts, coffee, and people standing around smoking cigarettes. Even though they may not be drinking alcohol, the damaging, often unconscious, sugar addiction in recovering alcoholics continues. Alcoholics are typically what I refer to as "carbovores," eating diets largely consisting of carbohydrate-rich foods, relentlessly craving sweets, and additionally relying on stimulants such as caffeine and nicotine to constantly keep blood sugar levels up. The "sweet tooth" doesn't just go away with abstinence from beer, wine, and liquor, hence the ongoing vulnerability to relapse. Once the cravings for carbohydrates and the dependence on carbohydrates as the primary source of fuel are eliminated, so are the alcohol cravings. Training the body to depend on ketones rather than sugar for fuel is key to this equation. This essentially means eliminating sugar and starch from the diet entirely.

For those having a greater difficulty adapting to a fat-based metabolism, supplements such as L-glutamine (which the brain can use in lieu of glucose) can help the brain transition away from sugar (sort of like training wheels) while the body adapts to its new, more stable, and long-sustaining source of fuel. Botanicals such as *Gymnema sylvestre* can help knock out carb cravings when taken in more-concentrated doses of between 4 and 8 g, three times per day for a month or so while dietary changes are being made. Supplying additional nutrients that have been greatly depleted by alcohol and carbohydrate abuse is also essential to recovery.

One might get a burst or a ball of flame with respect to energy from many carbohydrate sources, but no one can get long-term, *sustainable* energy. As soon as the flame starts to die out, which doesn't take long, you're stuck with cravings for fuel or stimulants again. It can be quite a roller-coaster ride.

This is why some dietary experts are always telling you to eat every two hours or to eat "numerous small meals throughout the day." If you're sugar dependent—and almost everyone in this culture is victim to that unnecessary reality—then frequent small meals become necessary to maintain an even keel.

If you have ever heated your home with a woodstove, then you know what I mean with the following analogy: If you had to heat your home with that woodstove using paper, twigs, and lighter fluid all day, you'd be a slave to that fire, and you'd need a mountain of fuel handy to constantly feed that hungry beast. You'd be forever preoccupied with keeping that fire going, and you'd have little other life. In effect, most people in this culture are similarly enslaved by the preoccupation with where their next meal or snack (or caffeinated boost) is coming from. The food industry and big agribusiness are only too happy to support that enslavement and the perpetuation of the notion that glucose is essential as a primary source of fuel and that frequent eating, snacking, and carbohydrate intake are somehow important to maintain healthy blood sugar levels. This even gets taught in medical schools. It is a lie. Nature would never have intended for us to constantly live this way. It is a terribly impractical metabolic state to maintain, particularly if you view this from the primitive perspective of ongoing survival in a less certain world where food wasn't constantly available. Our primitive (particularly ice age) ancestors would never have made it this far if carbohydrates were essential to the diet or if glucose (an anaerobic source of rocketlike fuel) were necessary as a primary source of energy all of the time. Nature isn't that crazy or stupid.

Mind you, it *is* possible to live in a state of primary glucose dependence. People do it all the time. The idea that we are *necessarily* dependent on sugar as our primary source of fuel is *true only conditionally,* only if we've metabolically adapted ourselves to that unnatural dependence. Most people in this culture *are* metabolically adapted to that very state. And you *can* go on managing your blood sugar levels all day with frequent meals, snacking, and the eating of more complex carbohydrates (i.e., piles of twigs, "eleven servings a day") to keep the fire burning more steadily, but I personally have far better things to do than live my life tending to that woodstove. It isn't necessary or essential at all, and it *will* age you faster (and cost you much more in grocery bills and health care costs). There *is* a far better, healthier, and more natural way to live and eat.

Dietary fat, *in the absence of carbohydrates,* is like putting a nice big log on the fire. Fat's flame burns at a regular, even rate, and is easily kept going. Protein, consumed in moderate quantities, is mainly diverted toward structural repair and maintenance. Only in excess does it convert to sugar. Fat's even flame keeps the hormone leptin under control, keeps insulin quiet, and keeps our appetite satisfied. Blood sugar, when one learns to depend on this steadier source of fuel, becomes a trivial concern. You become free to live your life instead of being constantly preoccupied with where your next meal or snack is coming from. One can go many, many hours on this longer-burning type of fuel without experiencing any discomfort or cravings at all. You may eventually get hungry if you really go a long time without eating, which is normal, but you are far less likely to experience irritability, dizziness, brain fog, cravings, fatigue, jitteriness, or mood swings because of it.

This is the way it's supposed to be!

What We Have Here
Is a Failure to Communicate

Less than 1 percent of the pancreas is devoted to insulin production. Excessive demands for insulin can initially result in gradually reduced sensitivity of insulin receptors, leading to more and more insulin release needed to accomplish the same job.

This is what is termed *insulin resistance.* In the earlier stages of the pathogenesis of glucose dysregulation, a tendency toward hypoglycemia may be the result. Over time, however, one's cell receptors become increasingly resistant to insulin's constant message, and type 2 diabetes becomes the problem. In more advanced cases, the overtaxed pancreas may ultimately lose its ability to produce sufficient amounts of insulin, and one may actually end up requiring insulin injections. Once thought to be a disease of older adults, type 2 diabetes is increasingly becoming prevalent in young children.

In fact, type 2 diabetes is really a disease not of blood sugar, but of insulin resistance—meaning the breakdown of communication between insulin and glucose. This is important to realize, as drugs that are designed to manage diabetes completely fail to address this issue and instead focus on lowering blood glucose, typically stimulating more storage of sugar as body fat. This does nothing to restore healthy cellular communication or reduce mortality from the disease. Diabetes drugs, though they may lower blood glucose levels initially, ultimately worsen the progression of the disease.

The recent Action to Control Cardiovascular Risk in Diabetes (ACCORD) study was published in *The New England Journal of Medicine* (Gerstein et al. 2008). Researchers who were following the effects of using insulin to lower blood glucose levels in diabetic patients were surprised to find that increased insulin use (to lower blood sugar levels) caused an *increase* in death from heart attack and stroke. The study was actually stopped short due to these alarming findings. This unfortunately continues to be the standard in diabetic care—a focus on blood sugar instead of insulin resistance.

Obesity, in many ways, can be viewed as the price we pay for our body trying to stave off diabetes. In the end, however, the issue is one of communication breakdown and insulin resistance. *The key is the restoration of insulin sensitivity and cellular communication.*

So, how do we do that, you ask?

If you want to change the way any organization works, first you have to go talk to the boss . . .

14
Leptin

■ ■ ■ ■ ■ ■ ■ ■ ■ ■ ■

The Lord and Master of Your Hormonal Kingdom

Back in 1994, a discovery was made that shook medical science down to its core. Scientists discovered a major hormone they didn't previously know existed. Moreover, it wasn't just a major hormone; it was the major hormone that ultimately influences all other hormones and controls virtually all the functions of the hypothalamus, in the brain. They found it in the last place they would have expected to: in our fat cells.

The name of the hormone is *leptin*.

Until the discovery of leptin, scientists believed that body fat was just an unwanted, ugly mass of excess, cumbersome energy storage. This view of fat has been changed forever. Body fat is now understood to be a complex, sophisticated endocrine organ.

A primary purpose of leptin is to coordinate the metabolic, endocrine, and behavioral responses to starvation, which, of course, is as fundamental to basic survival—our number one priority—as it gets. As such, it powerfully impacts our emotions, cravings, and behavior. **Everything** is secondary to survival. It turns out, in fact, that leptin isn't the only hormone secreted by adipocytes (fat cells) and that dozens of other hormones are produced there as well. Many of them are proinflammatory in nature. In fact, leptin itself is an inflammatory cytokine and has a major role to play in the body's inflammatory processes as well. It additionally mediates the production of other inflammatory compounds in your adipose tissue throughout your body. It's also one reason why overweight and obese people are so much more prone to inflammatory issues.

Who Knew the New Kid on the Block Ran the Whole Neighborhood?

If you haven't heard of leptin, even if your doctor hasn't heard of it, don't be surprised. Drug companies have yet to create any drug that can positively influence leptin function. *Diet is the only thing that can effectively do this.* (So much for fat pharmaceutical profits there.) Therefore, little about this important hormone is taught in medical schools or discussed in the media, despite its extreme importance. In all likelihood, you have either never heard about it or have only heard very little.

Leptin is a good hormone to get to know, though its function in the body is extremely complex. Understanding leptin is tantamount to understanding how to regulate the rest of your endocrine system, conquer your emotions, dramatically improve your health, and even prolong your life. In many ways, it's *the* single most important hormone in the body.

No other hormonal imbalance in the body, in fact, can ultimately be restored to healthy balance without leptin functioning normally. Keeping leptin levels healthfully moderated can prevent most diseases of aging and greatly extend the normal, healthy life span. Chronically excessive levels of leptin have been associated with most known degenerative diseases and inflammation as well as obesity and a short life span. The more you can increase your brain and receptor sensitivity to this critical hormone, by far the healthier you will be.

Leptin essentially controls mammalian metabolism. Most people think that is the job of the thyroid, but leptin actually controls the thyroid, which regulates the rate of metabolism. Leptin oversees all energy stores. Leptin decides whether to make us hungry and store more fat or to burn fat. Leptin orchestrates our inflammatory response and can even control sympathetic versus parasympathetic arousal in the nervous system. If any part of your endocrine system is awry, including the adrenals or sex hormones, you will never have a prayer of truly resolving those issues until you have brought your leptin levels under control.

This is a key thing to understand: The endocrine system is an exceedingly complex system of interrelationships that ultimately is regulated via an intricate hierarchical system of management.

At the top of the management pillar is leptin. Immediately below it is its subservient sidekick, insulin, which serves as somewhat of an antagonist to leptin. Beneath that are your adrenal hormones, adrenaline and cortisol. Then come the pituitary hormones, which regulate the thyroid and growth hormones (and others), then your thyroid hormones, then your sex hormones, and on down. It's a chain of command.

There is not a single endocrinologist in the world, no matter how brilliant or talented, who could possibly replicate the intricate and delicate balance that is orchestrated by the interrelationships of your own innate endocrine symphony, nor is there a single "bioidentical hormone" that can be prescribed that can truly replace what the body does naturally. Anything you do to micromanage a single hormone in the body affects them all—and often in unpredictable and unanticipated ways. This is not to say that bioidentical hormone replacement is never necessary or useful, but care must be taken not to reach blindly for this option instinctively without first seeking to comprehend the underlying mechanisms and foundational interrelationships involved. Sometimes a depressed hormone level is better treated as a *clue* to an underlying disorder than as a deficiency state requiring supplementation. Too often doctors (even natural doctors) assume that the body is somehow stupid and doesn't know how to function in its own best interest. Medical science is too often overly literal in its interpretations. Got high cholesterol? That must mean we need to artificially lower it with a drug (rather than look at why it might be elevated to begin with and address that). Got low testosterone? That must mean that your body is too stupid to make what it needs and we should supply it with more (rather than looking at the mechanisms that functionally regulate this hormone and determining the underlying problem).

Hormones, like a family, function together—and they dysfunction together!

JANET LANG, B.A., D.C.

Hormones are measured in nanograms and picograms—billionths and trillionths of a gram! Hormones are not supplements (despite what "Dr." Suzanne Somers says). They are extremely powerful substances that are used in minute amounts in the body in extremely intricate and complex ways to manage your entire physiology. If you want to improve the functioning of your adrenals, thyroid, or sex hormones, talk to leptin. Restoring healthy leptin functioning is the first major step toward ultimately restoring healthy endocrine balance, at any age, assuming your endocrine organs are intact and have not been destroyed, attacked by autoimmune processes, or removed.

Just what dysregulates leptin and upsets your entire endocrine applecart?

The most potent triggers of hormonal dysregulation are the blood sugar surges that result from chronic carbohydrate consumption.

It turns out that leptin and insulin are birds of a feather. The same things that tend to disrupt insulin also powerfully impact leptin. The worst offenders by far are dietary carbohydrates that are composed of either starch or sugar and the blood sugar surges they produce; this includes bread, cereal, potatoes and other starchy vegetables, pasta, rice, and alcohol (yes, unfortunately, even wine and beer). "Natural" sugars, like honey, lo-han syrup, agave (even more concentrated in damaging fructose than high fructose corn syrup), and maple syrup, as well as the refined versions, can all be similarly problematic. High fructose corn syrup, manufactured using a plethora of nasty synthetic chemicals combined with GMO-engineered corn, is deadly. Medications of all kinds also contribute to leptin and insulin signaling problems. Caffeine and other stimulants similarly cause blood sugar levels to surge. The consumption of these substances, in turn, causes leptin levels to surge, which overwhelms cellular receptors in a way that (not unlike insulin resistance), over time, causes them to stop hearing leptin's messages.

The next casualties in line are the adrenals and what is called the hypothalamic-pituitary-adrenal axis, which becomes dysregulated and may even additionally suppress thyroid function, effectively turning down the idle in an effort to preserve your overheated engine. The adrenals, constantly bombarded with the unnatural task of chronically regulating blood sugar extremes, become overburdened and may additionally tune down the thyroid to prevent total burnout during states of chronic stress.

That's where things start to unravel. The combination of leptin dysregulation, glycation, excess insulin, adrenal exhaustion, and glucose oxidation is a superhighway to chronic fatigue, degeneration, and disease. Toss in some trans fat to pound the last nail in the coffin.

> The only thing that can possibly restore healthy leptin functioning is a diet that is **very low in sugar and starch** (which includes eliminating grains, breads, pasta, rice, and potatoes as well as sweets) **and is sufficient in healthy natural fats.**

It's very simple and very cut-and-dried. Your ice age primal body and mind are ruled by leptin. Adequate, not excessive, dietary fat—in the absence of dietary carbohydrates—is the optimal key to unlocking its power and potential for controlling your health, your well-being, and your life span. Remember: *To our primal physiology, sufficient dietary fat means survival.*

How Do I Know if I Am Leptin Resistant?

Any, but not necessarily all, of the following symptoms (borrowed from *The Rosedale Diet,* by Ron Rosedale and Carol Coleman) can indicate that you are leptin resistant:

- being overweight
- fatigue after meals
- the presence of "love handles"
- high blood pressure
- constantly craving "comfort foods"
- feeling consistently anxious or stressed out
- feeling hungry all the time or at odd hours of the night
- having osteoporosis
- being unable to lose weight or keep weight off
- regularly craving sugar or stimulants (like caffeine)

- having high fasting triglycerides, over 100 mg/dL—particularly when equal to or exceeding cholesterol levels
- having a tendency to snack after meals
- having problems falling or staying asleep
- no change in how your body looks, no matter how much you exercise (Rosedale and Coleman 2004).

Any of this sound familiar?

15

Weight Management 101 and the Path to Type 2 Diabetes

■ ■ ■ ■ ■ ■ ■ ■ ■ ■ ■

Insulin is known as the fat-storage hormone. It is regulated by leptin, though the same dietary influences impact insulin and leptin much the same way, and people can become resistant to the messages of both insulin and leptin in the same way. Again, they are birds of a feather. Carbohydrates such as sugar and starch—as opposed to moderate dietary protein and fat—are the primary dietary macronutrients that stimulate insulin release and generate unhealthy leptin surges, which disrupt healthy communication and encourage hormonal resistance.

Ultimately, most unwanted body fat is made from dietary sugar and starch. The hormone glucagon is required for the mobilization of fat stores and allows them to be burned for energy. Glucagon does not operate in the presence of insulin. If one consumes enough carbohydrates to stimulate insulin secretion, glucagon cannot function and body fat cannot be burned.

Body fat cannot be burned as long as insulin is present. (Some things bear repeating!)

A twelve-week study in Sweden compared the effects of a prehistoric (very low-carb) diet with what was termed a Mediterranean diet that comprised whole grain cereals, low-fat dairy products, fruits, vegetables, and unsaturated fats. (True Mediterranean diets actually look nothing like this.) After twelve weeks, participants' blood sugar level peaks dropped 26 percent with the prehistoric diet and only 7 percent with the so-called Mediterranean diet.

Again, diabetes is a disease not of blood sugar but of excess insulin. High blood sugar levels are a symptom of diabetes, but not the root cause. A diet excessively high in carbohydrates, which invokes excess insulin and leptin production and faulty hormonal signaling, is. Type 2 diabetics who are made to take insulin are actually ultimately worsening their condition over time, though they may experience temporary relief or "improved" blood sugar values. This is a deeply flawed approach. Elevated insulin and leptin levels are highly associated with, and even causative factors of, heart disease, peripheral vascular disease, stroke, high blood pressure, cancer, obesity, and many other disease processes.

> Since most treatments for [type 2, insulin-resistant] diabetes utilize drugs which raise insulin or actual insulin injections themselves, the tragic result is that typical, conventional medical treatment for diabetes contributes to the manifest side effects and the shortened lifespan that diabetics experience.
>
> RON ROSEDALE, M.D., "DIABETES IS NOT A DISEASE
> OF BLOOD SUGAR"

Dietary carbohydrates are at issue here, along with, to a degree, excess consumption of protein, which ultimately gets converted to sugar and is stored via insulin as body fat. In fact, the more sugar dependent your metabolism is, the more readily your body converts other things, like protein, into sugar, too. In the end, fat cells are the last tissues to become resistant to insulin's messages. Becoming fat is your body's way of trying to delay the onset of diabetes.

A key point to understand is that **being fat doesn't come from eating fat; being fat comes from an *inability to burn fat*, which is a direct consequence of relying on carbohydrates—sugar—as a primary fuel source.**

Conversely, moderate protein consumption stimulates glucagon release and improves fat-burning efficiency via dietary-induced thermogenesis. It is important to note here, however, that a significant percentage of excess protein in the diet will ultimately be converted to sugar and stored as fat in the same way. Remember, the more you overeat carbohydrates and protein, the better your body gets at converting protein to sugar, *even if that protein is part of your own muscle and bones.* (Ever hear of osteoporosis?)

Most Americans do tend to overconsume protein, particularly from inferior sources. In the presence of excess carbohydrates, this is especially problematic, as the tendency toward glycation—the damaging reaction between protein and sugar—is greatly increased. (Remember those dreaded advanced glycation end products, or AGEs?) Waste products from excess protein metabolism, together with an increase in AGEs, burden and damage our eliminative organs and capacities.

Baaad juju!

The Downward Spiral

As various tissues proceed to become insulin resistant, the liver—the first organ to lose insulin sensitivity and proper insulin signaling—becomes prone, as a consequence, to overproduce blood sugar from glycogen, which raises blood sugar levels even further. Eventually, other tissues lose sensitivity, also. Your fat cells are the last tissues to become insulin resistant. Your brain is unable to effectively hear leptin's messages, and your hypothalamus keeps sending you the signal to eat more, even when your fat stores are full. Your metabolism seeks to conserve fat in its state of perceived famine. Weight loss seems impossible. When your fat cells are finally no longer able to respond to insulin, there's no place for the sugar to go. It builds up in your bloodstream, and you become diabetic, even if your insulin levels are still very high.

If it goes on long enough, you may even burn out your pancreas's ability to produce insulin anymore at all.

Other tissues unfortunate enough to lack the capacity for insulin resistance become chronically bombarded with excess tissue-damaging insulin and glucose. Among these, nerve cells are extremely vulnerable and become readily damaged by glycation, eventually developing neuropathy. Brain cells similarly are extremely vulnerable here, and deteriorate, rapidly glycate, and oxidize, creating cognitive and memory problems and setting the stage for Alzheimer's disease. The arterial endothelium gets increasingly damaged and scarred by the effects of insulin and the oxidation of glucose. Surges of insulin and leptin stimulate sympathetic (fight-or-flight) nervous system activity, causing the body to rapidly lose magnesium and the vessels to constrict, raising blood pressure and impairing cerebral and all vascular circulation. Vulnerable constricted blood vessels, clogged with glycated and oxidized plaques, and smaller vessels that supply the eyes and kidneys begin to become compromised, impairing blood supplies there. Vision and the function of organs such as the kidneys may become impaired or seriously damaged. Hearing loss with advanced age is now being understood as a frequent outcome of advanced glycation of the auditory nerves (Gopinath et al. 2010). Men with impaired peripheral circulation start seeking Viagra prescriptions . . .

In the end, you can be left blind and deaf, wind up on dialysis, and have your limbs amputated. The risk of heart attack, all degenerative diseases, autoimmune disease, and cancer is substantially elevated. It is not a pretty picture, and it is epidemic.

Hint: Osteoporosis Isn't Necessarily about Low Calcium Levels

Again, a person predisposed to burning sugar as his or her primary source of fuel, particularly if that person is a diabetic, will have the tendency to more efficiently convert protein to sugar. Bones are largely composed of protein and collagen, which give them their strength and flexibility. Calcium gives bone their hardness. Hardness without the strength and flexibility afforded by a protein matrix leads essentially to weak, brittle bones.

If a "sugar burner" should attempt to starve himself, go too long without eating, or overly restrict calories, then his body will tend to convert its own protein stores from muscle and even bone to sugar to burn for fuel.

It's easier for your body to make sugar from protein than fat. This effect is also at play while you are asleep at night, when your blood sugar level lowers because you can't eat. This leads to a breakdown of vital tissues at night to support your sugar habit. These low blood sugar levels, particularly in the presence of stressed-out adrenal fatigue and depressed cortisol levels, also commonly stimulate nighttime catabolic (tissue breakdown) adrenaline releases as the body desperately seeks to stimulate elevations in blood sugar levels. This leads to nighttime waking forms of insomnia and even to middle-of-the-night cravings in some people. Under extremes of stress, this can even result in muscle wasting, significant bone loss, immune system dysfunction, and possibly even organ damage. The same process, by the way, can result in a person who looks scrawny or emaciated all the time, seems nervous, and has trouble gaining weight. The result of dysglycemia isn't always obesity. Food sensitivity issues—particularly gluten sensitivity—can also drive these catabolic blood sugar level highs and lows or even trigger autoantibody production that targets the breakdown of virtually any tissue—including bone and even the brain. Appropriate testing for food sensitivities should be sought by anyone who has experienced bone loss or degeneration (see www.cyrexlabs .com or www.enterolab.com).

The loss of lean tissue mass in this way, however, can contribute further to obesity and chronic fatigue in many people as the majority of mitochondria, our cells' own little energy-producing, fat-burning factories, are largely in our muscles. Inflammation generated by excesses of omega-6 fatty acid, glycation, the effects of insulin and leptin, or anything else readily destroys mitochondria. Carbohydrate consumption promotes inflammation. The less muscle and the fewer mitochondria you have, the less is your ability to burn fat and produce energy. With fewer and fewer mitochondria, you are sapped of your vital energy and can't lose weight. It is a vicious cycle. Even if you're thin, you're flabby.

Gluten sensitivity, too, is a major contributor to the incidence of osteoporosis. According to studies in both *The Lancet* and the *British Medical Journal*, the prevalence of celiac disease with osteoporosis is so high that it has been recommended that all people with osteoporosis be tested for celiac disease. An article in *Clinical Rheumatology* stated, "Diffuse musculoskeletal pain, muscle weakness, and even osteoporosis may be the only symptoms of wheat allergies (gluten) and are completely relieved or reversed on a gluten free diet" (Kozanoglu et al. 2005).

The Solution?

First, eliminate the sugar, starchy carbohydrates, and gluten from your diet; this includes bread, pasta, grains, hidden sources of gluten, rice, beans, potatoes, and all sweets and sweeteners. Limit the amount of fruit, and stick mostly to berries when you do eat fruit (berries are lower in sugar, higher in fiber, and much richer in antioxidants than other sources of fruit). Second, consume just enough dietary protein to meet your immediate daily needs for rebuilding and regeneration from high-quality, nutrient-dense sources of *complete* protein, such as grass-fed meat, wild-caught fish, and pastured eggs. This may be as *little* as 44 to 56 g per day for most adult people (the approximate RDA), which translates to six or seven ounces (just a few) of meat, eggs, or fish—preferably in divided amounts. (See the protein content of foods chart in appendix C, at the back of this book.) Another method of calculation would be to shoot for 0.8 g of actual protein per kilogram of ideal body weight per day. Extremely large or active individuals—short of being an Olympic athlete or a professional bodybuilder—or individuals in a particularly nutritionally depleted state may need 10 g or so more (all relative to lean-body composition and one's activity level). That's really about all. Elite athletes and bodybuilders may need closer to 1.5 g of actual protein per kilogram of body weight to meet their daily needs. Amounts in excess of this will likely suppress ketosis, however (Phinney 2004). **Pregnant women, children, and teens, however, should not have their protein intake overly restricted.**

High-protein diets are not advisable or necessary to be healthy and slim and can lead to numerous problems. The trick is in maximizing the quality of the food source, the digestibility of the protein (or quality of your digestion), and what you combine it with so that you can make the best use of this precious commodity. This is not about inducing starvation in any way. In fact, if you go about it correctly, you should never be hungry. It's about improving the *efficiency* with which you use the quality, nutrient-dense foods in your diet.

Digestion takes more energy to perform than any other daily human activity. Eating more of optimally sufficient amounts of *complete* protein—particularly when not overly cooked or combined with starches—actually greatly helps improve the digestion and assimilation of your food, and you will expend much less energy doing so, so you will have more energy to do other things! In fact, you may be utterly shocked to discover how much energy it is possible for you to have.

Two of the other common causes of osteoporosis are poor digestion and nutrient deficiencies. Among these are hydrochloric acid insufficiency (remember, hydrochloric acid is needed to digest both protein and minerals, including calcium) and biliary (gallbladder) problems, leading to poor absorption of the fat-soluble nutrients that are needed for the absorption and use of minerals, particularly vitamins D_3 and K_2. Taking vitamin D_3 for healthy bones without also supplementing with vitamin K_2 can, according to *The Nurse's Health Study,* actually double your risk of hip fracture! Roughly a dozen or more different nutrients are needed for the healthy formation of bone matrix. Eating a quality, nutrient-dense, whole-food diet—and being able to properly digest it throughout life—is key to healthy, *quality* bone density

Hormonal imbalances in aging women, particularly inadequate levels of progesterone, can also contribute to bone loss. Maintaining healthy adrenal function is essential for healthy female hormonal balance, particularly at menopause.

Finally, bone density has as much to do with physics as with chemistry. A sedentary lifestyle will result in significant bone loss over time. Weight-bearing exercise is needed to generate and maintain healthy bone density. Many people aren't aware that astronauts who spend time in space usually come back with significant bone loss, sometimes so severe that they are unable to stand or walk. The departure from the earth's gravitational pull causes bone to rapidly weaken.

Being a couch potato can have the same effect over time. Taking calcium pills is no more likely to build your bones than eating a side of beef is likely to make your muscles look like Arnold Schwarzenegger's. Bone develops (or shrinks) by the same principle that muscle does: Use it or lose it.

In a Nutshell . . .

In sufficient amounts, without added carbohydrates, dietary fat is satiating and calms the hormone leptin, which in turn helps control hunger and sends the message to the hypothalamus that "the hunting is good," whereby fat stores become more expendable and are more freely burned for energy. Fiber from vegetables and greens can be additionally filling, which may help, but it is dietary fat that actually satisfies the appetite and curbs overeating.

The more that dietary fat serves as your primary source of fuel and not carbohydrates, the better you will become at fat burning, the healthier—and naturally slimmer—you will ultimately be, *and* the longer you will live. It turns out, in fact, that the very thing we have been told is our worst possible enemy actually may be our very best friend, if not our salvation. The idea here is not to eat a diet that is excessive in fat, but one that is *sufficient enough* to meet the physiological demands for essential fatty acids and fat-soluble nutrients and to satisfy the appetite. Using dietary fat in this way, while eliminating insulin-provoking carbs and moderating protein intake as demonstrated by the very newest longevity research, is the deceptively simple and ultimate secret key to unlocking your health and longevity.

> The key lies in minimizing calories while maximizing nutrient density.

Overcoming Weight-Loss Myths

Contrary to popular belief, healthy weight loss is not about increasing metabolism but about increasing the *efficiency* of metabolism. Why would you want the engine in your car to run hotter? People seeking to improve fitness and lose weight often exercise vigorously for prolonged periods of time in the hope that exercise will boost their metabolic rate. While this can burn calories slightly more rapidly, it also accelerates the production of dangerous free radicals and may also simply make you hungrier. According to a prevailing theory of aging, oxidative damage at the level of the mitochondria is responsible for much of the inflammation and degeneration associated with aging (Heilbronn et al. 2006).

What you want is for the engine in your car to run more *efficiently*. Again, it's all about improving communication and signaling between cells and tissues via optimizing hormonal function plus using the right type of fuel, and this is accomplished by minimizing the need for insulin and keeping leptin levels optimally low. This is best accomplished by eliminating sugar, starch, and excess protein from the diet, and by satisfying hunger by eating enough fat to satiate the appetite, thereby teaching your body to burn fat rather than sugar for fuel, thus maximizing your metabolic efficiency.

The idea that eating fat can help you lose fat may seem counterintuitive. It certainly conflicts with everything you hear or read in the media or get lectured about from your doctor or a conventionally trained nutritionist or dietician. Yet the most dramatically effective weight-loss approach ever researched involved a diet that consisted of little more than one thousand calories a day divided into five two-hundred-calorie feedings every four hours of *almost pure fat* (90 percent). Two British researchers, Gaston Pawan and Alan Kekwick, developed this diet after researching many different alternatives and macronutrient ratios (Kekwick and Pawan 1956). They took subjects who were overweight and placed them in three groups.

Each group received one thousand calories per day. One group was fed 90 percent carbohydrates, the second group 90 percent protein, and the third group 90 percent fat. The group receiving 90 percent carbohydrates **gained** an average of 0.24 pound per day of the study. The group receiving 90 percent protein lost an average of 0.6 pound per day of the study, and the group receiving 90 percent fat **lost** an average of **0.9 pound per day** of the study. The results demonstrated the overwhelming superiority of a fat-based caloric regimen to even total fasting in burning body fat. No other weight-loss regimen researched has ever come close to matching this diet's ability to burn off stored fat. There's no question about it; the best way to burn fat is to eat fat, but **only** in the absence of carbohydrates.

In this (or any similar) dietary approach, with no source of sugar to burn, the body is forced to burn fat. The adequate presence of dietary fat lowers leptin levels and assures the hypothalamus that "hunting is at least okay," which keeps the metabolism running efficiently. Caloric restriction then accelerates the weight loss. There is *just enough* fat to convince the brain you aren't starving, but not enough to actually meet all your energy needs, so your own internal fat stores get used to make up the deficit. As long as fat is coming in, your metabolism doesn't shut down. Of course, the particular one-thousand-calorie-per-day, pure-dietary-fat approach used in the Pawan and Kekwick study is not a practical, advisable, or sustainable diet in the long term for anyone; it's woefully restrictive and lacks adequate protein and other nutrients. However, the research underscores the superior impact of eating fat (not carbohydrates) to burn even more fat than would be possible even with a total fast. There's a hint here, folks.

Again, don't go crazy and try this one at home, kids, at least without appropriate medical supervision. The point here is that eating fat—in the absence of carbohydrates—does, in fact, help burn more fat, and lots of it. You get good at anything by doing more of it. You don't get good at burning fat by constantly burning sugar.

For a practical, sustainable, and healthy version of this unwanted-fat-loss approach, the focus should be on nutrient-dense, animal-source foods containing rich sources of natural, healthy fat and moderate amounts of protein. **Quality nutrient density is key here.** Adding bulk with sufficient quantities of fibrous, antioxidant-rich vegetables fills out most nutrient requirements nicely and staves off deficiencies, feelings of deprivation, and hunger. Done correctly, this approach to diet actually maximizes your body's repair and regenerative potential, boosts your healthy immune function, allows for easy loss of unwanted weight, and eliminates hunger.

> *Most people mistakenly believe that low-fat diets are the only way to lose weight. They do not realize that the right fats, such as coconut oil and other healthy oils in synergistic combination, not only encourage weight loss but also help you heal.*
> SALLY FALLON AND MARY ENIG, PH.D., *EAT FAT, LOSE FAT*

Fats and Carbs Together: A Bad Combo

> *The deleterious effects of fat have been measured in the presence of high carbohydrate. A high fat diet in the presence of high carbohydrate is different than a high fat diet in the presence of low carbohydrate.*
> RICHARD FINEMAN, PH.D., PROFESSOR OF BIOCHEMISTRY,
> STATE UNIVERSITY OF NEW YORK DOWNSTATE MEDICAL CENTER,
> AND FOUNDER OF THE NUTRITION AND METABOLISM SOCIETY

The impact of dietary fat on insulin release is negligible, except in great excess or in the presence of dietary carbohydrates. When fats and sugar or starch-based carbohydrates are eaten together, the body will burn the sugar preferentially for fuel, storing more of the fat for later.

Sugar is such a damaging substance to the body that the body will race to rid itself of excesses as quickly as it can. The body does this first by rushing as much sugar as possible to cells, with the help of insulin, as a means of producing immediate anaerobic, turbo-charged energy— the equivalent of putting rocket fuel in your car. If this is not immediately needed (in other words, if you don't happen to be trying to outrun a charging rhino), then much of the sugar is converted to glycogen and stored in the liver and muscle tissue. Once this very limited capacity for storage is filled, your body proceeds to convert what is left to triglycerides in the liver and stores whatever is left in your fat cells.

Obesity is not the *cause* of metabolic problems; it is only an outward indicator. If one is insulin resistant, energy or glucose can't get into cells for fuel and must be converted to fat and stored for another time. This is all a very inefficient and energy-intensive process that tends to generate fatigue or sleepiness after meals as a person gradually becomes increasingly insulin and leptin resistant. Fatigue after meals, incidentally, is one fairly strong indicator of insulin and leptin resistance (note that food sensitivity reactions can generate this symptom, also). In this state, you are basically unable to make use of the energy in your food. Dietary fat that isn't otherwise used elsewhere in the body and can't get burned for energy is incorporated into fat tissue.

Feel tired all the time, by any chance?

The Slippery Slope

By increasing the amount of stored body fat, leptin levels automatically rise. With chronically elevated levels of leptin, an inflammatory cytokine, inflammation increases throughout the body. This is one major reason why overweight and obese people are so at risk for degenerative illness, heart disease, and cancer—raging chronic and systemic inflammation. Furthermore, these surges of insulin and leptin increase sympathetic overarousal, anxiety, and the actions of stress hormones. (Know anyone with chronic anxiety or trouble sleeping?)

Stress hormones, when being produced in such a damaging cycle, catabolize, or break down, tissue as well as weaken the immune system. A protective substance lining our gastrointestinal tract and lung tissue known as *secretory IgA,* which is the first defense we have in our immune system, is broken down under chronically high (or excessively low, as occurs in adrenal burnout) cortisol levels. This leaves the small intestine vulnerable to something known as *leaky gut syndrome.* This is where undigested proteins and other substances that normally are not allowed across the semipermeable intestinal barrier are able to get across and trigger antibody responses that can elicit allergic, physical, emotional, or cognitive food sensitivity–based reactions. As the vicious cycle continues and the levels of cortisol, adrenaline, insulin, and leptin climb, what is known as the TH-2 (T-helper cell 2) antibody immune response can be up-regulated (increased) and the TH-1 (T-helper cell 1) humoral immune response can be down-regulated (decreased), leading to more-exaggerated food sensitivities as well as other antigenic responses. The suppression of TH-1 leaves one more vulnerable to contagions and illness or infection. (Know anyone who gets colds all the time and has allergies or food sensitivities?) This cycle can be very difficult to bring under control and tends to be self-perpetuating. Food sensitivities can contribute to unwanted cortisol and insulin levels and can be a very common source of weight gain and resistance to weight loss for some.

The excesses of fat being generated by insulin and cortisol also more readily secrete enzymes (such as *aromatase*) that stimulate the excessive conversion of testosterone to estrogen in men (the number one cause of so-called testosterone deficiency in men) and the conversion of estrogen to toxic DHT testosterone in women, making weight loss extremely difficult in both men and women and mimicking in women many symptoms commonly associated with low thyroid function.

This can make one appear testosterone or estrogen deficient in blood or saliva tests. Lower testosterone levels also make men more prone to dopamine neurotransmitter deficiencies, as depressed testosterone activity also depresses dopamine receptor activity. Excessively lower estrogen levels in women suppress serotonin receptor activity and increase the proneness to depression and other issues. Good times.

The answer here is almost never hormone replacement, even with bioidentical hormones, which only temporarily alleviate the symptoms and can eventually greatly exacerbate the problem. You may feel temporarily better with supplemental estrogen, or even feel like Superman, at least for a while, on supplemental testosterone, but in the end, you are only making the problem worse. The underlying answer is in controlling this whole cascade of events by basically doing what is necessary to manage your levels of leptin, insulin, and adrenals (which usually means starting with addressing your blood sugar issues). The excessive conversion of hormones is an extremely vicious cycle and is at the heart of syndrome X, or metabolic syndrome.

Metabolic syndrome and its other related negative hormonal influences cannot ever be effectively micromanaged in the long term by hormone replacement. Bioidentical hormones have their rightful place in medicine, but their overuse often causes many more problems than they ultimately solve. The practice of functional medicine should have its foundation in respect for the complexity of the human organism and the intricate, interrelated web of endocrine function. One must peel back the layers of the onion to find the source of the problem and not simply persist in treating the symptoms.

Why Calorie Counting Doesn't Work

It seems everyone who wants to lose weight becomes fixated on one common pastime: counting calories. It becomes an obsession for some. The whole principle behind the concept of dietary calories lies in the potential of a given food to generate energy or heat. Using this as a measure of which foods should and shouldn't be eaten presupposes, however, that the human body is mainly a "heat engine" and that we consume food solely for the purpose of producing energy or heat.

This simply isn't so and makes for a deeply flawed approach, destined for bigger problems. The human body is, in fact, a complex "chemical factory." Different food substances are eaten, used, and processed in many different ways, and the use of different macronutrients is far from equal. Energy is far from the only thing extracted from what we eat. Protein, for instance, goes largely to building, rebuilding, or maintaining structures in the body, including skin, bones, hair, lean tissue, hormones, neurotransmitters, and innumerable other cellular components. It is estimated that the human body manufactures over fifty thousand different proteins in various forms for ongoing metabolic processes and various aspects of the physical structure. In the case of dietary protein, it is only excess amounts that get significantly converted to sugar and stored as body fat or unwanted calories.

Since we are fairly efficient at recycling our protein stores, only a few ounces of concentrated, complete protein per day are actually needed by all but the most active or depleted individuals. The problem with trying to meet protein needs with vegan sources of protein lies in the incomplete amino acid profile and the high starch content of nearly all vegan-source protein-containing foods. Without having four stomachs or an herbivore's metabolic system, we're just not designed to pull it off. We are capable of manufacturing hydrochloric acid (unlike herbivores) for a *reason*. Even trying to combine proteins to obtain a complete amino acid profile (which would mean a necessary calculation and balancing act at every meal), one usually ends up with a lack of sufficient actual protein. A vegetarian or vegan diet is almost always ultimately a starch-based diet, and we're not cows; we can't just do it all with veggies in the long term. *We need the fully digestible nutrient density.*

But I digress.

Dietary fats also have a complex, profound, and varied role to play in physical structure and function. Dietary fat—arguably the most important macronutrient, with the possible exception of water—serves the needs of innumerable physiological processes: building, rebuilding, and maintaining cellular membranes and nerve tissue; manufacturing hormones and neurotransmitters; facilitating cellular communication and absorption of critical fat-soluble nutrients; stabilizing the nervous system; supporting the immune and lymphatic systems; creating proinflammatory and anti-inflammatory compounds; supporting the proper use of proteins; and fueling the brain, heart, and other muscles. (Whew!) This alone should help underscore the fundamental insanity of low-fat diets.

Most fat gets absorbed, not into the bloodstream, but into the lymphatic system. Again, only *excess* fat (or fat in the presence of dietary sugar or starch) goes to body fat for storage. Certain shorter-chain fats, however, such as those found in butter (butyric acid) and especially in coconut oil (medium-chain triglycerides, sometimes referred to as MCTs) have potent antimicrobial activity, are similar in caloric value to carbohydrates, are nearly always burned preferentially for energy, and do not easily store as body fat, if at all. These short- and medium-chain fats can, in fact, even help energize and fuel weight loss!

Carbohydrates, on the other hand, have a minimal role to play as any sort of structural compound in the body. Less than about 2 percent of bodily structure is composed of carbohydrates, and *all* of this can be manufactured without the presence of dietary carbohydrates. Certain *glyconutrients* serve as components of joint tissue and cartilage. Certain other glyconutrients play a unique role in immune function. Fiber—a nonusable carbohydrate—essentially serves as bulk in the diet and may help facilitate waste elimination in the colon (though it is not essential for that) and serves to bind excess conjugated hormones and better allow for their proper excretion. Apart from this, the body uses only minute amounts of sugar to fuel red blood cells and is able to store all of about two thousand calories' worth as glycogen in the liver and muscles for emergency use for major exertion. *All the rest*—every single calorie of carbohydrate consumed that is not immediately required for turbocharged, anaerobic effort—is converted in a limited way to glycogen, or is eventually converted to triglycerides by the liver and stored as body fat, for at least as long as insulin is willing to keep facilitating the effort.

Once one is insulin resistant from constant bombardment of dietary carbohydrates, for which there is a *zero* dietary requirement, sugar simply begins to build in the bloodstream. There, it accelerates glycation of red blood cells and endothelial tissue, forming AGEs, which results in increased numbers of free radicals, untold oxidative damage, and rampant systemic inflammation. The body undergoes activation of genes that up-regulate certain enzymes to better facilitate burning of sugar as a primary source of fuel (which is unnatural as a prolonged metabolic state) *in an effort to simply get rid of it.* And fat burning comes to a screeching halt.

You are one of two things: you are either a "fat burner" or a "sugar burner." If you are overweight, crave carbohydrates (and stimulants), or are insulin or leptin resistant, then you are a sugar burner. It's that simple.

It also should be noted that stress, food sensitivity issues, caffeine and other stimulants, alcohol, sleep deprivation, aspartame, tobacco, and drugs of all types further aggravate and exacerbate excess insulin production (Schwarzbein and Deville 1999).

For people who are unconcerned about dietary carbohydrates from a weight-gain perspective because of higher metabolic levels or athletic activity, the caution is this: *Although it is possible to burn off the excess glucose, one cannot burn off the excess insulin.* Excess insulin production, no matter how thin you are, wreaks metabolic havoc and invariably yields unhealthy consequences over time and accelerates aging.

It is also possible to be thin and diabetic.

The Hidden (and Not-So-Hidden) Ravages of Blood Sugar Dysregulation

Glucose dysregulation and excess dietary carbohydrates can ultimately manifest as a vast array of disorders including, but not limited to:

- frequent illness and immune disorders
- serotonin depletion
- candidiasis
- fatigue
- dizziness
- irritability
- depression
- anxiety
- confusion and memory problems
- night sweats
- weight problems

- alcoholism
- nervous habits
- mental disturbances
- insomnia
- heart disease
- adrenal insufficiency
- thyroid disorders
- pituitary disorders
- kidney disease
- pancreatitis
- chronic liver failure
- diabetes and hypoglycemia
- cancer

Among the simplest telltale signs of insulin and leptin resistance are the appearance of love handles, cravings for carbohydrates or sweets or stimulants (such as caffeine), and sleepiness or fatigue after meals.

Ensuring moderate amounts of quality dietary protein and sufficient natural fats (including omega-3 fatty acids) in the diet, along with eliminating the consumption of sugar and starchy carbohydrates, vegetable oils, and margarine, can help restore insulin sensitivity and reduce or eliminate many associated symptoms of insulin resistance or glucose dysregulation. Also important is *limiting or eliminating the use of caffeine and other stimulants, alcohol, tobacco, artificial sweeteners, all recreational drugs, and unnecessary over-the-counter and prescriptive medications* (Schwarzbein and Deville 1999).

Engaging in stress-reduction activities and exercise helps further. Numerous supplements can also help accelerate the improvement of insulin function. Over time, insulin sensitivity can be restored through careful attention to these important dietary principles, some appropriate supplementation, and a reduced-stress lifestyle.

But What about Exercise? Won't That Make Up for It?

In a word, no.

Exercise is certainly "something better than nothing" toward helping the situation. It can help in restoring insulin sensitivity and can burn off some excess carbohydrates and fat, depending on the type of exercise done, but not all exercise is created equal or is necessarily always beneficial. If you are a carbovore, however, you may never get around to effectively burning your fat stores—or fully reach your physical or performance potential.

Exercise can never compensate for a lousy diet any more than drugs or supplements can. At least 70 percent of your health equation depends on your diet. Most of the other 30 percent is a combination of appropriate supplementation, stress reduction, positive attitude, and exercise. Exercise is a helpful component of healthy weight loss in tandem with a healthier diet. The key is the *quality* of exercise, not a great quantity of exercise.

Although the details of this topic are best saved for a separate book, suffice it to say that brief bouts of peak anaerobic exertion are essentially superior for expanding the health of the heart and lungs and facilitating weight loss and lean tissue development. More exercise is not necessarily better, contrary to the common tendency of those people who endeavor to jog endlessly on their treadmills or spend hours in the gym lifting weights.

Our ancestors would never have bothered with such wasteful and wearing expenditures of energy! Consider that, apart from walking, exercise for our Paleolithic ancestors consisted mainly of brief bouts of running to catch things they were hunting or running away from things that wanted to eat or trample them. These brief, intense bouts of exercise or exertion served to expand heart and lung capacity, challenged and developed the strength of skeletal muscles, and rapidly used blood glucose and glycogen stores. Now, you might be thinking, "That doesn't burn any fat!"

Au contraire.

Consider what message you send your body when you spend hours jogging on a treadmill. After about the first twenty minutes of exercise, when the body changes over from the predominant use of glucose to the predominant use of body fat, we go into that "fat-burning mode" that aerobic exercise pundits tell you is "the zone." But what is this really telling the body when we spend extended amounts of time in this so-called zone? It is saying, "Hey, we're being asked to do this ridiculously tedious and demanding thing and it's going to require *a lot of fat.*"

Make no mistake about it, you will burn some fat doing this, but remember that fat to our physiology means survival, and if it's going to take a lot of that precious commodity to fuel what you're doing, your body is going to work at becoming more efficient at making this fuel available. It will become better at converting everything you eat into fat and will burn it more efficiently and sparingly over time so that it becomes harder to use up your stored fat. God forbid you should fall off your exercise wagon. You will rapidly gain back whatever you may have lost (and then some) while your body's energy stores prepare for the next marathon. (Yes, fat and ketones are vastly better, more efficient, and longer-lasting fuels for a marathon than carbohydrates. "Carb loading" for marathons is more than a myth; it's a big, big mistake.)

A study by metabolic researcher Stephen D. Phinney titled "Ketogenic Diets and Physical Performance" demonstrated the superior effects of ketogenic diets on athletic performance and endurance once metabolic adaptation to burning fat as the primary source of fuel is in place (Phinney 2004). Other studies in the works by Phinney are serving to support the superiority of ketogenic states, even in strength training and other anaerobic challenges! Simply consider for a moment the strength and prowess of our ketogenic, cave-dwelling ancestors (who likely would have run circles around today's most elite athletes and put their physical development to shame).

Prolonged aerobic exercise (instead of brief bouts of anaerobic exertion) does little to improve body composition in the long term and, if anything, diminishes your heart and lung capacity. Consider that all the while you're plodding along on your treadmill, you are also effectively telling your heart and lungs they don't have to be any stronger or more capable than what you're asking them to do. You will actually lose cardiopulmonary capacity over time, even weaken your heart. (Remember Jim Fixx, the founder of the jogging craze who dropped dead of a heart attack? He isn't remotely the only long-distance runner to do so.) Furthermore, exercise is a form of stress on the body. We can tolerate—and are well designed to tolerate—*brief* bouts of peak effort, from which our adrenals require a certain amount of time, a good twenty-four hours, to fully recover. Our body strengthens in response to peak effort in a way that makes us stronger and faster the next time. That's the way we were designed.

There's no question our primitive ancestors would have had superb endurance and that certain "persistence hunters" would have been able to follow prey for miles and for days if necessary, running the prey to exhaustion. They would never have been able to accomplish this without also exercising peak cardiopulmonary effort at intervals, however, which would have generated much greater and more neceessary cardiopulmonary capacity, something jogging at a constant pace on a treadmill simply cannot accomplish. Also, the advantage of shorter bouts at high intensity is less stress hormone excess. In other words, just because they could do it doesn't mean they would necessarily want to. Our ancestors were certainly designed for a mixture of both strength and endurance challenges, and so are we. There's nothing wrong with walking long distances, but for peak strength and cardiopulmonary fitness (and optimal fat burning), nothing can beat high-intensity, shorter-duration, interval-style training.

So what actually happens when we pound or lift away, unnaturally, for long exercise periods in the gym? We produce a lot of cortisol, our primary stress hormone, and cortisol in turn raises blood sugar levels and is catabolic in nature. In other words, *cortisol eats muscle and other tissues for lunch.* (Remember, too, that your heart is also a muscle.)

You are making one sweaty step forward and two big, wasted (or worse) steps back. Chronic cortisol production suppresses the immune system and breaks down your muscles as fast as you're trying to build them. The elevations in blood sugar stimulated by cortisol also stimulate more insulin production, which is not necessarily a desirable thing for improving insulin sensitivity or healthy blood sugar levels, and little of positive value is accomplished.

Furthermore, once you've finished your extended bout of aerobic exercise, the fat burning more or less stops, or substantially slows. This is an extremely inefficient means of losing body fat.

With brief, intense anaerobic training, however, there is a residual fat-burning effect that can last up to *two days!* In the first couple of minutes of any intense exercise, your body uses pure adenosine triphosphate (known as ATP), and immediately after that's exhausted, your body uses its glycogen stores. It takes a good fifteen to twenty minutes to burn off the glycogen and start using fat. If you maximize your efforts within that twenty-minute window, your body actually learns to store energy increasingly in your muscles as glycogen instead of layered on your waist and thighs (and who knows where else) as unwanted body fat.

There is an aftereffect with this interval approach to exercise that is known as *excess postexercise oxygen consumption,* or EPOC (a sort of afterburn), that in effect ramps up the weight loss for extended periods of time—even while you're sleeping! Your body has to work hard to repair and restore spent energy levels after an intense workout, and this takes a lot of calories. It can take up to a full day for a full recovery. Think of it as a bonus calorie-burning workout within a workout. A scientific study that was done by Laval University in Quebec, Canada, proved that short, intense workouts burn up to **nine times more fat** than traditional aerobic training (Tremblay et al. 1994). In another study, at Colorado State University, subjects exercised for twenty minutes in sets of two-minute intervals, followed by one full minute of rest in between. Even at rest, their rate of fat oxidation was up **62 percent,** and they continued to burn fat for a full sixteen hours following the exercise (Osterberg and Melby 2000)!

Work out harder and smarter for less time, lose more fat—and live longer.

Finally, recent evidence shows, too, a longevity-enhancing effect from high-intensity exercise. An article in the journal *Mechanisms of Aging* looked at the association between telomere shortening with age and the effects of VO2 max exercise. The authors' write:

> The results of the present study provide evidence that leukocyte telomere length (LTL) is related to regular vigorous aerobic exercise and maximal aerobic exercise capacity with aging in healthy humans. LTL is not influenced by aerobic exercise status among young subjects, presumably because TL is intact (i.e., already normal) in sedentary healthy young adults. However, as LTL shortens with aging it appears that maintenance of aerobic fitness, produced by chronic strenuous exercise and reflected by higher VO2 max, acts to preserve LTL. . . . Stepwise multiple regression analysis revealed that VO2 max was the only independent predictor of LTL in the overall group. Our results indicate that leukocyte telomere length (LTL) is preserved in healthy older adults who perform vigorous aerobic exercise and is positively related to maximal aerobic exercise capacity. This may represent a novel molecular mechanism underlying the "anti-aging" effects of maintaining high aerobic fitness. (LaRocca et al. 2010)

What these guys are referring to as aerobic exercise, by the way is not jogging. Note that they speak of "chronic **strenuous** exercise" and "**vigorous** aerobic exercise" and "higher VO2 max." It is pushing your lungs to the max in a way that challenges and develops greater lung capacity (another important true longevity marker). What most people think of as aerobic training has nothing to do with this. If you don't feel winded afterward, you haven't accomplished much with respect to enhancing the capacity or health of your lungs and heart. In addition, it is exclusively this form of exercise that is well known to stimulate the release of human growth hormone, or HGH, which is long associated with preserving youth and vitality. A study published in the journal *Sports Medicine* found that "exercise intensity above lactate threshold and for a minimum of 10 minutes appears to elicit the greatest stimulus to the secretion of HGH" (Godfrey et al. 2003).

So, what do you do?

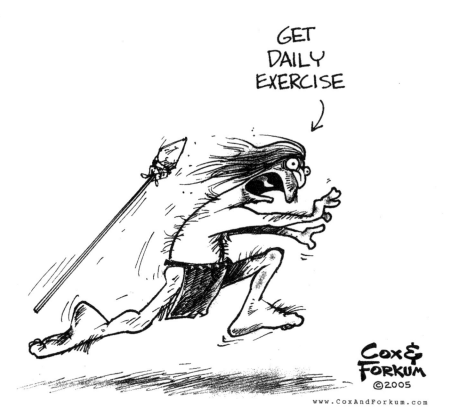

Fig. 15.1. "Getting your daily exercise"

First, limit intense exercise to no more than about twenty minutes in duration and focus on brief bouts of significant anaerobic exertion, interspersed with brief periods of recovery at a slower pace that is sufficient for a return to the resting heart rate. This can be done via sprinting, cycling, rowing, elliptical machines, and many other methods. Or, it can be done using kettlebells (my personal favorite), weights, or calisthenics in which muscles are, after warming up, challenged close to their peak capacity for a very few sets. Strength or resistance training reverses the reduction in muscle fiber size that accompanies aging and inactivity and has been shown conclusively to increase insulin sensitivity. Study after study has shown that resistance training is superior to what is commonly termed aerobic exercise in improving insulin receptor sensitivity and even aerobic capacity! It also lowers actual insulin levels.

Once each muscle group has had its neural recruitment capacity sufficiently challenged and has performed at its peak exertion level, you are done for the day. This may take no more than ten or fifteen minutes of challenging exertion, total. Another way of going about it can be sprinting (when biking, rowing, swimming, or elliptical training) for four or five sets of up to a minute each, allowing for heart-rate recovery in between. This exercises and expands heart and pulmonary capacity as well as honing strength. Talk about a time-saver, not to mention a lifesaver!

Done appropriately, this style of exercise can be adopted by anyone, regardless of age or fitness level, with or without a gym. Changing your routine and type of exercise daily is another means of enhancing your gains and eliminating plateaus. Don't let your body get too used to any one routine. Also, working muscles in groups or doing whole-body exercises is infinitely more efficient, effective, and natural than exercising as a collection of individual body parts using isolation exercises or machines. Following these brief bouts of *anaerobic exertion*, critical building and rebuilding mechanisms can immediately take place over the next day or two to make you ultimately better and stronger than you were before. Remember, you don't build strength or regenerate healthy tissue *during* exercise; it is accomplished during recovery. You must allow sufficient recovery between intense bouts of exercise!

This is how evolution designed us to achieve fitness, not by running marathons or standing around all day doing bicep curls.

In exercising in brief, intense bouts, you become more readily efficient at storing future sources of carbohydrates as glycogen in muscle, which increases the size and definition of the muscle and better fuels it for the future, instead of simply converting the carbohydrates to body fat for marathons. You also become much more efficient in using those glycogen stores. You better preserve your precious adrenal health. Enhanced muscle strength, stimulated by growth hormone during peak effort, increases the number of mitochondria in the body—our body's little fat-burning factories (hint, hint), found almost exclusively in muscle—and thus inherently enhances our use of fat as fuel and consequently as our primary energy source as well. This also ensures that your body more comfortably releases fat stores for fuel, since no undue demands are being placed on endurance capacity. You become a lean, mean, fat-burning machine!

For advanced, excellent, and possibly the best-detailed information regarding this general approach to cardio fitness and bodybuilding or strength training, get Dr. Al Sears's book *PACE: The 12-Minute Fitness Revolution* (Sears 2010). (*PACE* stands for "progressive accelerated cardio-pulmonary exertion.") You can also visit his website, at www.alsearsM.D. .com/pace. For other related reading and information on additionally effective approaches that are compatible, Lawrence E. Morehouse, Ph.D., and Leonard Gross's book *Maximum Performance* is excellent (Morehouse and Gross 1977). For people interested mainly in bodybuilding, read the book *Body By Science* by Doug McGuff, M.D., or anything by Mike Mentzer, and for general fitness and strength training, see information on Robb Wolf, Mark Sisson, Art DeVang, Frank Forencich, and Erwan LeCorre. Pavel Tsatsouline, former physical training instructor for the Soviet Special Forces, author, and no-nonsense fitness-training expert, has good books on strength and kettlebell training, something I happen to love. Tsatsouline also has several DVDs. Former U.S. Navy Seal and kettlebell training coach and expert Michael Skogg has a newly available world-class and cutting-edge kettlebell training system on DVDs that I highly recommend (for more information, check out Skogg's website, at www .Skoggsystem.com).

For people who are not in need of weight loss but who just want to develop their strength and flexibility, yoga and other core-strengthening exercises may be useful. Some anaerobic training for improving cardiopul-monary capacity is *always* a good idea, though, unless contraindicated by your health care provider.

Increased lung capacity, possibly more than any other single physical factor, is tantamount to greater longevity (Schunemann et al. 2000).

16

Taming the
Carb-craving Monster

■ ■ ■ ■ ■ ■ ■ ■ ■ ■ ■ ■

Note: **It is not necessarily suggested that you need to take all the supplements presented below.** This list is merely a guide to many actions and substances that are known to be additionally helpful to the basic dietary guidelines presented.

- Eliminate sugars and starches from the diet. (*Note:* If you are extremely insulin resistant or diabetic, it may take you a longer time to undergo the metabolic conversion allowing for the use of fat as a primary source of fuel, which may best be facilitated by and accomplished in tandem with the use of additional supportive supplements.)
- Consume moderate amounts of nutrient-dense protein and enough natural dietary fat to satisfy your hunger. This greatly helps normalize blood sugar levels. Be sure to get adequate amounts of essential fatty acids, particularly EPA, DHA, and GLA.
- Regularly take a B-complex supplement with meals (preferably one that is whole food complex–based or coenzymated). B vitamins assist in improving carbohydrate metabolism. Vitamin B_1 and especially its fat-soluble derivatives allithiamine and *benfotiamine* can greatly help reduce glycation. From 100 to 250 mg or more per day is the common dosage.

- L-carnosine is an amino acid that can serve as a powerful neuropro-tective, antiglycating nutrient. From 500 to 1,000 mg, one or two times daily, is a typical dose.

- L-carnitine (not to be confused with L-carnosine) is a quaternary ammonium compound and an amino acid derivative, not an actual amino acid, and is necessary for transporting fatty acids into the mitochondria, where they can be burned for energy. It can reduce the time it takes to convert from sugar burning to fat burning in resistant individuals. From 2,000 to 5,000 mg per day may be helpful.

- Acetyl-L-carnitine is fat soluble and is better able to protect and aid in fueling the brain than regular L-carnitine. It is ultimately antiglycating and, especially in tandem with R-lipoic acid, has been shown in studies to markedly reverse neuropathy. From 500 to 2,000 mg per day may yield beneficial results.

- Chromium is a trace mineral essential to the normalization of glucose metabolism and is commonly deficient. From 200 to 400 mcg per day of chromium picolinate or GTF chromium is usually sufficient.

- R-lipoic acid, which functions as an antioxidant, is uniquely effective against both fat-soluble and water-soluble free radi-cals, can prevent and even help reverse glycation, can improve blood sugar metabolism, and can improve cellular energy pro-duction. From 50 to 250 mg per day or more may be needed by some people.

- Benfotiamine is a powerful, fat-soluble version of vitamin B_1 that is known to significantly inhibit the formation of AGEs and help prevent damage to nerves and small blood vessels caused by glucose. Its fat solubility also gives it better overall bioavailability and aids its passage to the interior of the cell so that it can prevent glycation within the cell, where our vulnerable DNA lies. Doses of from 100 to 250 mg per day have been used in studies, often with dramati-cally positive effects.

- Pyridoxamine is a unique form of vitamin B_6 that specifically interferes with toxic glycation reactions. It is among the most potent natural substances for inhibiting AGE formation. Doses of from 50 to 100 mg have commonly been used in studies that reported beneficial effects. It is so effective, in fact, that the FDA has blatantly sought to reclassify this natural nutrient as a *drug*. I'll spare you my colorful comments on this.

- *Trans*-resveratrol is found in grape skins and red wine. This compound has shown itself to potentially have many dramatic and exciting benefits to health, among them significantly improving insulin sensitivity. The downside is its exorbitant cost. Recommendations include taking no less than 100 mg per day to supposedly relatively mimic the benefits seen in laboratory animals. Be especially careful of sources. The cis form of resveratrol is completely ineffective but is widely sold in commercial resveratrol supplements simply labeled "resveratrol." Read the label carefully. Only the *trans* form of resveratrol is known to be of benefit.

- CoQ10 (in the form of ubiquinol) helps support healthy mitochondrial function, serves as a powerful fat-soluble antioxidant, and can greatly improve oxygen and energy use. It is found in every major organ, especially the heart, and is dramatically and dangerously depleted by the use of statin drugs. Common dosage ranges from 50–300 mg (note: err on the higher dose if you hae a history of statin drug use).

- Omega-3 fish oil or Antarctic krill oil has something to offer to almost everyone. Getting adequate amounts is *critically important*. This vital nutrient often calms or eliminates carbohydrate cravings and can greatly enhance insulin sensitivity, as well as help curb inflammation and enhance mood and cognitive function.

- L-glutamine, an amino acid, can stop cravings for sweets, starches, and alcohol instantly as the brain is able to use L-glutamine temporarily for fuel. It is also the number one food for enterocytes, the cells lining the small intestine, and can greatly help regenerate the gastrointestinal mucosa. It usually comes in 500 mg capsules and needs to be taken on an empty stomach for best effect. Start with the lowest dose and increase as necessary. It can also be absorbed sublingually (sprinkled under the tongue) for a more immediate effect. Up to 5 g (5,000 mg) or even more may be necessary. Loose powders are widely available and quite palatable if larger doses are needed. (*Caution:* Refrain from using L-glutamine if you knowingly have cancer, as L-glutamine can serve to fuel certain types of tumor growth.)

- Candida overgrowth can create severe carbohydrate cravings in some people. Addressing this issue can be key for them. Numerous supplemental and detox approaches exist for candida problems.
- For people who crave carbohydrates under stress, gamma-aminobutyric acid (GABA, an amino acid) or GABA-enhancing compounds such as L-theanine can be helpful.
- For people who are addicted to carbohydrate comfort foods due to a lack of adequate endorphin production, the amino acid D-phenylalanine can be helpful in enhancing endorphin levels and subsequently reducing cravings.
- For some people, what appears to be a simple case of "carb cravings" may, in fact, be related to an addiction to the exorphins (morphine-like compounds) in grains and to hidden gluten sensitivity. Getting tested for gluten sensitivity through either Cyrex Labs (www.cyrex-labs.com) or EnteroLab (www.enterolab.com) can be the first step to getting to the bottom of a much deeper problem.
- The herb *Gymnema sylvestre,* taken in 4 g (4,000 mg) increments three times a day, can usually eliminate most, if not all, cravings for sweets. In extremely addicted individuals, twice this dose may be needed to successfully eliminate cravings. This is a great tool that can be likened to using bicycle training wheels while dietary modifications are being made. After a time, the herb will no longer be needed, once healthier eating habits are adopted. It also possesses compounds that can support the restoration of insulin sensitivity.
- Eliminate the use of caffeine and other stimulants. Stimulants aggravate blood sugar problems and deplete two important neurotransmitters, serotonin and norepinephrine, adversely affecting mood and energy.
- Sometimes a person craving carbohydrates is merely starved for adequate protein and, more specifically, L-tryptophan, the least abundant amino acid in our food supply. Supplementing with appropriate doses of L-tryptophan can calm these cravings and help restore healthy neurotransmitter (serotonin) function. Start with one 500 mg capsule on an empty stomach and increase the dose by one capsule each half hour until a feeling of increased well-being is achieved. **Do not use L-tryptophan if you are currently**

taking antidepressants such as selective serotonin reuptake inhibitors (SSRIs) or monoamine oxidase inhibitors (MAOIs), except under the guidance of a knowledgeable health care practitioner.

- Try adding some pancreatic lipase on an empty stomach. Deficiencies of lipase are common in people who have trouble managing blood sugar, and supplementation can improve your ability to digest and use fats instead of sugar for fuel! (Pancreatic lipase is found typically as part of a pancreatic enzyme–complex supplement.)
- Seek to reduce or eliminate the unnecessary use of over-the-counter and prescription medications.
- Stop smoking. Duh!
- Eliminate the use of alcohol.
- Avoid alternative, "natural" sweeteners such as honey, rice syrup, lo-han syrup, fructose, agave nectar, and maple syrup.
- Stevia is a carbohydrate-free sweetener derived from a South American herb. It is anywhere from two hundred to three hundred times sweeter than sugar and is therefore used only in very small amounts. Extracts containing steviosides (active herbal compounds) have been shown to benefit blood sugar stability. It is the only sugar substitute I am comfortable recommending for all but the most sugar-reactive individuals. Stevia is widely sold in health food stores and many supermarkets. It works very well in beverages and can be used in cooking. It can be purchased in refined form in packets, in liquid extracts, and as a powdered herb. The brand of stevia I've found that is the least refined (short of growing it yourself in an herb garden, which many people do) is Stevita, which can be purchased at www.stevitastevia.com. *Caution:* Sweet tastes can foster sweet cravings.
- Eliminate the use of aspartame (Nutrasweet), sucralose (Splenda), acesulfame-K (Sweet-One), saccharin (Sweet-n-Low), and all other artificial sweeteners. *Period.* Avoid them like the plague. Studies show these substances are more likely to make you fat than thin and can increase your risk for cancer and numerous other health problems.
- Eliminate all MSG. It is an excitotoxin that has been shown to directly cause leptin resistance and induce obesity in addition to being markedly toxic and readily damaging to the brain.

- Identify and eliminate foods to which you may be allergic or sensitive. This can be an extremely problematic source of cortisol-induced, unwanted insulin production and weight gain. Elimination/ provocation diets are the gold standard and the most affordable method of diagnosis. Grains (gluten) and dairy (casein) are the most common offenders, followed by soy, peanuts, and corn. Chicken eggs are also commonly problematic for many people. Cyrex Labs (www.cyrexlabs.com) has extremely accurate testing. A stool antigen test by Enterolab (www.enterolab.com) can be reliably diagnostic of several common food sensitivities as well.
- Get a good night's sleep. Don't be a night owl. Studies repeatedly show sleep deprivation as strongly correlated with decreased insulin sensitivity and unwanted weight gain, along with other problems. Try to get at least six to eight quality hours of sleep every single night, as we were designed to do!
- Exercise daily, or at least three to five times per week. Short bouts of high-intensity interval training or exertion-and-resistance training are most effective. Exercise has been shown to decidedly help improve insulin sensitivity. Exercise such as this immediately following a meal containing carbohydrates also can help burn off some of the sugar.
- Give special attention to stress management. Increased levels of stress hormones (e.g., cortisol) may significantly elevate blood sugar levels and insulin production, as well as suppress the immune system. *Actively cultivate stress-reduction habits*—or else!

Note: Cravings for sugar, alcohol, or carbohydrates, as well as cravings for stimulants such as caffeine, may be an indication of serotonin depletion. Chronic use of these substances actually depletes serotonin over time and can lead to low levels of this important neurotransmitter. This lack of serotonin can either generate or exacerbate cognitive deficits, as well as depressive, labile, or anxious states—particularly in susceptible individuals (Schwarzbein and Deville 1999).

Eleven More Reasons to Cut the Carbs
(If You Aren't Already Convinced)

The following list of reasons to cut your carbs is adapted from *The Carnitine Miracle,* by Robert Crayhon, M.A. (Crayhon 1998).

1. High-carbohydrate diets lower HDL cholesterol and, more important, raise triglycerides—an independent risk for heart attack.
2. You are much more likely to have a heart attack following a high-carbohydrate meal than a high-fat meal.
3. Carbohydrates raise your level of insulin, which makes you fat and increases your risk for metabolic disorder, diabetes, and worse.
4. A high intake of carbohydrates and sweetened beverages is associated with an increased risk of breast cancer (Witte et al. 1997).
5. Carbohydrates eaten in excess raise levels of plasminogen activator inhibitor-1, which increases the risk of heart attacks and strokes.
6. Eating too many carbohydrates makes LDL particles smaller and denser, generating lipoprotein(a), which in turn raises the risk of heart and artery disease. No statin drug can modify or reduce your production of lipoprotein(a); only diet can through reduction of insulin-provoking carbohydrates.
7. Eating a lot of starches and sugars raises the levels of triglycerides and blood fats following a meal, creating a condition called *postprandial lipemia,* which is another risk factor for heart disease.
8. Eating a lot of starches and sugars can increase the likelihood of yeast overgrowth, toxic bowel, and an impaired ability of the liver to remove toxic materials from the body, all of which increase the risk of disease.
9. Pregnant women who eat diets high in carbohydrates form a smaller placenta (Godfrey et al. 1996). This has ominous implications. The formation of the placenta dictates how well the mother will be able to transfer nutrients to the fetus.
10. A diet high in grains like wheat or legumes, which contain mostly starch, will contain phytates that reduce the absorption of valuable nutrients such as calcium, iron, and zinc. Such a diet will also increase your exposure to highly allergenic compounds such as gluten, which is found *primarily* in wheat, rye, and barley, potentially even leading to autoimmune diseases.

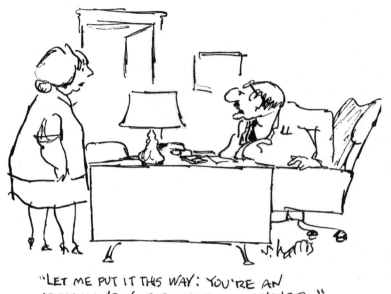

"LET ME PUT IT THIS WAY: YOU'RE AN ADDICT AND YOUR GROCER IS A PUSHER."

Fig. 16.1. The sugar addiction

11. Excessive intake of carbohydrates, especially sugar, will weaken immune function. Too many carbohydrates also increases the damage that stress can do to the body (Holman 1996).

Why You Shouldn't Use the Glycemic Index as Your Guide

The glycemic index was established as a means of gauging how rapidly the sugar in various foods enters the bloodstream as compared with pure glucose (or white bread). Pure glucose (or white bread) is assigned an arbitrary value of 100, against which all other foods are measured. Other foods are assigned a number that reflects a percentage of that glucose rating. The higher the percentage, the bigger the surge in blood sugar the food causes, the more it raises insulin levels, and the more potentially problematic it may be.

Seems like a useful thing, right?

Well, the problems with this method of measuring the effect of sugar in food are many. For example, there are two different ways in which a food can be "low glycemic." First, it can be like fiber, which simply doesn't have any sugar content or convert to sugar in the body. Second, it can be like fructose, which doesn't have much impact on insulin but is an extremely glycating—or, more properly in this instance, "fructosilating"—substance that can do immeasurable damage to your arteries and tissues. In fact, fructose is twenty to thirty times more glycating (i.e., damaging) than is glucose.

Interestingly, some foods actually have a higher glycemic index score than glucose. Puffed rice, corn flakes, Rice Krispies, and instant white rice all rank higher. (Run, don't walk away from these foods, and don't look back.)

The glycemic index is always based on 50 g of a particular carbohydrate. So, although a carrot may have a rather high glycemic index, this does not take into account the fiber, water, vitamins, and minerals in that carrot. It actually boils down to being a fairly modest amount of actual sugar per carrot; this varies further depending upon whether the carrot is cooked. Cooked carrots are significantly more glycemic than raw carrots—another thing the basic glycemic index may not take into account. If you wanted to get the effect from raw carrots that is reflected by the glycemic index, you'd need to eat twelve or thirteen carrots in a sitting. That's a lot of carrots, although the glycemic effect is something more easily jacked up if you happen to be juicing those carrots.

Another thing the index does not take into account is what other foods you are eating with a particular food; the other foods can greatly alter a specific food's glycemic effect. Finally, the glycemic index is based on a limited window of only three hours and does not take into account certain foods, such as, say, alcohol sugars, that have a delayed glycemic effect and impact blood sugar much later—something not understood until more recently.

The glycemic index doesn't really tell you how much usable carbohydrate exists in a particular food, which leads to it being a very misleading gauge. Using another method of gauging the carbohydrate content of a food, a food's *glycemic load,* is a bit more useful. The glycemic load still takes the glycemic index into account, but is based instead on a per-serving standard, which is far more realistic and practical. The glycemic load is calculated by taking the assigned glycemic index number, dividing it by 100, and then multiplying it by the actual grams of carbs in a particular serving size.

This is a slightly better approach, though it's far from perfect. It still won't take into account the impact of fructose, alcohol sugars, cooking methods, or other foods that can be combined with the food in question. For that, you are on your own and must simply use your own awareness and best judgment. Avoiding usable carbohydrate as much as possible should be the default rule. This isn't to say you shouldn't be eating carrots, but it's better not to overdo them. The lower the sugar and starch content of your veggies, the better!

17

High Fructose Corn Syrup

■■■■■■■■■■■■

A Sticky Wicket Best Avoided

Today, the number one source of dietary calories in America comes from a corn-based industrial sweetener known as high fructose corn syrup (sometimes abbreviated as HFCS). It is an ingredient used to sweeten almost everything, including sodas, cookies, soups, yogurt, salad dressing, bread, cereal, iced tea, "health bars," ketchup, bacon, peanut butter, mustard, even beer. It is prevalent in nearly *all* processed foods. Ninety cents out of every dollar in America spent on food is spent on processed food. The food industry uses high fructose corn syrup more than any other sweetener because it's **cheap** to produce, transport, and store. As always, follow the money.

It is among the most dangerous and damaging food additives ever created.

High fructose corn syrup has been shown to interfere with a key enzyme in the body that delivers copper to your vital organs. This effectively results in a copper deficiency for many people, adversely impacting a wide range of organ systems, including the heart, testes, and pancreas, and damaging the liver, generating inflammation and cirrhosis. It has been strongly linked to the sharp rise in both obesity and diabetes. Furthermore, fructose is twenty to thirty times more glycating than glucose. It turns anyone into a raging AGE-producing factory. Animals fed a high-fructose diet in laboratory studies developed livers that looked a lot like those of hardcore, aging alcoholics—inflamed and shot through with dead cells and scar tissue, the condition known as cirrhosis.

High fructose corn syrup has been linked to:

- diabetes
- heart disease
- cancer
- obesity
- gout
- weakened immune system
- cirrhosis of the liver
- osteoporosis
- elevated cholesterol levels
- anemia
- mineral deficiency

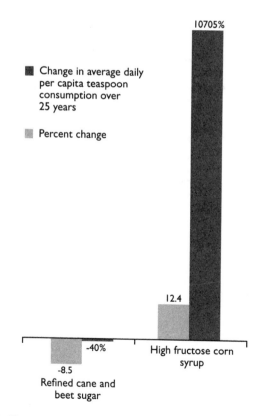

Fig. 17.1. Change in use of high fructose corn syrup, 1970–2005.
Source: USDA/Economic Research Service, 2006.

The Corn Refiners Association insists, "Research confirms that high fructose corn syrup is safe and no different from other common sweeteners like table sugar and honey. All three sweeteners are nutritionally the same." This, of course, is all part of the Corn Refiners Association's twenty- to thirty-million-dollar advertising and public relations campaign to counter the overwhelming scientific evidence to the contrary. Research findings since 2004 have been extremely damaging to the high fructose corn syrup market, and justifiably so.

High fructose corn syrup is metabolized into fat faster than almost any other sugar, and that speed is augmented when the syrup is in liquid form, as found in soft drinks. Chemical tests among eleven different carbonated soft drinks containing high fructose corn syrup found them to have "astonishingly high" levels of *reactive carbonyls*. Reactive carbonyls are undesirable and highly reactive compounds associated with unbound fructose and glucose molecules and are believed to cause tissue damage (via AGEs) that is known to cause diabetes, according to evidence found by a research study and reported at the 2007 national meeting of the American Chemical Society. Based on the study data, the researchers estimate that a single can of soda contains about **five times** the concentration of reactive carbonyls found in the blood of an adult person with diabetes!

Additionally, all high fructose corn syrup is manufactured from genetically modified corn, which has been linked to a much higher incidence of corn-related allergies, among other, more insidious problems potentially associated with any GMO food.

Finally, it has also recently been revealed that high fructose corn syrup contains significant traces of mercury, an extremely powerful and damaging neurotoxin (and, yes, the FDA knew and did nothing).

Read all labels. Avoid high fructose corn syrup like the plague that it is, and beware of cheap, processed foods. The price you pay may be much higher than you think!

What about Artificial Sweeteners?

Be wary of all the chemicals in your life.

Andrew Weil, M.D.

Chemical substitutes for sugar such as aspartame (Nutrasweet), sucralose (Splenda), acesulfame-K (Sunnette), neotame (made from aspartame and containing a toxic substance that can be found on the EPA's most hazardous chemical list) and saccharine (Sweet-n-Low) have all been implicated in innumerable serious problems and symptoms and should not be used by anyone who cares about his or her health. More consumer complaints have been filed against Nutrasweet alone than any other substance governed by the FDA, and a study conducted from the Duke University Medical Center and published in September 2008 in the *Journal of Toxicology and Environmental Health* indicates that Splenda reduces the amount of good bacteria in the intestines by 50 percent, increases the pH value in the intestines, contributes to increases in body weight, and affects the P-glycoprotein in the body in such a way that crucial cancer- and HIV-related drugs can be rejected and critical nutrients in general may not be absorbed (Abou-Donia et al. 2008). This is only one recent study among many illustrating considerable reason for concern and avoidance of these sugar substitutes. Also, both aspartame (Nutrasweet) and neotame can increase insulin and leptin levels in people who consume them and thus contribute to obesity.

Here's a fun aside (you'll want to be sitting down for this): The researchers who created aspartame and saccharine discovered their usability as sweeteners when, while doing research that had nothing to do with food or sweeteners, they *decided to taste* these chemicals and liked the sweet taste. No lie. (What were these boneheaded idiots thinking by tasting a laboratory experiment?) The researchers who developed sucralose, also known as Splenda, **originally started out in an attempt to create an insecticide.** (Yes, you read that right.) An assistant (obviously a genius) who was asked to test the compound mistakenly thought he was being asked to *taste* it (Coffey 2009). The rest, as they say, is food-industry history. *You* do the math with respect to how beneficial these substances are likely to be for your health.

All artificial sweeteners have been implicated in cancer (among many other unpleasant things), and none is a naturally occurring substance in nature. They should all be avoided by everyone. The only sugar substitute that seems to be entirely safe is the South American herb stevia. Stevia is as much as three hundred times sweeter than sugar, has no carbohydrate or caloric value, has been safely used by primitive South American cultures for centuries, and may even have some beneficial glucose-regulating and insulin sensitivity–restoring effects. Stick to pure stevia, though, and avoid some of the newer commercial sweeteners (such as Truvia) that combine stevia with other chemicals and additives. The Stevita brand, in both liquid and granules, is the most unrefined brand I've found, and it is composed entirely of the juice of stevia leaves preserved with a little grapefruit seed extract. It also seems to have a better taste than many more refined brands of stevia.

> Remember: If it comes out of a test tube,
> it's not food.

The Agave Myth

Last, beware of what amounts to the new "yuppie" form of high-fructose syrup being sold as a natural, even exotic-sounding product called agave nectar. Agave is actually much richer in damaging fructose and, as such, potentially much worse for you than industrial high fructose corn syrup (with the exception of the fact that the industrial high fructose corn syrup is made using synthetic chemicals and GMOs). High fructose corn syrup contains about 55 percent fructose content. Agave nectar, by contrast, contains anywhere from **70 percent to 97 percent pure fructose!** Yes, agave has a supposedly low glycemic index. Big deal. So do antifreeze and Nutrasweet. The marketing for this highly processed substance has been brilliant, however, and many so-called organic food products now add cheap agave as a supposedly healthy sweetener. Don't fall for it . . . please.

18

What about Fiber as an Essential Carbohydrate?

On January 20, 1999, *ABC World News Tonight* with Peter Jennings reported that a newly released, massive study revealed that fiber was shown to be "worthless" in helping to prevent colon cancer. The study had just been released in *The New England Journal of Medicine.* The report found that fiber, once thought to be a panacea for preventing colon cancer and the be-all and end-all for colon health, provides *no protection at all* from the disease. Yes, you heard right. The massive nurses' study, involving eighty-eight thousand people and spanning sixteen years, found conclusively that consuming a high-fiber diet makes no difference whatsoever in the prevention of colon cancer.

The *New York Times* had the similar headline "Fiber Does Not Help Prevent Colon Cancer, Study Finds" (Stolberg 1999). The once widely accepted hypothesis by British missionary surgeon Dr. Denis P. Burkitt, who had studied certain groups in Africa seemingly resistant to colon cancer and speculatively concluded that high-fiber intake was the protective factor, was decisively shot down once and for all. The *New York Times* article said, "He spread his thesis as dietary gospel, prompting millions to change their diets. Now, the largest study ever to examine Dr. Burkitt's theory has found that, at least when it comes to preventing colon cancer, all those fruits, vegetables and cereals do not do any good." The senior author of this study, Walter Willett, M.D.,

Ph.D., professor of epidemiology and nutrition at the Harvard School of Public Health, stated, "The hypothesis that fiber intake is important in reducing colon cancer risk was interesting, but the reality is that the data have not provided much support for that." He went on to say, "Our study was the longest follow-up study done, and we could use multiple measurements of diet. We looked at adenomas as well as colon cancer and there was no hint at all that fiber was reducing the risk."

You'd think that all of this would have resulted in modified nutritional recommendations by dieticians and doctors, but it seems they all missed the news that evening and failed to read the morning paper. The myth that fiber prevents colon cancer seems to doggedly persist, nonetheless, even though high-fiber grains, for instance, have been repeatedly linked to many forms of gastrointestinal disease, including colorectal cancer.

Cultures such as the Inuit, as well as ice age humans, consumed little or no dietary fiber. This isn't to say that certain antioxidants and nutrients found in fibrous vegetables and fruits aren't of value to us or that fiber has no useful role at all to play. Clearly, great varieties of fibrous vegetables and fruits have been typically abundant in healthy, neo-Paleolithic, primitive hunter-gatherer societies, and their antioxidants and phytonutrients are probably more important to us now than ever. Fiber does not appear to be a critical part of the equation, however, and vegetables and especially fruits are not the be-all and end-all.

It is clear from other anthropological evidence and other studies that fiber from vegetables and fruits may not be as central to our health and longevity as nutritional pundits, particularly vegetarians and vegans, would have us believe. In fact, excess dietary fiber can serve to overly bind minerals in the diet, irritate the colon (particularly fiber from grains), and generate significant mineral deficiencies.

On the plus side, *soluble* fiber (found in nuts, seeds, fibrous vegetables, and fruit) can serve to feed healthy bacteria in the gut (assuming, of course, that one has healthy bacteria in the gut to feed), and the bacteria can then convert that fiber to useful nutritional substances such as butyric acid, which is the primary fuel for colon cells and the number one substance for preventing colon cancer, along with vitamins A and D. Incidentally, butyric acid is also richly found in grass-fed butter, which is partly where butyric acid gets its name. Grass-fed butter (or its casein-free alternative, ghee), which is also a superb source of true vitamin A, may in fact be a greater preventive food for colon cancer than dietary fiber ever could be. Who knew?

The sun and vitamin D3, however, may be the best colon cancer preventive of all. Dr. Gordon Ainsleigh, a sunlight advocate, encourages sunbathing to foster healthy vitamin D levels to fight cancer. In 1992, Ainsleigh reviewed fifty years' worth of medical literature on cancer and the sun. He reported in the journal *Preventive Medicine* that widespread, regular, moderate sunbathing would lower the incidence of breast and colon cancer death rates by a whopping one-third.

Fiber can be useful in helping bind spent, conjugated hormones in the gut and eliminating them before they can be reabsorbed. In a world that's full of dangerously excessive amounts of estrogen and the estrogen-like compounds termed *xenoestrogens,* fiber has probably never been more useful in this regard than it is now.

When it comes right down to it, though, probably the best thing about fiber is that it doesn't convert to sugar.

So go ahead and eat your veggies—and plenty of them—with melted butter, ghee, or olive oil to help better absorb the minerals and fat-soluble nutrients in them. Lightly sautéing or steaming can also help break down cellulose, improving digestibility. Eat some raw, too. Limit fruits because of their sugar content (some antioxidant-rich berries are okay). Fibrous vegetables are nicely filling, and we need the extra antioxidants and phytonutrients they can provide us, especially in today's toxic world. Just remember, fibrous vegetables may just be a side dish, but they are an important one in modern times—probably more now than ever. Toss the bran flakes in your nearest compost heap.

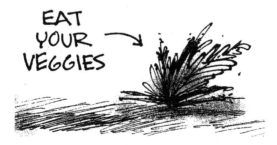

Fig. 18.1. Eat your vegetables.
Cartoon by Cox & Forkum

What about Juicing:
Isn't That Really Good for You?

The whole idea around juicing seems healthy enough: get more servings per day of fruits and vegetables into yourself by juicing them and getting rid of the less appealing pulp. It's all the rage in health food stores and health clubs, and it's a fad that borders on prescriptive dogma among devout health nuts and vegans. Nice plan, on the surface of things, but what are you actually doing? *Think!*

For starters, our ancestors would never have done such a thing. They always ate the whole vegetable or piece of fruit, discarding mainly any woody stems or seeds. The idea of extracting and discarding the pulp and drinking the liquid from vegetables or fruits is quite unnatural and makes a very flawed assumption: that the bulk of the nutritional content of these foods exists in the juice.

Unfortunately, that's just wrong.

Consider, for instance, that the skin of any fruit or vegetable is what actually protects the vital interior components from the ravages of the environment, including radiation. As such, *the greater concentration of antioxidants in any fruit or vegetable is almost always in the skin.* The pulp also contains numerous bioflavinoids, pigments, and phytonutrients, which also typically get discarded in juicing. So, what are you left with in the liquid? *Mostly sugar water* mixed with a few vitamins, minerals, and diluted amounts of other nutrients. Tasty, but the negative impact of the sugar will outweigh whatever benefits are received from the other nutrients in the juice almost every time.

It's not that some of what lies in the juice isn't good for you; it's just that the sugar is always worse. Juicing low-glycemic, fibrous vegetables and greens, on the other hand, is perfectly okay—even potentially quite beneficial—because their sugar content is minimal. Steer away from sweetening the mix with too much carrot juice, though. It's better just to eat those carrots whole and raw. Add something like stevia, if you have to.

If you want to juice your fruits, that's great. Just throw out the sugar water and eat the pulp instead!

19
Adrenal Exhaustion

▪ ▪ ▪ ▪ ▪ ▪ ▪ ▪ ▪ ▪ ▪ ▪

A Uniquely Modern Epidemic

Among the most common modern-day afflictions, both diagnosed by holistic practitioners and undiagnosed, is what is known as *adrenal exhaustion*. This is brought about by chronic or severe stress; chronic exposure to foods that trigger sensitivity reactions; exposure to electromagnetic frequency (EMF) pollution from cell phones, cordless phones, Wi-Fi routers, and other electronic sources; and especially excess dietary carbohydrate and blood sugar dysregulation. Adrenal stress, dysregulation, and exhaustion can leave you feeling completely worn out and depleted and can greatly interfere with normal sleep patterns. The symptoms of low adrenal function are varied, depending upon severity and individual factors. They commonly include:

- trouble staying asleep
- being a "slow starter" in the morning
- afternoon fatigue
- feeling run down or overwhelmed
- cravings for salt and sweets
- experiencing dizziness when standing up too quickly
- afternoon headaches or headaches with stress or exertion

Adrenal dysregulation can also include adrenal "hyperfunction" (not to be confused with Cushing's disease), which can eventually also lead to some stage of adrenal exhaustion. Among common symptoms of adrenal hyperfunction are:

- feeling constantly stressed out
- trouble falling asleep
- irritability and anxiety
- high blood sugar levels
- tending toward weight gain under stress
- excess perspiration or perspiring, even while inactive (in normal temperatures)
- waking up tired, seemingly no matter what

Adrenaline is the hormone secreted by the adrenal medulla, and it is associated with acute states of the fight-or-flight mode. Once released, it mobilizes blood sugar to fuel the emergency, dilates pupils, shuts down digestion and other nonessential or nonsurvival-oriented bodily functions, constricts blood vessels and raises the blood pressure, and increases the heart rate. Cortisol, secreted by the adrenal cortex, is produced in response to more-chronic states of stress and as a blood sugar–management hormone. Individuals with chronic stress or dysglycemia may exhaust the adrenal cortex's ability to produce adequate amounts of cortisol (see Adrenal Stress Index example 1, figure 19.1), which results in what can be termed adrenal exhaustion.

Because leptin rules the endocrine roost, as it were, and insulin stands firmly second in command, the adrenal hormones, adrenaline and cortisol, are next in the line of authority over your moods, energy, and well-being. The health of your thyroid depends upon the health of your adrenals. In fact, no thyroid issue can ever fully resolve or significantly improve without the restoration of adrenal health.

Women must depend on healthy adrenals to ease the transition of menopause. Exhausted adrenals are unable to take the "baton" from the ovaries, as they are supposed to at this time, to continue producing needed hormones. If your adrenals are shot, that transition called menopause can be pure hell. Women with healthy adrenals at menopause barely even notice anything has happened, which is how it is supposed to be. Hot flashes and other menopausal symptoms are not remotely normal simply because they are commonplace.

Your adrenals are often the first obvious casualty of blood sugar dysregulation. Stymied adrenal function can lead to chronic feelings of stress or being overwhelmed, fatigue, weight gain, insomnia, mood disorders or instability, headaches or migraines, and eventually thyroid problems. (Down the road, problems with sex hormones can develop, too, via an endocrine metabolic phenomenon known as the *pregnenolone steal*). *You will never correct a problem with your thyroid or sex hormones without first correcting adrenal imbalance.* And in order to correct that, of course, you must determine and address your main adrenal stressors and address issues around insulin and leptin.

Common adrenal stressors can include blood sugar dysregulation (the big one), chronic use of stimulants, chronic high levels of EMF exposure, chronic infections, food-sensitivity issues, prolonged life stress or chronic trauma, chronic lack of adequate sleep, and excessive exercise.

Apart from excess dietary carbohydrates and lifestyle issues, the next most common cause of adrenal problems is easily food sensitivities. (See chapter 28, "What about Food Allergies and Sensitivities?") Consuming food substances to which you are sensitive will automatically generate a stress response in the body that involves both cortisol and insulin. Even if your diet is low carb or low cal, it is possible to gain undesirable weight and generate systemic inflammation if you are chronically eating foods to which you are sensitive.

There are several vicious cycles that can be commonly generated from adrenal dysregulation and these are difficult to correct. The hypothalamic-pituitary-adrenal axis can become dysregulated, leading to many other hormonal problems. The hippocampus of the brain (found at the temporal lobes, just above the ears), which is needed for emotional and neurological stability, short-term memory, and memory consolidation, among other things, can begin degenerating as the result of excess cortisol saturation and excess excitatory activity, which can be from chronic stress, EMF pollution (a topic covered in part 3), not getting enough sleep, excess dietary carbohydrates, and food sensitivities. Also, the gastrointestinal tract can develop impaired regenerative capacity and mucosal erosion as the result of either insufficient or excess cortisol levels, which can lead to leaky gut syndrome, allergies, immune system vulnerabilities, and food sensitivities, among other things. The popular use of progesterone creams can also easily create or exacerbate cortisol excesses.

Excess leptin and insulin surges generated by chronic carbohydrate consumption can get this problematic adrenal ball rolling in no small way and create a self-perpetuating nightmare.

Suffice it to say, it ain't pretty. These vicious cycles can unravel anyone.

Cortisol levels shift throughout the day naturally and follow a predictable daily rhythmic pattern that can become dysregulated by stress. These pattern disruptions (see Adrenal Stress Index example 2, figure 19.2) can be readily managed by the use of *adaptogens,* which are stress-mitigating herbs that can help reset these erratic patterns on a brain-communication level and help restore healthy cortisol rhythms. The Adrenal Stress Index, or ASI, as it is commonly referred to by natural health care practitioners, is a salivary hormone panel from Diagnos-Techs Inc. that is offered by many certified nutritional therapists, nutritional therapy practitioners, naturopaths, and other holistic practitioners, and it can be used to accurately evaluate adrenal function and cortisol rhythms. (*Note:* Efforts to support adrenal recovery may be entirely futile with individuals who are anemic. The presence of anemia must first be ruled out or properly addressed when seeking to support adrenal issues.)

Examples of Adrenal Stress Index Results

The chart in figure 19.1 shows the results of an Adrenal Stress Index test. The dark black line connected by squares shows the person's actual pattern (in this case, depressed cortisol levels and stage 7 adrenal exhaustion), while the dotted lines reflect the upper and lower limits of the normal, healthy cortisol range at various points during the day, from early morning through nighttime. This person experiences chronic fatigue and regularly craves caffeine.

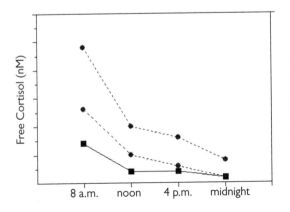

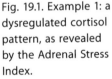

Fig. 19.1. Example 1: a dysregulated cortisol pattern, as revealed by the Adrenal Stress Index.

The pattern in example 2 (figure 19.2) reflects a markedly dysregulated cortisol rhythm throughout the day and night that may respond well to supplementation with adaptogens. This person experiences extreme fatigue in the morning (craving caffeine) and problems with restless sleep and winding down at night.

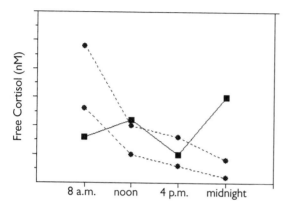

Fig. 19.2. Example 2: a dysregulated cortisol pattern, as revealed by the Adrenal Stress Index.

Once a person's level of adrenal imbalance has been properly evaluated, steps can be taken to appropriately support the specific adrenal issues and help bring the person back into balance. Beware of recommendations that include hormone replacement, however. Hormones such as dehydroepiandrosterone (DHEA) and pregnenolone should be considered only in cases of what is known as stage 7 adrenal exhaustion, taken in only very minute amounts as a liquid sublingual preparation, and taken for only very short periods of time.

Otherwise, please resist direct hormonal supplementation, even with bioidentical hormones, unless there is absolutely no other choice. This should only be considered a last resort. Remember: *Hormones are not supplements.*

Addressing the body functionally, as a whole, taking into account the extreme complexity of its biochemical and hormonal interrelationships, is the most effective way to actually correct the underlying problems and achieve long-term restoration of health. Dealing with each component of health, endocrine function or body function, as a separate compartmentalized entity only leads to more imbalances in the long run—and potentially big bank accounts for the practitioners who subscribe to this archaic and outmoded approach. Functional, restorative medicine and nutritional therapy that takes into account the intricate complexity of human systems and evaluates from a *foundational* standpoint is the clear and necessary future of positive health management.

When addressing adrenal issues, always first consider the endocrine chain of command and be aware that in order to correct imbalances, you must always look first "upstream" and consider what may have caused the initial imbalance in the first place. Modern conventional medicine practitioners, often even holistic medicine practitioners, are quick to micromanage hormonal issues that they are willing to recognize by prescribing hormone replacement. (Note that medical doctors tend not to recognize adrenal imbalances that are not an actual, full-blown, rare condition such as Addison's disease or Cushing's disease.) Even bioidentical hormone replacement can be extremely problematic when used in this way. This is not to say that bioidentical hormone replacement is never necessary, but it also shouldn't necessarily always be the first step in resolving imbalances. Interrelationships with other hormones must also be carefully considered.

Look to the source. Go to the foundations first—always.

20

A Word about Water

■ ■ ■ ■ ■ ■ ■ ■ ■ ■ ■

Chronic cellular dehydration painfully and prematurely kills. Its initial outward manifestations have until now been labeled as diseases of unknown origin.

F. BATMANGHELIDJ, M.D.,
YOUR BODY'S MANY CRIES FOR WATER

Next to oxygen, water is the most important substance we put into our bodies. Most of us fail to get enough of it. It is used in every metabolic process in the human body and is utterly essential to the function of the human brain and nervous system. The human body mass is composed of roughly 55 to 60 percent water at minimum and the human brain of 70 to 80 percent water. The human body can produce about 8 percent of its water needs from its own metabolic processes. That leaves 92 percent that must be obtained through diet. Caffeinated beverages and alcohol cause dehydration, as do stress and physical activity. Replenishing the body with substantial amounts of pure, clean water is critical. No nutrient in the body can function without water. And the body's bioelectrical system is nonexistent without it.

Gerald H. Pollack, Ph.D., University of Washington professor of bioengineering and author of the book *Cells, Gels and the Engines of Life* (Pollack 2001), has studied the intricate and central role of water in cell biology and is currently developing advanced theories associated with this that are being recognized as nothing short of revolutionary, not the least among these being that water may actually be more like *liquid crystal* than a simple fluid. Crystals soon to be engineered for computers are said to radically enhance information-storage capacity and computation and communication speed. The metaphorical extension to the human brain (our own internal computer—the most powerful on Earth) here is apparent. In his thirty-second Annual Faculty Lecture, "Water, Energy, and Life: Fresh Views from the Water's Edge" (accessible through YouTube), Pollack talks about the idea that water forms a structural, negatively charged crystalline interface between and within your cells that functions in part like a battery. The extra fascinating element of his research shows that what actually charges this battery is either UV sunlight or infrared photonic energy (light). Sunlight essentially builds order within water and enhances its surface interface negative charge, magnifying its effects. Exposure of our cells to penetrating UV or infrared light results in improved water structuring and energy production at the cellular level. We all need to spend more time outdoors in fresh air and sunshine.

Pollack also suggests, based on the available research, that consuming water that has been *structured* may also be of considerable health benefit. Numerous products and devices already exist on the market to make structured water available to the consumer, some of which can be quite expensive. In an interview with Dr. Joseph Mercola, Pollack also suggested that cooling water to 39°F (10°C) or exposing it to a created vortex, thereby adding surface area and bubbles to its makeup, may also result in inexpensively enhanced structured water (Pollack 2011). The described "light effect" may also help explain why exposure to UV and infrared light (including saunas and cold-laser therapies) seems to improve one's state of health and well-being and help generate healing.

Microstructured water, which reduces "clumping" of water molecules into smaller, five-molecule and six-molecule arrays, more easily penetrates cell membranes. The whole concept of water being referred to as H_2O is actually somewhat in error, as water does not appear in nature this way. In nature, the *minimum*-sized array found (typically in places like remote mountain springs, some deep artesian wells, and unique places such as Lourdes) is "$5\text{-}H_2O$" or "$6\text{-}H_2O$." Most tap water has much larger clumping arrays of "$20\text{-}H_2O$" or "$30\text{+-}H_2O$" (owing to the presence of contaminants, which make water "stickier" and cause molecules to glob together). This leads to water that is less easily absorbed and more likely to unpleasantly slosh around in your stomach and hydrate your cells less efficiently (though it's still better than other beverages). Contaminants and other substances combined with water ultimately make water less hydrating. This is why pure water from almost any source is always more hydrating than, say, juice or tea. Sweetened "sports drinks" may enhance the *retention* of water (through extracellular bloating), but they are inefficient at actually rehydrating the *inside* of your cells, where water is most needed. Save your money on these heavily marketed products and stick to pure, clean (or possibly ionically enhanced) water instead.

Without ample purified water, life is not possible—nor is health or optimal brain function. We are only in our infancy with respect to our scientific comprehension of what water actually is and what it does within and surrounding our cells. One thing we know for certain is that it is essential to critical cellular communication on all levels and is the single most important substance for life.

Often, what may seem like a complex physical or emotional issue is little more than chronic dehydration. Losing as little as 2 percent of your body's water content through diuresis or dehydration can result in noticeable fatigue. A drop of 10 percent can cause problems ranging from musculoskeletal issues (e.g., joint pain, back pain, cramps) to digestive problems (e.g., heartburn, constipation), immune problems or allergies, and even cardiovascular symptoms or anginal pain.

The importance of this foundational substance, which is essential to all life, should never, ever be underestimated.

Save your money by avoiding sodas, juices, and other unnatural, unnecessary, and sugary beverages. Water is always best. And it's affordable. Among dehydrating beverages are caffeine, alcohol, some herbal teas, all juices, and sodas. Be sure to add another 12 to 16 ounces of pure water to your daily intake for every 8 ounces of diuretic beverage consumed. For further excellent information, look for the book *Your Body's Many Cries for Water,* by F. Batmanghelidj, M.D. Also see the Water Cure website, at www.watercure.com.

Symptoms potentially associated with chronic dehydration include:

- depression
- stress
- dyspeptic pain
- colitis pain
- false appendicitis pain

- hiatal hernia
- rheumatoid arthritis pain
- low-back pain
- neck pain
- anginal pain
- anxiety
- headaches
- high blood pressure
- high blood cholesterol levels
- excess body weight
- excess hunger
- asthma and allergies
- chronic fatigue
- irritability
- constipation
- cognitive impairment

Feeling symptomatic? If in doubt, try drinking a tall glass of pure, clean water! But please make sure it's properly purified and filtered first.

An article in *National Geographic News* stated, "Around the world, scientists are finding trace amounts of substances—from sugar and spice to heroin, rocket fuel, and birth control pills—that might be having unintended consequences for humans and wildlife alike" (Dell'Amore 2010). Even the best-quality water-treatment facilities in the country don't actually test for more than about two hundred compounds (U.S. Environmental Protection Agency regulations require testing for only about one hundred), even when there are potentially over one hundred thousand toxic chemicals—not including pharmaceuticals, viruses, parasites, bacteria, and heavy metals—affecting our water supplies worldwide. The same article also stated, "In a 2008 study scientists discovered a by-product of cocaine in 22 of 24 samples of drinking water at a Spanish water-treatment plant—despite a rigorous filtering and treatment process."

The Washington Post in December 2010 reported, "An environmental group that analyzed the drinking water in 35 cities across the United States, including Bethesda and Washington, found that most contained hexavalent chromium, a probable carcinogen that was made famous by the film *Erin Brockovich*" (Layton 2010). This is a shocking, very real, and very dangerous problem.

I personally would never habitually drink regular, unfiltered tap water. A high-quality water-filtration system for your home drinking water (if not also your shower water) is a critical investment everyone should make. Reverse-osmosis systems are a potential option (though if you choose this option, I recommend remineralizing your water prior to drinking it, using Himalayan or Celtic sea salt or using ConcenTrace Trace Mineral Drops by Trace Minerals Research). Reverse-osmosis drinking water is quite acidic in pH, however, and completely lacks any inherent structure or electrolyte content (though the process does remove most impurities, except possibly bacteria).

A surprisingly affordable option for quality home and emergency filtration and purification is a countertop gravity-powered (nonelectrical) unit called a Berkey Water Filtration System (www.directive21.com). The value and quality are exceptional, as is its elegant simplicity. The Berkey filtration system effectively removes viruses, pathogenic bacteria, cysts, and parasites as well as undesirable chemicals and toxic heavy metals to nondetectable levels, leaving beneficial minerals intact—all by using a simple gravitational, microporous, long-term reusable, ceramically based filtration system. Each filtration element is able to purify (not just filter) up to three thousand gallons of water. The very-long-lasting ceramic filtration element also adds quite a bit of alkalinity to the water, which may have some potential detoxification benefits.

Finally, deep-artesian springwater is some of the purest and healthiest water available on the planet. You can locate one near you by going to www.findaspring.com. Just don't expect to get the real stuff from bottled water companies.

The Myth of "Healthier" Bottled Water— Caveat Emptor

Over the past several years, bottled water has been recalled due to contamination by arsenic, bromate, cleaning compounds, mold, and bacteria. Additionally, bottled water has been found to contain chlorine, fluoride, aluminum, arsenic, disinfection by-products, and pharmaceutical substances. This industry is very poorly regulated, and many brands—up to 40 percent of them—are virtually no more than regular municipal tap water with a fancy label and a steep price tag attached to it. In fact, municipal water supplies are much more tightly regulated than the bottled water industry. All concerns (and more) about tap water unfortunately apply to bottled water. The plastic bottles, themselves, leech toxic *Bisphenol A* (BPA), a potent and toxic estrogen-mimicking chemical, into their contents. Molecule for molecule, BPA is more potent biologically than estradiol. There are more than one hundred independent studies linking BPA to serious health and cognitive problems in humans. Endocrine-disrupting *pthalates* are also readily leeched into water from plastic containers. Save the environment and save yourselves: avoid bottled drinking water like the plague. Get a reusable glass bottle and bottle your own purified water at home instead. You'll save a fortune (and maybe even your health) along the way!

Finding That Happy Medium between Dehydration and Drowning

How much water should we drink daily? Well, it's certainly arguable that our ancestors did not walk around carrying water bottles or conscientiously drink "eight full glasses a day." That said, our ancestors also didn't face the levels of stress or environmental contamination that we now do or drink dehydrating sugary or caffeinated beverages. It makes sense to hypothesize that our need for this life-giving substance is likely greater today than ever before. Then again, overconsuming water can lead to something called *water intoxication* and overdilution of sodium in the body, also known as *hyponatremia,* leading to tissue swelling and cellular damage. Symptoms can include an irregular heartbeat, fluid backing up into the lungs, and even swelling in the brain and nerves, which ultimately mimic the effects of alcohol intoxication (without all the fun). It's a little like drowning from the inside out. Athletes tend to be the most susceptible to this problem, but anyone who is overzealous with water consumption can succumb to the ill effects of hydration excess. True water intoxication is fairly rare. Most people really do fail to drink enough water, but watch out for going too far the other way.

Also, keep in mind that it's less about how much you drink than how fast you drink it. The human body (and kidneys) can process only so much water at a time. Drinking water more slowly (in sips) improves absorption and utilization considerably. A good analogy is likening drinking water to watering a dry houseplant. If you just dump a huge cup of water over an arid potted plant, you only flood or drown the plant and create useless runoff. If, instead, you slowly trickle the water in, the plant can far better absorb the water you give it. Same thing with us.

The rule of thumb I follow is this: Take your body weight (in pounds) and divide by 2 to get the rough number of ounces of pure water to drink daily. I generally recommend keeping this under a gallon per day. If dehydrating beverages are consumed, follow the aforementioned guidelines. If you are exposed to prolonged heat or exercise, obviously your need for water will be greater, and more is fine. I avoid drinking distilled water, and I often prefer to add ionic trace minerals to much of the water I drink to further enhance its electric potential and nutrient value on a cellular level.

Bottoms up!

21

Understanding the
Role of Protein

■ ■ ■ ■ ■ ■ ■ ■ ■ ■ ■ ■

Protein is essential to life and, unlike carbohydrates, is essential to the diet. Although we are able to synthesize and recycle many proteins and amino acids—the body is made up of more than fifty thousand different proteins—there are eight amino acids, the building blocks of protein, that are known to be essential: leucine, isoleucine, valine, lysine, phenylalanine, L-tryptophan, threonine, and methionine. The term *essential* basically means these amino acids cannot be made in the body and must be derived from dietary sources and be fully present for normal protein synthesis to occur in the body. Without the presence of *complete* protein in the diet, normal and healthy protein synthesis in your body is brought to a screeching halt.

Quality complete protein is found exclusively in animal-source foods. Combining vegetarian protein sources, such as beans and brown rice, for instance, to create complete protein still makes for a dominantly starchy food, yielding far more starch than protein, despite the combined, more complete amino acid profile, and in no way does this imply protein sufficiency. To accomplish actual daily protein sufficiency with rice and beans, the trade-off would be excessive caloric intake to meet the protein demand from a more carbohydrate- or starch-based food source. The result would yield disastrous implications for blood sugar regulation, together with excess insulin and leptin surges.

Hot off the Press

In just the past couple of years, a brand-new and extremely important metabolic pathway was discovered. Researchers were studying a naturally occurring substance known as *rapamycin,* which is synthesized from soil bacteria, as it was able to demonstrate some fairly powerful cancer-inhibiting properties. Drug companies were extremely interested in finding out how it worked and accidentally stumbled across this new, previously unknown metabolic pathway, now referred to as *mTOR,* which stands for "mammalian target of rapamycin."

Much as insulin serves as a sort of default sugar sensor and leptin serves as the body's fat sensor, mTOR (it turns out) serves as the *body's protein sensor,* monitoring the availability of protein, or amino acids (particularly the branched-chain amino acids, most notably leucine, as well as methionine), for growth and reproduction. It is also influenced by insulin levels, impacting IgF-1 activity, and is part of a related metabolic pathway. When protein levels are detected that exceed our basic maintenance requirements, the excess levels up-regulate the activity of the mTOR pathway, stimulating cellular proliferation and adverse (from a longevity standpoint) mitochondrial effects. Increased insulin also has this effect, and the mTOR protein belongs to what is known as the *P13K pathway,* which is activated by insulin, nutrients, and growth factors. mTOR has a central role in the regulation of cell growth and protein synthesis. It essentially activates our reproductive and cell-proliferating capacity. It makes sense that dietary protein in excess of what is needed for maintenance and repair would send a message that it might be a good time to reproduce or make more cells. It is well known that animals in the wild whose diets are restricted by reduced food availability also typically have fewer young or may even fail to reproduce in a particular year, depending upon the available energy supply. Protein availability seems to be the key limiting factor. What is less stimulating of reproductive processes, however, is ultimately more stimulating of individual regeneration, repair, and enhanced mitochondrial function. This is where it gets interesting.

A recent study stated, "It has been shown that limiting dietary amino acids, specifically methionine, inhibits signaling through mammalian target of rapamycin (mTOR) thereby decreasing mitochondrial damage and protein translation" (Rosedale et al. 2009). The effect, in plain language, is slowed aging and improved health.

Again, cellular proliferation occurs mainly under three circumstances: reproduction (DNA replication and pregnancy); growth, as, for example, in children; and cancer. A presentation on April 14, 2008, at the American Association for Cancer Research annual meeting revealed that modified caloric restriction may offer a protective effect against the development of epithelial cancers. Epithelial cancers, also known as *carcinomas,* arise in the tissue that lines the surfaces and cavities of the body's organs, and they make up 80 percent of all cancers. "Calorie restriction and obesity directly affect activation of the cell surface receptors' epidermal growth factor and insulin-like growth factor," explained study coauthor Tricia Moore, a graduate student in the Department of Carcinogenesis at the University of Texas's M. D. Anderson Cancer Center. "These receptors then affect signaling in downstream molecular pathways such as Akt and mTOR. Calorie restriction, which we refer to as negative energy balance, inhibits this signaling, and obesity, or positive energy balance, enhances signaling through these pathways, leading to cell growth, proliferation, and survival."

If, however, the dietary protein level stays below this threshold, ancient mechanisms kick in that are designed to help us outlive an apparent famine, which then shuts down cellular proliferation and up-regulates, instead, repair and regeneration. This process signals an effort to keep us healthy enough, long enough, so that our cells can reproduce another day. Our energy is conserved through maintaining our own cellular repair instead of making new cells. That's what we want! We want just enough protein to meet the demands of our own repair, regeneration, and basic maintenance needs that can extend our own longevity, enhance our own health, and possibly even reverse signs of aging, but not so much that we up-regulate mTOR. And we always want to keep insulin levels as low as possible.

So, how much is just enough? For most adults the RDA, roughly 0.8 g per kilogram (2.2 pounds) of *ideal* body weight (e.g., 150-pound ideal body weight (68 kg) × .8 g = 54 g), is probably sufficient for 97.5 percent of the adult population (one of the rare RDAs worth paying some attention to). The average would lie somewhere between 45 and 60 g of actual protein per day for the majority of adults. One study noted that the amount of protein needed to effectively retain lean tissue mass and quality physical performance in athletes was closer to 1.2 to 1.7 g/kg daily, translating to 60 to 80 g of protein per day, assuming adequate mineral intake (Phinney 2004). **The same study also noted negative effects if this level of daily protein was exceeded by more than 25 percent of the daily energy expenditure, citing a drop in performance and suppression of ketogenesis.**

Note: Keep in mind that when we're talking about grams of protein, we're not saying grams of meat or fish. Protein is only a part of what makes up meat or fish. Fat, water, and many other nutrient components make up a piece of meat or fish. I've provided a chart in appendix C to help translate the protein content into ounces of food to make figuring this out easier. You can either have your butcher or fishmonger cut the meat or fish into the weight portions you want or you can purchase a digital food scale (these aren't at all expensive) to help take the guesswork out of things at mealtime. Eventually, you will probably just be able to eyeball it, but until then, it might make sense to monitor the amounts more closely to get into the habit of protein moderation.

Research published in the journal *Aging Cell* stated, "Reduced function mutations in the Insulin/IGF-1 signaling pathway *increase maximal lifespan and health span* in many species. Calorie restriction (CR) decreases serum IGF-1 concentration by ~40%, protects against cancer and slows aging in rodents." The study showed that "protein intake is a key determinant of circulating IGF-1 levels in humans" and suggested that "a reduced protein intake (no more than 0.95 g/kg of body weight per day) may become an important component of anticancer and anti-aging dietary interventions" (Fontana et al. 2008).

In another study, titled "Clinical Experience of a Diet Designed to Reduce Aging," the authors stated, "It has been demonstrated that the longevity effects of calorie restriction can be partially attributed to the reduction in protein intake." They added, "It has been shown that limiting dietary amino acids, specifically methionine, inhibits signaling through mammalian target of rapamycin (mTOR) thereby decreasing mitochondrial damage and protein translation" (Rosedale et al. 2009).

The broader range of a low of 45 to 50 g of protein (roughly the RDA) for people of low-average weight and metabolic demands to a high of 80 g of protein for the leanest, most muscular, and most metabolically demanding athletes amounts to a range of 6 to 8 ounces of concentrated, complete protein (meat, fish, eggs) per day, which is best consumed in divided amounts. (See the chart of protein content in foods in appendix C.) **It isn't a good idea to exceed roughly 25 g of actual protein in a meal, however, as this is the mTOR-stimulating threshold.** Just as an example, a single tin of sardines in olive oil yields about 27 g of protein (plus lots of high-quality fats, including EPA and DHA), just over half of an average person's total daily need! That's about all. It's not a lot, and it's far fewer grams of protein than many people regularly consume—even per meal. In this country, we really do have an unnatural access to an unnatural abundance of food and have come to expect big portions as a matter of course. Bigger portions do not lead to a longer life, however.

Important note: Pregnant women, growing children, and teens should not have their protein or fat intake overly restricted. Carbohydrates (sugar and starch) are not at all required by people in these populations, but caloric restriction in general is not particularly advisable. Embarking on a carbohydrate-elimination diet to which one might not be accustomed during a pregnancy is also not advised. In the case of pregnancy, seek consultation with a qualified medical practitioner before embarking on any big change in diet. Simple rule of thumb: Where reproduction and growth are needed or desired, extra protein is needed.

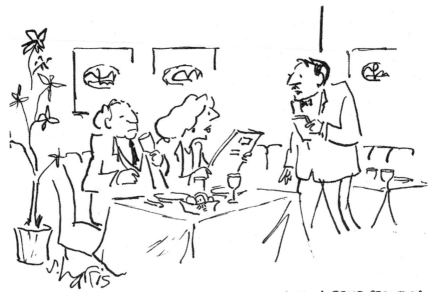

"WOULD YOU LIKE THAT TO BE A STEAK WITH A BROAD-SPECTRUM ANTIBIOTIC, OR ONE WITH A VARIETY OF THERAPEUTIC PROTEINS?"

Fig. 21.1. Getting the best-quality protein

The central idea here where optimal health and longevity are concerned is nutrient density per calorie. The quality and the digestibility of the protein source are key and ultimately matter more than greater quantity. This healthy modification to your diet alone can readily save you thousands of dollars on grocery bills while still allowing you to afford the best-quality nutrient-dense sources of protein (e.g., fully grass-fed, organic, or wild-caught meat and fish).

Keeping protein consumption to a much more moderate level also makes digesting it far less challenging. You are more apt to easily digest and make better use of a small amount of protein at a meal as opposed to a large slab of meat or fish in your gut that your body has to struggle to break down and assimilate. Many people lack sufficient hydrochloric acid and pancreatic enzymes to do so; lesser amounts of protein ease the digestive burden. Protein digestion is also very energy intensive—in fact, digestion demands more energy than anything else we do—and moderating intake may improve energy levels and help minimize fatigue. Furthermore, the digestion of protein yields nitrogen by-products that the liver must process, which also burdens the eliminative system somewhat. Minimizing this also helps your body's eliminative processes function more efficiently, allowing for better detoxification overall.

But Isn't Eating Lots of Lean Protein What Our Ancestors Did?

Protein—and food, in general—was not always as unnaturally abundant as it is in our modern world today. In more primitive times, we expended a fair amount of energy procuring it, and there were times we had to live without adequate food for days, weeks, and even months. Everything in the wild is feast or famine. We also had to share whatever we found with family groups or tribal members when we were lucky enough to get it. Fat, as a key nutrient-rich energy source, was always greatly coveted for its nutrient density and energy value. Protein has always been treated by the body as a precious commodity and is allocated carefully within our metabolic framework. Adequate dietary fat, by the way, is absolutely required for protein to be properly used in the body. A diet of excessively lean protein can be somewhat toxic, and the negative effects of this have been referred to by the Inuit (as reported by Arctic explorer Vilhjalmur Stefansson) as something called *rabbit starvation,* which causes extreme fatigue, general malaise, cardiac dysfunction, and headaches; the remedy for this was always added dietary fat. The fat-free liquid protein diets in the late 1970s even resulted in death for some people. Protein in the absence of dietary fat just isn't a good idea and isn't remotely natural. Also, more isn't necessarily better.

Nothing is ever wasted by our bodies. We have the ability to recycle a significant amount of protein in our bodies day to day, but we still need a few ounces of complete (i.e., animal-source) protein in our daily dietary intake to be optimally healthy.

If dietary protein is *overly* abundant, then a significant quantity of the dietary excesses is readily converted to sugar and stored as fat as a means of surviving what could be a future famine, and our mTOR metabolic pathways governing growth and reproduction are up-regulated, allowing for growing new tissues, having children, or storing fat. At the same time that these reproductive pathways are up-regulated, **our own internal repair and maintenance pathways are down-regulated.** It's out with the old and in with the new, as it were. Understanding this science gives us modern humans more of a choice and a chance for an even longer, healthier life than our ancestors had.

When food is overly abundant and we eat that way, our ancient reproductive mechanisms recognize a window of opportunity for reproduction and basically sacrifice existing cellular repair and our own individual longevity interests for the sake of creating something new, and energy diversion toward cellular proliferation ensues. But when food (protein) appears to the body as being more limited or scarce, it's like saying, "Building a new house is too expensive right now, so let's fix up the one we've got." The body up-regulates repair and regeneration so we can stay healthy enough long enough to better reproduce at another time when the conditions are riper and food is more plentiful for that. It's a means of basically beating Mother Nature at her own game (something that modern research can help us with that our Stone Age ancestors didn't know about). There are two nutrients that directly mitigate this primordially based biochemical decision-making process: carbohydrates (sugar) and protein. The pathways that regulate them are insulin and mTOR.

Why, you ask, is that?

22

Our Primordial Past

■ ■ ■ ■ ■ ■ ■ ■ ■ ■ ■

*Understanding Mother Nature's Plan
and Where We Fit In*

Floating somewhere near the center of our Milky Way is a gaseous interstellar cloud made up mostly of an eight-atom sugar known as *glycolaldehyde*. It is believed that this may have been the chemical precursor to life on Earth. It can react with ribose, a three-carbon sugar, to form the basis of all life on Earth: RNA and DNA. The same ghostly cloud also contains a sweet compound called *ethylene glycol* (basically antifreeze), a very close relative of sugar. Sugar was life's first fuel on Earth, and the memory of this is all still a part of our most primal genetic makeup and the makeup of every other living organism on the planet.

In ancient times, when life in the form of single-celled organisms first appeared in the primordial seas, before there ever was an oxygen-based atmosphere, there were only two nutrients available: sugar and protein. The genes of every living organism on Earth still remember this. Sugar and protein have been regulating reproduction and life span ever since the first single-celled organisms appeared in the earliest primordial seas. All energy production in the earliest primordial times was fermentative and anaerobic. These two nutrients eventually established the basis and driving force behind reproduction for all organisms, and, consequently, behind aging and life span.

The first living cells were *prokaryotic* in nature; each one was identical to the next, much like bacteria, lacking a nucleus and feeding anaerobically on sugars.

Later, development of an oxygen-based atmosphere allowed for evolution into *eukaryotic* cells (possessing a nucleus), which allowed for cellular differentiation into organs, eyes, skin, and other tissues, making higher organisms possible. The developing presence of oxygen—essentially among the first waste products of Earth's earliest life-forms—eventually allowed for the use of fat as a nutrient for the first time. Eukaryotic cells are fueled aerobically and use fatty acids and ketones for this purpose, just as most human and other mammalian cells do today. Fat is an aerobic nutrient and forms the basis of aerobic metabolism. Herein lies the distinction between the two energy sources: aerobic and anaerobic forms.

One theory of how cancers develop involves the idea that an excessively fermentative, acidic, sugar-rich, and anaerobic environment (known to be friendly to cancer growth) somehow simulates our earliest primordial environment and stimulates the reversion of some cells to their primordial, prokaryotic state. Tumors are basically masses of undifferentiated, identical cells with a weak protein matrix that feed exclusively on sugars. In other words, when the environment is ripe—when the availability of sugar is high and a fermentative, acidic, and anaerobic environment is allowed to take hold—this primordial component of our genetic makeup is somehow triggered and stimulates cells into an unhealthy, abnormal, and exceedingly primitive form of cellular proliferation. Healthy cellular differentiation cannot occur in a fermentative environment. This certainly presents a plausible model for carcinogenesis as well as other unhealthy forms of cellular proliferation.

The development of an oxygen-based atmosphere eventually allowed for the use of fat as an important energy source. In the evolution of more-complex organisms such as mammals, it is fat that serves as the primary, most efficient source of fuel. Leptin, which is the key fat sensor in the body, then controls and regulates all our energy stores via the hypothalamus, which manages the signals given to every other hormone in the body.

Sugar and protein are the nutrients that regulate the three parallel pathways that control aging in humans: leptin, insulin and mTOR.

RON ROSEDALE, M.D.

The Part That Evolution May Not Have Intended

As fundamentally primal beings, we have a well-developed survival instinct. We have an innate, vested interest in our own personal longevity and well-being. But we also harbor within us other influential entities with their own selfish agendas: our genes. Our genes are guided and essentially driven by nature's ultimate agenda (the big "A"), which is the perpetuation and continuity of life (the big "L") as a whole. This imperative also drives us to reproduce, which is the primary focus of those genes, whose sole purpose is simply to replicate.

Nature, it turns out, is not necessarily so interested in the things that constitute the individual components of life, such as you or me. We, as individual life-forms, are but infinitesimal and ultimately expendable specks of dust in Mother Nature's bigger equation. Just as we have a basic indifference to the various cells in our own bodies that regularly degenerate and die, making way for new ones (all we care about, after all, is our overall survival and continuation), so too nature is primarily interested in its own ongoing big picture. Not, specifically, our puny individual lives. Basically, nature wants us to live long enough and be healthy enough so that we can reproduce successfully. Once we have achieved this end or have arrived at the end of our useful reproductive life, well, it's not that nature wants us dead, necessarily. Nature sort of just loses interest. The body simply moves increasingly and unceremoniously downhill toward the deterioration and gradual loss of function we unhappily recognize as senescence—old age.

Nature isn't that interested in "innately and wisely" teaching each of us how to live with health and vitality into very old age. That's where our own innate personal survival instinct—and modern science—comes to the rescue (if we're willing to pay attention). We can't really count on nature's example to guide us here, or even the example of our ice age or hunter-gatherer ancestors, entirely. Eating foods that closely replicate the same diet that essentially shaped our physiological requirements, of course, makes inherent sense and must certainly play a foundational role. But nature does not necessarily guide us to instinctively manipulate these dietary nutrients with postreproductive longevity in mind. Our primitive ancestors ate what they could to survive. Whatever they ate consistently helped establish our present-day nutritional requirements—but they weren't focused on manipulating what they ate to optimize their health and longevity. With respect to enhancing our postreproductive longevity, we're basically on our own—without a fully natural compass.

What we are really seeking as individuals with our own personal drive toward survival, then, is to somehow find and exploit Mother Nature's loopholes for the benefit of our own individual postreproductive health, longevity, and expanded youth. For literally the first exciting time in our human history, we have the science available to tell us how to do exactly that.

Beginning back in the early- to mid-1900s, a number of experiments involving caloric restriction in animal models showed us that caloric restriction had a mysteriously universal effect of greatly improving health and extending life span. This research now spans some seventy-five years and is extremely well established and widely known.

Evidence of the effects of caloric restriction in slowing aging and extending youth can be found in its abilities to prevent the immune dysfunctions of old age, improve DNA repair abilities, reduce damaging free-radical activity, lower glucose and insulin levels, maintain fertility at advanced ages, boost energy levels, increase protein synthesis, reduce the accumulation of damaged proteins, inhibit the inflammatory responses of aging, lower the levels of cholesterol and triglycerides in the blood, counteract neural degeneration, and prevent the age-related decline in the health-building hormone dehydroepiandrosterone (DHEA).

Caloric restriction also prevents or postpones the incidence of and reduces the severity of diseases such as cancer, kidney disease, and cardiovascular disease (Masoro 2003).

It is also known today to be additionally important that adequate vitamins, minerals, and nutrients be supplied or added to caloric restriction approaches to avoid nutrient deficiencies. **The idea is to limit calories, not nutrients** (Nicolas et al. 1999). Therefore, nutrient density also plays a very important role.

Longevity enthusiasts who attempt to apply the earlier caloric restriction research by attempting to sustain themselves each day on a single kumquat and a tablespoon of oatmeal are gravely missing the point, to say nothing of living an unnecessarily stress-inducing, deprivation-oriented life. No such thing is necessary, nor is it really helping them arrive at their hoped-for objective. Recently popularized raw-food vegan diets can achieve temporary improvements by essentially down-regulating insulin and mTOR (and through such diets being generally detoxifying). The problem here is multifold, however. In addition to the fact that we as humans lack four stomachs and cud-chewing ruminant tendencies to maximize the use of plant-based foods to meet all our needs, such a diet completely fails to provide many essential animal-source nutrients needed for long-term maintenance of our health, our brain, our nervous system, and our vitality. Without adequate fat to normalize leptin (among countless other things) or complete protein sources to allow for critical rebuilding and maintenance, such dietary approaches ultimately do far more depletive harm than good in the long run. The addition of quality, raw animal food sources and fat and fat-soluble nutrients to these regimens would exponentially improve their long-term effectiveness. If you insist on being a raw foodist, then be sure to include more raw animal products and fats in your diet. The difference it will make in your health and the health of your brain and nervous system will be immeasurable.

To depict the more modern-day caloric restriction concept in science more accurately, the term *caloric restriction with optimal nutrition* (also known as CRON) has been suggested. This process of "undernutrition without malnutrition" has been shown to consistently lengthen life span, postpone the onset of aging, and prevent the development of cancer and degenerative diseases. Only carbohydrates and protein need to be limited (in that order), while fat and fat-soluble nutrients actually play a more nutritionally and energetically dominant and important role.

The addition of antioxidant nutrients has been shown to have a potential longevity-enhancing effect on caloric restriction—something to additionally consider (Lemon et al. 2005). Antiglycating nutrients (e.g., benfotiamine, pyridoxamine, R-lipoic acid, acetyl L-carnitine, L-carnosine) may also be considered additionally helpful for some. Keep in mind that I'm not saying everyone **needs** to take these supplements, only that they might yield an extra advantage to those who can afford them and might be inclined to take things a step further.

Early on, it was believed (because of some flawed experiments involving macronutrient isolation) that caloric restriction *in general,* not any one specific form of nutrient restriction, was somehow responsible for the effect. Experiments in which lab rats were fed a diet exclusively consisting of carbohydrates led to rapid degeneration, accelerated aging, and death. Exclusive protein feeding also resulted in fairly rapid degenerative decline and death.

Then researchers fed their rats a diet consisting exclusively of pure lard, an unnatural food for rats. Something different happened. Instead of developing degenerative diseases and cancer like the others, these rats developed impacted colons and their little intestines ruptured. That, not any natural cause, is what killed them. Since the scientific community, as a whole, was on an active, rabid campaign of fat vilification during this time period, the fact that these rats died only confirmed what was essentially expected by the researchers, who just knew that fat was evil, anyway, and the actual cause of death was disregarded as insignificant.

This, of course, is outright lousy and fundamentally flawed science. Either the data concerning fat should either have been disregarded or some new experiment should have been devised. The flaws in this original research involving macronutrient manipulation have since been recognized, and we now know that fat factors differently into the equation. Until very recently, however, the mechanisms behind caloric restriction and *why* it actually worked were poorly understood.

Modern studies of healthy human centenarians, those people who are one hundred years old and older, have revealed the presence of a certain class of genes that seem to be activated in these individuals. Called *sirtuins,* they have come to be known as our longevity genes. In mammals, one of these genes is referred to as *SIRT-1* (in worms, it is called *SIR-2*). In certain fortunate people who appear to age unusually gracefully and remain vital to extremely old age, the *SIRT-1* gene just sort of seems to be inherently activated, for unknown lucky reasons. This is why certain long-lived people can claim not to have taken particular care of their health and still seem to make it to very old age. This is why were hear comments like, "Yeah, granny smoked cigars and drank a fifth of whiskey every day and lived to be one hundred." Such mysteriously fortunate individuals, of course, are the exception and not the rule. Recently, a nutrient found in red wine called *resveratrol* was shown to have the effect of activating this gene. It has also been clearly demonstrated that **caloric restriction similarly activates these genes in all organisms and has all the same beneficial effects.**

Reporting in the September 21, 2007, issue of the journal *Cell,* researcher David Sinclair from Harvard Medical School, in collaboration with scientists from Weill Cornell Medical College and the U.S. National Institutes of Health, discovered two additional genes in mammalian cells that act as gatekeepers for cellular longevity. When cells experience certain kinds of stress, such as caloric restriction, these genes rev up and help protect cells from diseases of aging (Yang et al. 2007).

The newly discovered genes are called *SIRT-3* and *SIRT-4*. Like SIRT-1, they are part of the larger class of sirtuins. The newly discovered role of SIRT-3 and SIRT-4 confirmed the particular importance of mitochondria as vital for sustaining the health and longevity of a cell.

Mitochondria, cellular organs that are found in the cytoplasm, are often considered to be the cell's battery packs or energy-producing factories. When mitochondria become compromised by particular stressors, energy is drained out of a cell and its days are numbered. This, in turn, compromises our energy production, health, and metabolic efficiency. Sinclair and his colleagues discovered that SIRT-3 and SIRT-4 play a vital role in a longevity network that maintains the vitality of the mitochondria and keeps cells healthy when they would otherwise die. **The most powerful method found of activating these life-saving and life-extending genes is caloric restriction.**

When cells undergo caloric restriction, signals sent in through the cell membrane activate an enzyme called *nicotinamide phosphoribosyltransferase* (NAMPT). As levels of NAMPT ramp up, a small molecule called *nicotinamide adenine dinucleotide* (NAD+) begins to amass in the mitochondria. This, in turn, causes the activity of enzymes created by the SIRT-3 and SIRT-4 genes—enzymes that live in the mitochondria—to increase as well. As a result, the mitochondria grow stronger, energy output increases, and the cell's aging process slows down significantly.

In laboratory experiments, certain animal subjects have had their healthy life span extended by 30–60 percent—sometimes even by 300–400 percent—using methods of optimized caloric restriction! The implications are staggering. The same basic mechanism seems to exist across all species studied, from yeast to even primates (like us).

But *Why* Does Caloric Restriction Work?

Why would mimicking starvation have such a profound effect on extending life span? It seems almost counterintuitive. The answer to this mysterious question had been the holy grail of longevity researchers for close to seventy-five years.

Now we know.

In the early 1990s, there was an unusual discovery made by a researcher, Cynthia Kenyon, Ph.D., professor of biochemistry and bio-physics at the University of California, San Francisco. She was studying an ancient species of worm (a nematode called *Caenorhabditis elegans,* also known by high school biology students as planaria). This particular little worm—from a species that has been around for millions and millions of years—developed a genetic mutation that, quite unusually, seemed to more than double the worm's life span. This was the most significant life extension that had been reported in any organism up to that point. In 1993, Kenyon and colleagues published a study in *Nature* that describes this life-extending genetic mutation (Kenyon et al. 1993).

Normally, mutations are not considered to be a particularly beneficial thing; they typically are more inclined to kill or greatly inconvenience an organism. This mutation was different. The researchers called this myste-rious, magical, and marvelously beneficial mutated gene the *DAF-2* gene. A few years later, the research team actually discovered what this gene did. It rocked the entire scientific world in the field of longevity research. They'd found their holy grail. The *DAF-2 gene essentially encoded an insulin receptor.* In other words, when insulin was down-regulated in this worm, the worm lived longer. Much longer.

Since when does something like a worm produce insulin, you ask? Insulin in these simple life-forms has nothing to do with blood sugar regulation, but instead is entirely designed to regulate reproduction and actual life span. Subsequent research has confirmed this role of insulin across *all* species, including primates.

How much insulin we produce over the course of our lives con-trols how long we live! And it turns out, the less insulin we need, the better.

Studies looking at the effects of insulin levels on human health and longevity are emerging, and the picture is quite clear. One study showed that over a ten-year period, the risk of dying was almost twice as great for people with the highest insulin levels than for those with the lowest lev-els. The study authors stated that excess insulin, or hyperinsulinemia, is associated with increased all-cause and cardiovascular mortality, indepen-dent of other risk factors (Dekker et al. 2005). High levels of serum insu-lin promote high blood pressure by impairing sodium balance. Prolonged exposure to excess insulin can severely compromise the vascular system. By acting as a catalyst in promoting cellular proliferation, excess insulin also increases the risk for and progression of certain cancers. High insulin levels promote the formation of beta-amyloid in brain cells and may contribute to the development of Alzheimer's disease. Overproduction of insulin even contributes to prostate enlargement by helping to promote the overgrowth of prostate cells. Insulin resistance, a by-product of chronic excess insulin production, is associated with the development of abdominal obesity and health problems such as atherosclerosis and impotence. Furthermore, insulin resistance and obesity are risk factors for type 2 diabetes mellitus. Hyperinsulinemia is, in fact, a predictive factor for type 2 diabetes mellitus.

It turns out that insulin is an extremely ancient molecule and exists in identical form in everything from yeast cells to humans. Far from its formerly perceived, limited role in nutrient storage or even blood sugar control (a trivial sideline for insulin), insulin is now being understood as something far more important and fundamental to the very underlying mechanisms of our health and longevity. In monitoring our energy availability, while leptin oversees the actual energy stores, it is insulin that switches on and off the extremely ancient mechanisms that allow us to outlive what our body thinks is an apparent famine.

That's the clue to as to how we beat Mother Nature at her own game. The down-regulation of insulin (and mTOR) triggers the up-regulation of repair and maintenance on a cellular level that allows us to remain healthy until food becomes more available and we can finally reproduce. Bingo.

That's our magic loophole. And it's not a drug, a supplement, or something that is expensive or complicated to implement. In fact, applying this simple loophole will even save you some real money—money on groceries *and* money on health care. You don't even have to feel hungry. Plus, you will discover a vitality and feeling of self-empowerment you never knew was possible for you to have. It's a win-win situation, all the way around.

What Do All the Longest-Living Individuals Have in Common?

If there is a known single marker for long life, as found in the centenarian and animal studies, it is low insulin levels.

RON ROSEDALE, M.D., "INSULIN AND ITS METABOLIC EFFECTS,"
PAPER PRESENTED AT *THE DESIGNS FOR HEALTH INSTITUTE'S
BOULDERFEST* SEMINAR, BOULDER, COLORADO, AUGUST 1999

Research across the board has shown that long-lived individuals (animals and humans) share the following characteristics:

- low fasting insulin levels
- low fasting glucose levels
- optimally low leptin levels
- low triglyceride levels
- low percentage of visceral body fat
- lower body temperature
- reduced thyroid levels

Low thyroid levels, you say? Isn't that a bad thing?

The idea here is that a reduced caloric load, which results in the almost exclusive use of fat for fuel and optimal nutrient intake, improves metabolic *efficiency*. As long as things are operating efficiently, higher metabolism isn't necessary or even desirable. Your internal engine runs less hot, and the engine therefore lasts longer (and your thyroid controls the idle).

This isn't to say that having low thyroid levels in a blood chemistry or salivary hormone panel is always necessarily good at all. It's a contextual thing. If your thyroid hormone T3 (triiodothyronine) level is low because you've been burning your adrenals out or because you've developed Hashimoto's autoimmune disease and are producing thyroid peroxidase antibodies and destroying your own thyroid cells, that's not so good. It's all relative. The *reason* why your thyroid levels are low is more important than the state in and of itself. In a person, however, who has all the rest of the laboratory markers for long-lived individuals listed above, a functionally lower level of T3 may be perfectly acceptable, even desirable! As long as there are no adverse symptoms, that is. In a human clinical study article titled "Clinical Experience of a Diet Designed to Reduce Aging," the authors remarked, "It has been stated that the reduction in T3 and body temperature could alter the aging process by reflecting a reducing metabolic rate, oxidative stress and systemic inflammation" (Rosedale et al. 2009).

One single longevity marker stands out among all long-lived animals and people above the rest, however, and that's *low insulin levels.*

"Sure," you say, "all this is good for a worm or a mouse, but how about me?"

In July 2009, the eagerly awaited results of a twenty-year study on the effects of caloric restriction on primates were finally published in the journal *Science,* see figure 22.1 (Coleman et al. 2009). Two groups of rhesus monkeys (selected for their strong similarity to us) were studied. The monkeys in one group were allowed to eat as much as they wanted, and the monkeys in the other group were given a sufficiently nutrient-dense diet with 30 percent fewer calories than they would normally consume. Twenty years later, only 63 percent of the monkeys that ate as much as they wanted were still alive. Thirty-seven percent of them had died from age-related causes. And the caloric-restriction group? Eighty-seven percent of them were still alive, and only **13 percent** had died of age-related causes. Throughout their lives, the calorically restricted group maintained superior health and aging-related biomarkers in every area: brain health, metabolic health and rate, insulin sensitivity, and cardiovascular vitality. *The monkeys in the caloric-restriction group enjoyed a threefold reduction in age-related disease!* Also, they lost fat weight but maintained healthy levels of lean tissue mass. They also retained greater brain volume, which normally shrinks with age and glycation, but more than that, they retained superior cognitive function. The cardiovascular disease rate of the caloric-restriction group was fully half the rate of the control group. Forty percent of the monkeys in the control group developed diabetes or prediabetes. *Not one single monkey in the calorically restricted group developed either.* Remarkable. The available photos from the study showing examples of age-matched individuals from the two groups are visually striking. Stunning, even. The caloric-restricted monkeys looked almost *half the age* of the control monkeys. (See figures 22.1 and 22.2 on page 212.)

The study was designed, of course, well before Kenyon's work or anything related to mTOR was published. Both of these studies have added richly to the understanding behind the mechanisms of just **why** caloric restriction is so effective, so one can only imagine how much more might have been accomplished with that awareness in mind.

FYI: Among the most common misconceptions about monkeys and apes, incidentally, is that they are vegan animals. They are better adapted to making use of plant foods in some ways than we are, but they also readily eat the same things we eat. *All* monkeys and apes are known to eat meat, and many even hunt for meat. The one notable exception is the mountain gorilla, and even it gets some insects in its diet. Monkeys and apes are omnivores and, like us, will eat whatever might be available to

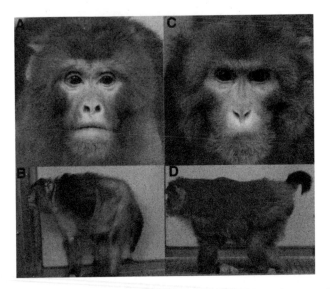

Fig. 22.1. A picture is worth a thousand words: both monkeys are the exact same age. Photo by permission: *Science,* "Calorie Restriction Delays Disease Onset and Mortality in Rhesus Monkeys."

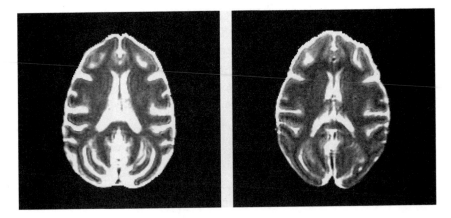

Fig. 22.2. Brain scans of two different rhesus macaque monkeys illustrate the findings of a landmark study of diet and aging at the University of Wisconsin-Madison. The image on the left shows the brain of an animal allowed free rein at the dinner table (control), while the image on the right shows the brain of a monkey that for two decades has been on a nutritious but reduced-calorie diet. The brain of the animal allowed to eat freely has less tissue volume and more fluid (bright areas) than the brain of the monkey on the low-cal diet. The images suggest less brain atrophy or cell loss with aging for animals that consume a diet with 30 percent fewer calories than if they were permitted to eat as much as they like. Photo courtesy Sterling C. Johnson and R. Coleman, www.news.wisc.edu/newsphotos/monkeydiet09.html.

them in their environment. Some even catch and eat fish (crazy, but true)! One of the reasons rhesus monkeys were selected for this particular study, in fact, is their pronounced similarity to us, even in terms of diet. For more reading about this particular aspect of things, I can recommend the book *The Hunting Apes: Meat Eating and the Origins of Human Behavior,* by Craig B. Stanford (Stanford 1999).

There are actually several more-recent studies, too, showing significant health benefits where caloric restriction in humans is concerned. The study by Rosedale and colleagues in *The Journal of Applied Research* demonstrated in the context of an outpatient medical clinic that a diet high in fat (unlimited quantity), **adequate in protein** (50–80 g per day), and **very low in carbohydrate,** with some added multivitamin and mineral supplementation (together with 2,000 mg L-carnitine, 400 mg alpha lipoic acid, 100 mg CoQ10, and 1 tablespoon of cod-liver oil per day) led to significant improvement in recognized serum factors related to the aging process (e.g., glucose, insulin, leptin, and triglycerides) (Rosedale et al. 2009). Patients were told to eat when they were hungry. The results also included a significant loss of body weight, a significant reduction in systolic and diastolic blood pressure, and a reduction in the levels of leptin, insulin, fasting glucose, and free T3 hormone (with levels of thyroid stimulating hormone, or TSH, and creatinine largely unchanged). Despite the predominance of fat in the diet, serum triglyceride levels were also greatly reduced.

Another area of human longevity research getting a lot of publicity these days involves manipulating the length of something called a *telomere.* Telomeres are sequences of nucleic acids extending from the ends of chromosomes that act to maintain chromosomal integrity. Every time our cells divide, telomeres are shortened, leading to cellular damage and cellular death associated with aging. Shorter telomeres have been associated with significantly higher cancer incidence. In fact, a recent Italian study showed that people with shorter telomeres have ten times the cancer risk of those with longer telomeres (and those with short telomeres were twice as likely to die from cancer) (Armanios et al. 2009).

Scientists at Geron Corporation discovered that the key element in rebuilding our disappearing telomeres is the "immortalizing" enzyme *telomerase,* an enzyme found only in germ cells and cancer cells. Telomerase appears to repair and replace telomeres, manipulating the "clocking" mechanism that controls the life span of dividing cells. In fact, the discovery of telomerase was considered important enough that is was awarded the 2009 Nobel Prize in Medicine. A therapy that is able to significantly activate telomerase, called the Patton protocol, has since been developed based on a plant extract. The resulting compound, known as TA-65, has shown some impressive antiaging, telomere-lengthening effects in clinical trials, though the cost to the average person wanting to purchase TA-65 for his or her own use is approximately four thousand dollars for a six-month supply. (Ka-*ching*!) Drug companies, of course, are looking for ways to enhance telomerase any way they can. In fact, look for other upcoming supplements and, possibly, life extension–related medications claiming to do just this. What they won't tell you, however, is that **caloric restriction also preserves and may even also reverse telomere length.** You don't have to wait for a questionable drug to come out or go broke buying hyped "designer supplements."

Certain supplements have also been demonstrated to preserve or even lengthen telomeres: Vitamins C and E and resveratrol have been demonstrated to slow telomere shortening. Both omega-3s and vitamin D (note that these are fat-related nutrients) have been shown to even *lengthen* telomeres! Intense cardiovascular exercise, too, has been shown to preserve telomere length (Puterman et al. 2010).

Also, where telomere length is concerned, it's important to keep your homocysteine levels as low as you can. Homocysteine is a toxic by-product of cellular metabolism that has been linked to heart disease, Alzheimer's disease, and Parkinson's disease. Primary methyl donors such as vitamins B_6, B_{12}, and folic acid as well as other methyl donors such as dimethylglycine (DMG), trimethylglycine (TMG), betaine, and S-adenosyl methionine (SAMe) have been shown to readily and successfully lower homocysteine levels. Good thing, too. Now there's yet another reason to monitor homocysteine levels and keep them in check: relatively recent research has shown that **high levels of homocysteine can triple the rate of telomere loss during cellular division** (Xu et al. 2000). Homocysteine rapidly ages you and significantly increases your susceptibility to disease! B-complex vitamins (particularly B_6, B_{12}, and folic acid) are cheap insurance in this regard, though I always make a point of getting at least some B_{12} in its methylcobalamin form sublingually to ensure absorption. Note that a high percentage of vegetarians have a tendency toward high homocysteine (Wadoa et al. 2004).

Of course, it's easy to restrict overall calories with lab animals, as they have no choice in the matter. It is quite another matter to try and restrict overall caloric intake when you're driving past fifteen fast-food joints on your way home, are surrounded by constant manipulative advertisements, and have a refrigerator and cupboards full of food at your ravenous fingertips. *Unless,* of course, you apply the caloric-restriction model in a way that does not leave you hungry, which is exactly what this book tells you how to do. Just follow the simple, most basic dietary guidelines outlined here to eat optimally well, and you will feel fully satisfied, live healthier and longer, and even save some real money along the way! Even while buying the best-quality produce, grass-fed meats, and wild-caught fish, you can find yourself saving considerable money on groceries. The basic guideline to remember is this: Greatly restrict or eliminate sugar and starch (preferably eliminating gluten completely); keep your protein intake adequate (roughly the RDA: 44–56 g per day or 0.8 g of protein/ kg of ideal body weight), amounting to a total of approximately 6 to 7 ounces of organic eggs, grass-fed, or wild-caught meat or seafood per day; eat as many fibrous, "aboveground," nonstarchy vegetables and greens as you like; and eat as much fat (from fattier cuts of meat or fish, nuts, seeds, avocados, coconut, butter or ghee, olives, olive oil, and other sources) as you need to satisfy your appetite. The bottom line here is that natural dietary fat is not at all our enemy and that, in the absence of dietary carbohydrate and with adequate protein, eating natural dietary fat can result in a far more satisfying, longer, and healthier life overall. It's simple, delicious, and satisfying. No hunger or feelings of deprivation are needed, and you get all the benefits of supporting a longer and healthier life while saving money. It's better for the planet, too.

If you do nothing from this book other than what was outlined in the last paragraph, your health and well-being will change remarkably, and chances are you will age much more gracefully and live longer, and you can do it all without going broke.

And that's no monkey business.

> *I don't want to achieve immortality through my work; I want to achieve immortality by not dying.*
>
> WOODY ALLEN

23

Using Insulin and Leptin to Our Advantage

■ ■ ■ ■ ■ ■ ■ ■ ■ ■ ■ ■

It remains true that leptin is actually what controls the bigger hormonal picture in humans (and other mammals). When leptin levels repeatedly surge in response to dietary elevations of starch or sugar, this has a numbing effect on the ability of the brain to "hear" leptin's message. We become leptin resistant. The brain assumes its leptin levels are too low and that we are starving, even though the image you see in your mirror tells a different story. This, in turn, compels our hypothalamus to send out a direct signal to eat more, causing insulin to increase and store more fat.

When leptin levels are optimally low, however, and our taste for fat is satisfied, insulin signaling also quiets, and fat burning, repair, regeneration, and maintenance are up-regulated instead, effectively increasing our health and individual life span.

How do we control leptin to our advantage? By eating just enough dietary fat, *in the absence of carbohydrates* and other insulin-generating stimuli, including excess protein, to satisfy our appetite and assure our hypothalamus that "hunting is good."

Since leptin controls hunger, leptin is the primary sensor for fat, and we are creatures of the ice age for whom fat basically means survival, and eating fat as our dominant source of fuel—the way we were actually designed—is the ultimate key to the mystery of health and long-term survival.

We don't need genetic manipulation or new longevity drugs. We can do it all with diet, easily, inexpensively, and very simply. By eliminating unnecessary carbohydrates (basically, all dietary sugar and starch) and effectively minimizing insulin, by consuming *just enough* protein to meet our basic maintenance and repair requirements and keep mTOR down-regulated, by "feeding the hypothalamus" with healthy signals from leptin, and by feeding our cells with the fat and fat-soluble nutrients that nourish and supply us with long, even-burning, nonglycating, satisfying energy, we can enjoy a level of health and vitality one might never have believed was possible.

It is all actually very simple. Using these exact same principles and controlling these same primal mechanisms, it may be possible to halt or even reverse many of the disease processes we have come to associate with aging, including cancer. A body focused entirely on its own repair, healing, regeneration, and maintenance will enjoy powerfully enhanced immune function, energy, and well-being—even reversing many of the signs and symptoms of aging.

How cool is that?

Is There Any Other Way?

Certain newly discovered nutrients such as trans-*resveratrol* (found in grape skins) have been shown also to have an activating effect on sirtuins, particularly SIRT-1, and have been additionally shown to preserve or even lengthen telomeres. *Trans*-resveratrol, the only active form of resveratrol, has been shown to increase immunity, control blood pressure, preserve red blood cells, inhibit fungal infection, protect the liver and the heart, improve insulin sensitivity, prevent blood clots, and inhibit inflammation. Studies suggest it could potentially be a cure for cancer, heart disease, and age-related brain disorders, among scores of other things. Some scientists feel *trans*-resveratrol could even help extend the human life span up to 70 percent (or up to an extra fifty years). It's pretty exciting stuff.

Resveratrol is found in minute amounts in red wine and is produced by a variety of plants when they are put under stress. By ingesting these "stressed" plant compounds, it is theorized that our physiology is then alerted to possible famine conditions and therefore responds by activating the same mechanisms triggered by caloric restriction. In 2003, resveratrol was first discovered to have antiaging properties, as reported in *Nature* by David Sinclair and Joseph Baur, other Harvard Medical School researchers, and their colleagues. This has resulted in the media and press promoting red wine as though it is the ultimate fountain of youth in a bottle. To match the benefits of resveratrol found in studies with mice, however, the average human would have to drink roughly one hundred to one thousand glasses of wine daily to obtain a similarly beneficial dose. (Oh, well, off to happy hour we go . . .)

Caveat emptor: Most commercial supplements sold as resveratrol contain only, or mostly, the cis-resveratrol form, which is largely inactive. *Trans*-resveratrol, the only active form, though available in some supplements, needs to be taken in relatively high doses; some researchers estimate the beneficial dose required to mimic caloric-restriction effects in humans is likely close to 100 mg or possibly more per day. This can be extremely expensive. Prepare to pay $75 to $150 a month or more for the "real thing." Also, beware of rip-offs. Many supplement companies will jump on this bandwagon, and only very few—mainly health care practitioner brands—will deliver the real deal, at a substantial price.

Thus far, the best proven, most cost-effective, and easiest-to-use tool most of us have to reverse many signs of aging and extend the quality and quantity of life is the minimization of insulin by minimizing insulin-provoking foods and substances—plus moderating a quality protein intake. The modified version of caloric restriction presented in this book can work for anyone, an approach that's far more affordable and sustainable than other dietary approaches. For people who can afford it, though, the addition of *trans*-resveratrol to this dietary approach could have some pretty exciting implications.

PART TWO

PRIMAL MIND

Your body is your subconscious mind!

CANDACE PERT, PH.D.

24

Feeding Your Brain RIGHT

■ ■ ■ ■ ■ ■ ■ ■ ■ ■ ■ ■

Why It Matters

Emerging findings suggest that dietary factors play major roles in determining whether the brain ages successfully or experiences a neurodegenerative disease.

MARK P. MATTSON, PH.D., "GENE–DIET
INTERACTIONS IN BRAIN AGING AND
NEURODEGENERATIVE DISORDERS,"
ANNALS OF INTERNAL MEDICINE, 2003

The myth, of course, is that there is a real distinction between body and mind. There is, in fact, no fundamental separation between mind and body. What happens to one happens to the other. They are both part of the same functioning or dysfunctioning system and must be understood together in context. You cannot have healthy cognitive or psychological functioning without a healthy, properly nourished body (and last I looked, the brain was part of the human body—in most people, anyway). The best psychotherapy, brain training, or medication cannot put a nutrient there that is not there or remove some damaging substance that doesn't belong. They cannot even begin to compensate for poor dietary tendencies.

Cognitive functional decline and underachievement in post-secondary education is 400% more likely with Gluten Sensitivity.

M. VERKASALO, "UNDIAGNOSED SILENT
CELIAC DISEASE: A RISK FOR
UNDERACHIEVEMENT," *SCANDINAVIAN JOURNAL
OF GASTROENTEROLOGY,* 2005

The brain and body need certain raw materials in order to function—*period.* Without proper and sufficient raw materials (i.e., proper nutrition), no amount of any quality therapy or intervention will ever have optimal or lasting results. Toxic stressors, be they sugar or starch, gluten, alcohol, heavy metals, excitotoxins, xenoestrogens, GMOs, contaminants, or EMF pollution, cannot be overridden with any amount of psychotherapy or the addition of more toxic stressors in the form of prescription drugs. Furthermore, all neurotransmitters and neuropeptides have receptors that exist in literally every organ and system in the body. Of the almost three hundred internal communication substances, nearly all are shared throughout the entire body and are anything but unique to the brain. Even neurons are not unique to the brain; they exist in abundance elsewhere in the body.

The mind (including memory and emotion) is not simply contained in the brain; *the mind exists as a "field" throughout the entire human organism!* What is done to the mind is done to the body, and vice versa. You simply cannot separate the two.

Prozac Nation

In 1985, the total annual sales for all antidepressants in the United States were approximately $240 million. Today, it is in excess of $12 *billion.* Between 1987 and 1997, the percentage of Americans in outpatient treatment for depression more than tripled. For those in treatment, the percentage of prescribed medication nearly doubled. Of the three hundred most commonly prescribed medications, *none actually serves to support natural physiological functioning.*

In an article published by the *Wall Street Journal* on December 28, 2010 (Matthews 2010), it was reported, disturbingly, that **more than 25**

percent of kids and teens are now taking prescription medications on a regular basis! In addition to taking drugs for conditions like ADHD and asthma, children are now taking things like sleeping pills, diabetes drugs, blood pressure medications, and even statin drugs, which are typically prescribed only for adults and carry with them unknown side effects for long-term use in young people. Dr. Danny Benjamin, a professor of pediatrics at Duke University, admitted to the *Wall Street Journal* that prescribing chronic medications to children is a serious problem. "We know we're making errors in dosing and safety," he said, noting also that parents must do more to question the safety of medicines their doctors prescribe. Gee, ya think?

Medications artificially manipulate biochemistry in an effort to ameliorate symptoms. All possess the potential for side effects and endocrine disruption. Exacerbation of nutrient deficiencies and endocrine disruption occur to some degree with most, if not all, drugs.

The fact is, **all psychoactive drugs act upon cellular receptors that are designed for our own naturally produced counterparts.** The very use of these psychoactive drugs can diminish our sensitivity to our own endogenously made chemicals over time and disrupt healthy cellular communication and functioning, ultimately making matters worse in the long term (even when there seems to be short-term benefit). Nutritional and dietary imbalances, food sensitivities, toxic influences, and neurological timing issues can affect virtually every disorder. There are natural solutions to virtually everything, as the human body and brain are miraculously equipped to heal themselves if facilitated by the presence of needed raw materials, the liberation from toxic burdens, and an appropriate, healthy attitude.

It takes a certain determination and willingness to take responsibility for one's own well-being. It takes a certain decision to take charge of discovering the answers for oneself. Sometimes (in keeping with human nature), it takes reaching the point where the pain of the problem is worse than the pain of the long-term solution to arrive at real, lasting change. Health is a choice we all make and a responsibility we ourselves shoulder. **No magic pill will ever take the place of a diet and lifestyle that honors our primal physiology.**

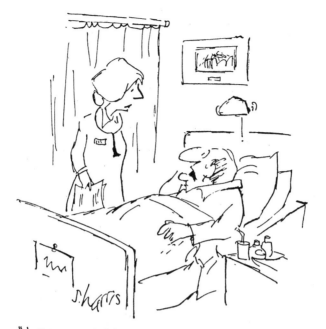

" I STOPPED TAKING THE MEDICINE BECAUSE I PREFER THE ORIGINAL DISEASE TO THE SIDE EFFECTS."

Fig. 24.1. When the cure is worse than the disease

My Own Clinical Experience

As a clinical neurofeedback specialist, my orientation is to approach the symptoms of cognitive and emotional dysregulation as, to some degree, dysregulations of arousal (together with improper functioning of neurological communications, phase relationships, and bioelectrical timing mechanisms). In comparison with the classifications in the ever-thickening *Diagnostic and Statistical Manual of Mental Disorders* (DSM-IV), the neurofeedback approach is infinitely simple. A nervous system can be functionally underaroused, overaroused, some combination thereof, or in a state of unstable arousal combined with either or both underarousal and overarousal.

Neurofeedback is not specifically a therapy, but is essentially a highly specific form of high-tech brain training. It is approached, at least initially, from one of these standpoints. (Of course, I'm oversimplifying quite a bit.)

Most presenting symptoms or issues fall into one of these related categories. The vast majority of clients that I see nowadays can readily be categorized as cases of either overarousal or unstable arousal. This has become increasingly the case in recent years. Brain training helps restore healthy communication, and the brain learns to regulate itself.

By far, the single greatest influence mitigating these forms of dysregulation that I see every day is diet, and most often blood sugar dysregulation—frequently together with insulin and leptin resistance. Food sensitivities and deficiencies are also extremely common and are overwhelmingly endemic as well, mainly in people with carbohydrate-based diets. Nothing can serve to compromise anything and everything to do with brain function or get in the way of the restoration of healthy brain function more than a lousy diet.

What are the implications?

> *Everything you have ever experienced, felt, or conducted in life is due to brain function. The ability to enjoy, perceive, sense, and experience life is dictated by the firing rate and health of your brain. It is impossible for a person to become healthy mentally or physiologically without a healthy brain.*
>
> DATIS KHARRAZIAN, D.H.SC., D.C., M.S., COURSE,
> "NEUROTRANSMITTERS AND THE BRAIN," PORTLAND, OREGON, 2008

Far and away, the people with the most damaged and intractably dysregulated brains and nervous systems I have seen or dealt with in my practice have all been vegans, with strict vegetarians a close second—*hands down.* I have numerous colleagues who have made the same independent observation. Anyone overly enchanted by the supposed findings of the book *The China Study: The Most Comprehensive Study of Nutrition Ever Conducted and the Startling Implications for Diet, Weight Loss and Long-Term Health*—by T. Colin Campbell, a vegetarian seeking to prove the superior healthfulness of a vegetarian diet—should read the exhaustively researched and objective analysis of those findings by researcher Denise Minger (http://rawfoodsos.com/2010/07/07/the-china-study-fact-or -fallac/). Her meticulous work is a research analysis masterpiece. It soundly puts the deeply flawed *China Study* to rest. Often, a diet of starch, sugar, lectins, phytates, and common allergens or sensitivity-generating foods is coupled with chronic problems, including deficiencies of numerous critical essential fats (EPA, DHA, healthy saturated fats), deficiencies of fat-soluble nutrients (preformed vitamins A, D$_3$, E-complex, and K$_2$), amino-acid imbalances, and deficiencies of other key animal-source nutrients, not the least of which is usable vitamin B$_{12}$ (and B$_{12}$ analogs from seaweed don't count). Such a diet, and its related deficiencies, leads to overarousal, anxiety-related disorders, memory problems, cognitive dysfunction, sleep disturbances, brain degeneration, neurological disorders, gastrointestinal disorders, and utter metabolic chaos. It is deeply problematic, and if maintained long enough, some of the damage may not even be reversible. These unnaturally restrictive diets, together with other carbohydrate-based low-fat diets, dysregulate insulin and leptin function to the extreme.

> Remember that the hormone leptin controls virtually all functions of the hypothalamus in the brain.
> That's a lot of control.

These issues concerning carbohydrate excesses, more than any others, underlie to some degree most of what I see as mood or behavioral issues, as well as a whole lot of other things, and play at least *some* role in all of them.

It is well established that elevated levels of insulin and leptin both generate and exacerbate sympathetic overarousal (the fight-or-flight mode). Surges of these hormones, driven mainly by chronic excess carbohydrate consumption, are both anxiety provoking and destabilizing to the nervous system. Diets lacking in adequate amounts of quality fat are further destabilizing. It is a vicious, often self-perpetuating cycle. Gluten sensitivity, and its far-reaching effects, is another overwhelmingly common concern. Neurofeedback can accomplish an incredible amount of progress with an individual all on its own, powerfully raising the internal stress threshold and training the person in self-regulation, but the combination of effective dietary measures with quality brain training is both synergistic *and* profound. I see this every day.

How We Get There in the First Place

Simply put, stress and trauma (whether physical, emotional, or biochemical) basically shove us off whatever cliff we happen to be standing next to. Wherever our vulnerability lies, in both our inherent makeup and our current state of health, that is the direction we go. The brain's timing mechanisms and phase relationships can become functionally deranged and help kindle certain tendencies at these points of vulnerability. Some people, when shoved, fall into a perpetual state of anxiety, others into depression, bipolar disorder, migraines, seizures, addiction, or some other condition. It's a long list. We are all individuals, and no two people respond exactly the same to any given stressor or trauma.

We see the world around us through the lens of our hormones, neurotransmitters, and, to the degree that we are dependent on it, our blood sugar. Unhealthy hormonal patterns generate unhealthy arousal patterns and, consequently, unhealthy emotional and behavioral tendencies. We wake up with low blood sugar due to insulin dysregulation and poor diet, and we feel lousy. We then proceed to interpret the lousy feeling through associating it with events and people in our lives, assuming they are to blame (and that life simply sucks) rather than recognizing that we are operating under distorted, biochemically induced misperceptions. We become hijacked by our dysregulated nervous system, behave in ways we abhor, and may even feel we are somehow fundamentally flawed as a person because of it. This is a *huge* source of self-esteem problems. We then continue to interpret the world around us through this warped lens and beat ourselves up (or blame others) for our own shortcomings.

At any given moment, we all have positive things and challenging things in our lives that we could be focused on as our reality. Why do we gravitate toward focusing on one thing versus another? *The functioning of our hormones, specifically insulin and leptin, to a very large extent influences the way we focus on and interpret the world around us and the events in our lives.* The secondary effects of blood sugar, insulin, and leptin dysregulation, which are a part of this, involve the disruption and depletion of neurotransmitter functioning. It is a huge issue, and it profoundly influences the way many people interpret and respond or react to their world. Is it any wonder that our society is in such a state of chaos?

Nothing will ever influence the functioning or dysfunctioning of your hormones or neurotransmitters (or your brain) more than the issue of blood sugar. Neurotransmitters are our main mood and brain regulators, and surges of blood sugar generate surges—and subsequent depletion or dysregulation—of the neurotransmitters serotonin, epinephrine, norepinephrine, GABA, and dopamine. Blood sugar surges also deplete B-complex vitamins, which are needed for the manufacture of neurotransmitters and a few hundred other things, and deplete magnesium, which is needed for parasympathetic (relaxed) functioning, liver detoxification, DHA synthesis, and another few hundred things.

Eating foods to which one is sensitive stimulates surges in cortisol or stress hormones, and subsequently in insulin as well as histamine, which acts as an excitatory neurotransmitter and can additionally agitate the nervous system. Insulin surges actually prevent the movement of L-tryptophan across the blood–brain barrier and block most all other neurotransmitter function. A brain that is dependent on glucose for its functioning will experience considerable compromise during these fluctuations, and moods, together with cognitive functioning, will tend to be unstable and at the mercy of blood sugar availability. A brain functioning instead on ketones, of course, would have no such vulnerability (though food sensitivities would still need to be monitored and deficiencies addressed).

Blood sugar surges stimulate accelerated glycation and an increase in the actions of insulin, leptin, inflammatory cytokines, and cortisol. These reactions collectively *contribute more than any other factors* to the degeneration of the brain and its functioning and are significantly disruptive to numerous bodily processes. The brain is enormously vulnerable to the glycating ravages (AGEs) of glucose, which induce aggressive oxidative processes, degrade its delicate structure, and diminish its functional capacity. Exposure to powerful antigens like gluten compounds also accelerates the damage. The more the brain degenerates, the more prone it becomes to chronic neurological sympathetic overarousal. The brain starts to lose its stress-mitigating capacity. Anxiety and anxiety-related disorders today are utterly epidemic.

By optimizing our dietary choices and our brain and minimizing our dependence on glucose for fuel, we alter the framework of our entire lives. It's about more than just staying healthy; it's about positively reshaping our internal experience toward what it truly means to be alive.

What could possibly be more important?

The Biology of Belief: The Real "Secret"

There is a great deal of attention being paid today to the new age concept that belief drives our reality, our biology, and our health. There is some real scientific validity to this, in fact, though forcing oneself to "think positive thoughts" while simultaneously suppressing or sublimating what one is actually feeling inside is not necessarily the fast track to better mental (or physical) health. If anything, it's likely to make things worse. Cultivating authenticity in one's experience of emotions is far healthier.

Very often the quality of our lives boils down to the quality of the questions we habitually ask ourselves, both consciously and unconsciously. Being more aware of this can make a big difference. Instead of asking Why do I always feel so lousy? make a point of asking yourself What can I do today—right now—to make myself feel healthier and happier? Your mind will *always* seek to answer any question you pose it. Ask a crappy question, and get a crappy answer. One type of question entrenches you in negativity and keeps you in a negative feedback loop; the other serves a far more constructive purpose. Take charge of your internal questions! If you're asking yourself Why does this always happen to me? your mind will probably answer you with something like Because you're such a loser (or something equally helpful). Remember: garbage in, garbage out. If you ask yourself a question that automatically inspires a **constructive** answer, then you've taken your first step toward self-mastery.

Fear, anger, and anxiety in the brain generate an erratic EEG (electrical brain signal pattern) along with a heart–mind incoherence pattern not at all compatible with intellectual processing or the higher-order thinking that one can associate with being functional in the world. Fear, anger, and anxiety effectively do away with clear thinking.

Choosing to focus on emotions such as compassion, appreciation, gratitude, empathy, and love (if, in fact, love can be relegated to so trivial and transient a thing as emotion) enhances healthy coherence, mental clarity, higher-order thinking, and expanded ability. Such higher-order thinking is also more directly associated with what are termed *anomolous human capabilities* and the extraordinary intuitive capacities studied by those dedicated to human potential research. The degree to which we can release (not simply sublimate) nonconstructive, self-limiting influences such as fear and anger and cultivate a focus on love, gratitude, and compassion is the degree to which we have greater access to our fullest resourcefulness and potential. This does not mean to deny possible dangers in our surroundings or to simply accept injustices, but rather to learn to confront them with greater clarity, coherence, and centered resourcefulness. The exhaustive body of research one can access through the Institute of HeartMath (www.HeartMath.org) shows conclusively the extraordinary benefit of cultivating heart–mind coherence, accessed through the highest human states of love, appreciation, gratitude, and compassion. This is not just "fuzzy-wuzzy new age thinking" here. Not by a *long* shot. The scientific evidence for this is overwhelming.

Additionally, learning to effectively release negative thoughts and feelings is actually much easier and more natural than trying to force positive thinking (check out *The Sedona Method* by Hale Dwoskin or go to www.sedona.com). By simply *letting go*—which is so simple it can seem difficult to some—you can instantly free yourself from a negative thought, belief, or habit, rather than trying to force positivity. When you release the negative (not simply suppress it), then what is left over is more naturally positive with a whole lot less effort. It can be as simple as unclenching and gently releasing a pebble from your hand. Try it; you might be surprised at just how easy it is.

"New age guilt" is rampant, but feeling somehow responsible for your own illness or tragedy in life and beating yourself up because you "harbored negative thoughts" is a pointless pastime. **If there is one single belief that people should cultivate, however, it's that we are ultimately responsible for our own health and that it is up to us to take this responsibility seriously and not simply entrust it to others who claim to have the answers but have their own agenda.** Let go of the pointless guilt and empower yourself with knowledge and positive action instead.

> No one will ever be more invested in your mental or physical health than you.

It has never been more important for us all to fundamentally understand how our body and mind work, and *it has never been more important to take our diet, mental state, and stress management seriously.* Take charge of your own mental, emotional, and physical health and recognize that anything is possible!

Given the appropriate raw materials (diet) and the removal of toxic burdens and unhealthy lifestyle factors, positive thinking and feeling becomes a *natural state* that doesn't need to be artificially cultivated. It simply flows.

It's our primal birthright.

25

How Important
Is Fat to the Brain?

■ ■ ■ ■ ■ ■ ■ ■ ■ ■ ■ ■

The brain is our single most expensive organ in the body, with respect to metabolic needs. It occupies only 5 percent of our total mass, but it uses at least 20–30 percent of our body's energy supply to meet its considerable demands. Many people assume that the brain needs glucose for this energy, but few are aware that the brain actually prefers ketones, the energy units of fat, for its dominant source of fuel!

The brain can and does use glucose, especially when a person consumes a diet that is dominated by carbohydrates or during an emergency, but glucose isn't as essential to the day-to-day functioning of the brain as is commonly presented and believed. In the absence of carbohydrates, once metabolically adapted, the brain will readily and naturally turn to ketones for its primary source of fuel.

The brain uses ketones in a state of ketosis. Cerebral ketone use is prevalent, for instance, in newborn infants nursing on fat-rich mother's milk. **The switch to dependence on glucose does not occur until carbohydrates are introduced into a child's diet.** The enzymes responsible for ketone metabolism, *d-beta-hydroxybutyrate dehydrogenase, acetoacetate-succinyl-CoA transferase,* and *acetoacetyl-CoA thiolase,* are present in brain tissue in sufficient amounts to convert ketones into acyl-CoA and to feed them into the tricarboxylic acid cycle at a sufficient rate to satisfy the metabolic demands of the brain (Siegell et al. 1999) Cerebral use of ketones is increased more or less in direct proportion to the degree of ketosis.

230

The body preferentially burns excess sugar whenever it is present, mainly to rid the body of this damaging substance any way it can. Sugar or glucose will also dominate as a source of brain fuel when turbocharged energy is in sudden demand, such as in an emergency. Sufficient carbohydrate stores in the form of glycogen in the liver are always available for this. No one ever needs to consume carbohydrates for glucose to be available to the brain or body when needed. Ever.

Depending entirely on glucose as a primary fuel for the brain and body is ultimately unnatural and problematic, in fact, but this is unfortunately the metabolic state in which the vast majority of people reside. Brain cells don't respond much to insulin and are therefore more vulnerable than just about any other tissue to the ravages of glycation and the oxidation or free-radical activity that glucose and glycation attract. There is no such thing as a safe, low level of glucose. Glucose and other sugars, such as fructose, *always* glycate and attract free-radical activity to some ongoing degree, no matter what. Although we need glucose to some extent for feeding our red blood cells, glucose is really what eventually kills many of us—a cruel irony. We do maintain some control over the rate of glycation and degeneration, though, through what we choose to eat and what supplements we take.

Glycation is the primary cause of brain degeneration in aging and also in Alzheimer's disease. (Alzheimer's disease is basically a state of brain neuropathy. Notice the sweet tooth in many patients with this condition.) Beta-amyloid proteins, or glycated tangles of proteins, clump and stick together in the brain and eventually cause the symptoms later identified as Alzheimer's disease. The same sort of damage that is done to the brain in alcoholism occurs at a slow but steady rate when a person consumes any form of a sugar- or starch-rich diet (even with so-called complex carbohydrates). Note that there are powerful associations with Alzheimer's disease and gluten sensitivity as well.

When the brain and body learn, instead, to burn ketones as their primary source of fuel, the brain is spared much of this damage and is fed with a far more sustainable, reliable, and abundant source of energy to meet its constant metabolic needs. One is far less subject to a "blood sugar low" and the mental, emotional, and physical symptoms associated with that state. Blood sugar is thus essentially eliminated from the mood and cognitive equation. The use of antiglycating nutrients can further protect from and help reverse, to at least some degree, these degenerative processes.

So, How Important
Is Fat to the Health of the Brain?

Immeasurably.

The brain is made up of more than 50 percent fat—up to 70–80 percent of its dry weight. In fact, the body's highest concentrations of omega-3 fatty acids are in the brain; up to one-quarter of the human brain's fatty acid stores are DHA, a component of omega-3 fatty acids commonly found in cold-water fish oils and meats of exclusively pasture-fed animals or wild game. Humans are unique among primates in this regard; the brains of chimps and other primates are dominated by omega-6 fatty acids. Omega-3 fatty acids, conversely, are entirely essential—vital—to the normal electrical functioning and the cardiovascular, joint, immune system, and gastrointestinal health of the human brain and nervous system. Omega-3 fatty acids are utterly vital for proper and efficient intercellular communication and anti-inflammatory processes. The consumption of usable carbohydrates and the presence of elevated levels of insulin, however, disrupt omega-3 metabolism and cause the body to lose magnesium, a mineral absolutely needed for the conversion of EPA to DHA, which is the storage molecule of omega-3 fatty acids in the brain and vital to all functions there. Insulin also tends to divert prostaglandin production to more proinflammatory omega-6 fatty acid pathways. It's also noteworthy that fully 50 percent of the fat found in the human brain is in the form of saturated fat, which is greatly needed for the protection and stabilization of the delicate, polyunsaturated omega-3 fatty acids. The brain also makes important use of arachidonic acid (which is much vilified). A variety of natural fats always work together to synergize and optimize functioning throughout the body and brain.

As much as 10 percent of human brain size has been lost in just the last century alone, likely as the result of decreased amounts of available dietary EPA and DHA and increased consumption of processed foods (Leonard et al. 2003).

Cholesterol, too, is downright critical for healthy brain function. Few people realize that the human body's richest repository for (eeeevil) cholesterol *lies in the brain.* The brain occupies only about 2 percent of the body's total mass, but it houses fully 25 percent of the body's total cholesterol! Cholesterol actually enhances signal transport and the functioning of the synapses of our brain cells and protects this bioelectrical signal from "leakage" in the myelin sheath. Cholesterol, functioning as an antioxidant, actually helps protect brain cells from oxidative damage and helps maintain the integrity of the delicate polyunsaturated fatty acids that compose it. Sufficient dietary and cellular cholesterol is critical for healthy cognitive and memory function. In fact, some of the more common side effects of statin drugs are impaired cognitive function and memory and even dementia-like symptoms!

The loss of magnesium through blood sugar surges, together with the absence of adequate dietary magnesium (or poor hydrochloric acid production and digestion), allows for the binding of structurally related but toxic elements, such as aluminum, to vacant receptor sites in the brain. Elevated aluminum levels in the brain, of course, have also been associated with Alzheimer's disease. Magnesium, in addition, controls over three hundred enzymes in the body and mind. It is critical for maintaining healthy parasympathetic functioning, which produces a calm, relaxed nervous system, and is commonly deficient in people consuming a high-carbohydrate diet.

Omega-3 fatty acids may be the single most commonly deficient nutrient in the modern human—particularly Western—diet. Supplementation with fish oils today provides the most reliable and affordable source of both EPA and DHA, which are omega-3 fatty acids' most important derivatives. Antarctic krill oil is another source of EPA and DHA, and it is potentially even more highly effective, though much more expensive. Antarctic krill oil contains unique phospholipids and antioxidants, which are not present in fish oil, that may better facilitate its absorption, preservation, and use, and it can be a viable alternative to fish oil for some people who are willing to pay significantly more. Our ancestors got preformed EPA and DHA by consuming large quantities of naturally and exclusively grass-fed wild game and organ meats and wild-caught, cold-water fish, where available.

Overcooking rapidly denatures and destroys these oils, as they are highly polyunsaturated. Deficiencies of omega-3 fatty acids are often particularly pronounced in people with depression, insulin resistance, obesity, bipolar disorder, cardiovascular disease, and ADD/ADHD, and supplementation has been shown at times to markedly benefit people with these conditions. *Fish oils are overwhelmingly preferable to flax oil,* as many individuals with learning disabilities and other mental, emotional, and cognitive disorders are known to lack the delta-6 desaturase enzyme necessary to create EPA and DHA from the parent form of omega-3 in vegetable sources, ALA. A mere 3–5 percent or less of the available ALA (in flax oil, walnuts, and similar sources) ever makes it to becoming EPA. Even less becomes the brain's vitally needed DHA (Enig 2001).

It is also known that trans fats in the body interfere with the prostaglandin metabolic pathway, as do magnesium deficiencies and excess amounts of omega-6 fatty acids (e.g., corn oil, sunflower oil, safflower oil), which compete for delta-6-desaturase enzymes biochemically.

The overconsumption of vegetable oils such as soy and canola, which are nearly always partially hydrogenated; safflower, sunflower, and corn oils (omega-6 fatty acids); cottonseed oil, which is extremely high in proinflammatory omega-6 fatty acids and not even a food-source oil; margarines and vegetable shortenings, which contain hydrogenated trans fats; and even excess olive oil (omega-9 fatty acids) can interfere with the body's use of omega-3 fatty acids. These vegetable oils can exacerbate insulin resistance, leading to obesity, atherosclerosis, and other conditions, and when overly processed or rancid can cause mutagenic changes, leading to numerous cancers. With the exception of olive oil, most vegetable oils are best avoided entirely. Olive oil is okay for salads, over steamed vegetables, and as an accent to various dishes, though I don't advise overusing it or actually cooking with it as it can easily become rancid when exposed to higher heat.

Hydrogenated and partially hydrogenated fats should never be used at all. Ever. Don't be fooled by claims of reduced trans fats in fast foods or processed food items or by packaging that claims it contains zero trans fat, then lists soybean oil, regular, nonorganic canola oil, or any other partially hydrogenated ingredient. Labeling laws currently allow a certain amount of trans fat per serving before it has to be disclosed. The food industry takes advantage of labeling loopholes everywhere it can. The more one can simply avoid processed or packaged products, the better.

The only safe amount of trans fat is zero.

Naturally occurring saturated fat and cholesterol do not compete with omega-3 fatty acids and, in fact, are mutually beneficial physiologically. In addition, saturated fat and cholesterol, unjustly vilified, provide both cell membrane integrity and *resistance to oxidation,* and make up at least 50 percent of cell membranes. Fully half of the fat in the human brain is saturated, in fact (Enig 2001). Naturally occurring saturated fat also assists in the absorption of vital nutrients; plays a vital role in bone

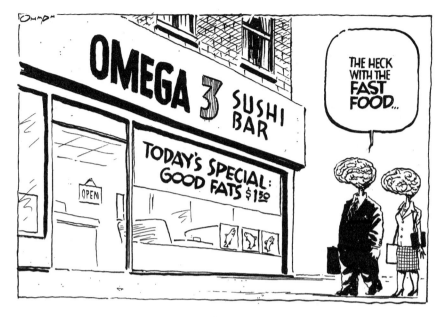

Fig. 25.1. Good fats lunch special

modeling; lowers the levels of lipoprotein(a), which is a marker for heart disease; protects the liver from alcohol ingestion; enhances the immune system, is needed for the proper use of essential fatty acids; and is used for energy production, normal hormonal production, and normal cellular metabolism. Shorter-chain saturated fatty acids (three to fourteen carbons in length) have potent antimicrobial and antiviral properties as well (Enig 2001).

> *It would seem that our glands effect control far above proportion to their size, and this is true. It is also true, however, that the glands have their master, probably the most remarkable creation in all of life's miracles—the human brain.*
>
> BERNARD JENSEN, PH.D.

26

Where Does ADD/ADHD Fit In to All of This?

■■■■■■■■■■■■

There is some inexplicably lingering, weak debate among scientists as to the effects of dietary sugar and carbohydrates on behavior in children. But sugar—and some other high-glycemic foods as well as artificial counterparts such as aspartame (Nutrasweet) and sucralose (Splenda)—enters the bloodstream quickly and has commonly been reported to induce hyperactivity and other behavioral problems in children. Gluten sensitivity is another epidemic problem generating behavioral difficulties, mood disturbances, and cognitive dysfunction in children and adults alike.

Other high-glycemic and insulin-generating foods, in addition to simple or refined sugars, include such things as pasta, breads (gluten-containing whole grain or otherwise), rice, and potatoes and other starchy vegetables. The consumption of high-glycemic foods, which cause a rapid rise in blood sugar, can trigger many behavioral, learning, and mood problems. When a child or adult is glucose dependent and does not eat frequently enough, eats foods to which he or she may be sensitive or allergic, or has a diet that is high in carbohydrate-rich foods, blood sugar levels can rise and drop dramatically. To pull these levels back to normal, the body releases adrenaline. Adrenaline triggers sympathetic nervous system activity: basically the fight-or-flight response. *It can be good to have high adrenaline levels if one's life is in immediate danger (that's what adrenaline is for), but it is extremely difficult to sit, listen, and behave when adrenaline release occurs while in the classroom* (Block 1997).

Avoiding excess carbohydrates is obviously key, as is the regular consumption of protein- and fat-rich foods throughout the day. Protein and fat consumption normalizes blood sugar levels and also provides a vital source of amino acids and other key fat-soluble nutrients that are needed for normal and stable neurological functioning.

Essential fatty acids, particularly in the form of omega-3 fatty acids, are known to be widely deficient in the modern diet and especially in people who manifest cognitive or affective disorders, ADD, and other learning disabilities.

The ultraprevalent trans fats found in most processed cereals, salad dressings, condiments, snacks, commercial vegetable oils, breads, and fast foods in many cases constitute up to 20 percent of our daily caloric intake. And they interfere with the absorption and use of all essential fatty acids and lead to additional cognitive impairment, inflammation, and disease. *Elimination of these unnatural fats from the diet is essential.* The elimination of these substances from the body once they are ingested and incorporated into one's cellular structure, however, may take time—*up to two years* (Enig 2001).

Read all labels carefully. When in restaurants, always ask what fats are being used in cooking and salad dressings. Restaurant owners need to be made aware that this stuff matters, too!

Among other foods commonly reported to cause problems are conventionally produced milk, chicken eggs, chocolate, soy, gluten-containing grains, corn, and peanuts. Also included as problematic are preservatives, artificial colors, pesticides, and other synthetic compounds found in processed foods. A Paleolithic-oriented diet would be naturally free (mostly) of such dietary inclusions. All of these foods can be considered fairly recent (i.e., ten thousand years ago or less) additions to the human diet. The one food sensitivity most commonly associated with ADHD is overwhelmingly gluten—the granddaddy of them all. Some researchers estimate that 70–80 percent of all people with ADHD are gluten sensitive, with many people's conditions commonly advanced to celiac disease. A study reported in the *Journal of Attention Disorders* stated in conclusion, "The data indicate that ADHD-like symptomology is markedly overrepresented among untreated Celiac Disease (CD) patients and that a gluten-free diet may improve symptoms significantly within a short period of time. The results of this study also suggest that celiac disease should be included in the list of diseases associated with

ADHD-like symptomology" (Niederhofer and Pittschieler 2006).

Also, the same article stated, "All ADHD patients or their parents report a significant improvement in their behavior and functioning after 6 months on a gluten-free diet." Take special note of the word *all* in this last sentence! Celiac disease and gluten sensitivity impact frontal and prefrontal lobe perfusion in the brain, affecting the part of our brain that is needed for planning, short-term memory, focus, and higher functioning.

In another study, it was found that "the presence of regional cerebral blood flow alteration in celiac disease (gluten sensitivity) patients could play a pathogenic role in psychiatric and neurologic manifestations, including the more common problems such as migraine headache and learning disabilities" (Abenavoli et al. 2004).

Elevated levels of an enzyme called *zonulin* have recently been found in individuals with ADHD as well as in people with autism, multiple sclerosis, and numerous psychiatric disorders. Zonulin is known to regulate intestinal permeability and is known to be associated with gluten sensitivity, including celiac disease. Tissue samples from patients with symptomatic celiac disease had higher levels of zonulin and antizonulin antibodies than samples from either patients on gluten-free diets or people without the disease. "People with celiac have an increased level of zonulin, which opens the junctions between the cells. In essence, the gateways are stuck open, allowing gluten and other allergens to pass [through]," wrote Alessio Fasano, professor of pediatrics and physiology at the University of Maryland School of Medicine. "Once these allergens get into the immune system, they are attacked by the antibodies" (Fasano 2000).

Researchers believe that the higher levels of zonulin may explain how a molecule as large as gluten can cross the intestinal wall and incite the creation of antibodies. Zonulin also helps regulate the permeability of the blood–brain barrier and could be a factor in other food sensitivities, neurodegeneration, and autoimmune diseases. The implications of this are very serious, and the problem can be remedied *only* by strict adherence to a 100 percent gluten-free diet. One can test for gluten sensitivity, as well as sensitivity to casein, soy, and eggs, using a proprietary stool antigen test anyone can order from EnteroLab (www.enterolab.com). Cyrex Labs offers the most accurate gluten sensitivity testing available anywhere with its own proprietary arrays. Ask your health care provider about this testing.

In an open study of seventy-eight children with ADHD who were referred to a nutrition clinic, fifty-nine improved on a few food trials that eliminated foods to which children are commonly sensitive; for the nineteen children in the study who were able to participate in a double-blind, cross-over trial of the suspected food, there was a significant effect for the provoking foods to worsen the ratings of behavior and to impair the psychological test performance (Kemper 2007). It's not all kids, either.

Another study stated, "Cognitive functional decline and underachievment in post-secondary education is 400% more likely with Gluten Sensitivity" (Verkasalo 2005). In this intriguing study, 2,427 subjects aged twenty-four to thirty-nine were followed, beginning in adolescence for twenty-one years. The author wrote, "The subjects with silent celiac disease did not differ from the rest of the cohort in age, gender, stature, weight, medical diagnoses (autoimmune, malignant), health concerns, use of alternative medications, physical activity, or their parents' cause of death. Fewer Celiac subjects had a university or college degree (5.3% vs. 22.8%). Fewer Celiac subjects worked in managerial or professional positions (28% vs. 45%). Employment rate, as well as occupational classification and socioeconomic status, suggested a uniform tendency to underachievement by the sCD (silent Celiac Disease) subjects. In children and adolescents with sCD, we found a significant increase in disruptive behavioral and depressive disorders. The underachievement in education and working life observed in subjects with silent CD is a new and intriguing finding. It may be related to the increased prevalence of disruptive and depressive behavioral disorders described in teenagers with untreated CD."

In yet another study, reported in the *Journal of Attention Disorders,* the authors wrote, "All ADHD-like symptomology patients should be tested for CD with serum screening tests, as CD could be one of the causes of these neuropsychiatric symptoms. We are convinced that untreated CD may predispose to important mental and behavioral disorders" (Niederhofer and Pittschieler 2006).

Food sensitivies—and especially gluten sensitivity—must always be considered when addressing ADHD or any other form of cognitive or learning disability.

Note: Do **not** rely on the results of allergy tests or standard blood or salivary tests that tell you that you don't have a gluten problem and assume everything is okay—*please.* False-negative results in blood, regular salivary, and conventional antigen tests are rampant for a wide variety of reasons. For just one out of many examples, there are **twelve** different fractions of gliadin, and the **only one** routinely tested for is *alpha-gliadin*. **If** you do happen to get a **positive** result on one of these tests, however, you can take that to the bank. Also, don't be lulled into some sort of complacency if a certain test tells you that your sensitivity to gluten or gliadin is "only mild." Immune system imbalances of TH-1 and TH-2, which can be quite common (especially among people with autoimmune issues), routinely impair immunoglobulin responses in antigen tests. And many people under chronic stress (know anyone like that?) have impaired or nonexistent IgA production, which results in false-negatives in routine stool and saliva analyses. Also, note that no currently available test is entirely foolproof, but newer testing through Cyrex Labs is as accurate as it gets. EnteroLab's proprietary stool antigen test is more accurate than available blood tests and can be ordered by anyone.

It's not a matter of degree of gluten sensitivity, any more than it can be a matter of being a certain degree pregnant. You either are or you're not. If you are, then take this very, very seriously. If you're not, don't assume you're out of the woods. Zonulin increases whenever *anyone* eats gluten, not just those sensistive to it. **If in doubt, eliminate gluten altogether.** You simply can't go wrong with that.

Other Dietary Considerations

Supplementation with fish oils in small quantities—only 1–2 percent of caloric intake—not only enhances the functioning of the brain and nervous system as well as the cardiovascular and immune systems, but also tends to help eliminate unhealthy cravings for sweets once adequate levels of protein and essential fatty acids are replenished.

Remember: **If EPA and DHA aren't in your diet, then they're not in your brain!** It is also critical to note that saturated fat is an essential factor in the protection, transportation, and use of these important and fragile oils and should not be overly restricted in the diet, particularly in children. Cholesterol, too, is utterly vital to the neurological functioning of children and adults alike.

B-complex vitamins, in general, are especially important for cognitive functioning and are readily depleted with carbohydrate consumption. Methyl donors such as B_6, B_{12}, and folic acid, as well as betaine, s-adenosyl methionine (SAMe), dimethylglycine (DMG), and trimethylglycine (TMG), are especially important for healthy brain function and metabolism. Regular use of a sublingual methylcobalamin vitamin B_{12} supplement can be especially helpful in this regard. Vitamin B_{12} may be less well absorbed from food, or even in pill or capsule form, by many people with compromised digestion. There is no toxicity associated with vitamin B_{12} at any dosage. It is far better to err on the side of supplementing with more than less. Vitamin B_{12} deficiency is becoming increasingly common, even among meat eaters. Regular supplementation with a sublingual form is good and inexpensive insurance.

A more recently recognized and tragically overlooked factor in many cases of ADHD involves **iodine deficiency.** Iodine is needed and used by each and every cell in the body. It can make for a night-and-day difference in many cases of ADHD and is a likely deficiency in many cases of the disorder. It is also needed for the proper functioning of each and every single hormone, to say nothing of normal thyroid function. The absence of iodine in most of our soils and foods today is only part of the problem. Iodized salt (containing iodide and not elemental iodine—only half the necessary form of total iodine for optimal functioning), which is useful mainly for minimizing the incidence of goiters (and is typically filled with undesirable additives, including aluminum), is of little use in providing sufficient tissue levels of **both** forms of iodine needed in the body for optimal functioning (Brownstein 2008).

One study reported in *The Journal of Clinical Endocrinology and Metabolism* in December 2004 followed sixteen women who were living in an iodine-deficient area and eleven other women who were living in an area that was known to be iodine sufficient. At the ten-year follow-up, ADHD had been diagnosed in eleven of the sixteen women in the iodine-deficient area compared with none of the eleven in the iodine-sufficient area. Also, the women's IQ was at least ten points lower in the iodine-deficient area (Vermiglio et al. 2004).

The rampant and ubiquitous overuse of halogens (a family of related elements in the periodic table) such as bromine/bromide, chlorine/chloride, and fluorine/fluoride in processed foods, medications, processed vegetable oils, bread, pastas, cereals, pesticides, drinking water, and innumerable other daily household items adds dramatically to this problem by displacing iodine in our body and brain and preventing its absorption. The result to our brain and metabolic functioning is insidiously devastating. The process of restoring healthy iodine levels can take several months or even years for some people, and it should be well and carefully understood. High doses of iodine, particularly when improperly administered, can induce uncomfortable detoxification reactions as the iodine displaces toxic halogens and heavy metals such as mercury, aluminum, and arsenic. A cautious and gradual building up of the iodine dosage in a proper and readily usable form is very important.

It's important to note that improperly applied iodine supplementation can worsen symptoms and accelerate glandular destruction in people with diagnosed (or undiagnosed) autoimmune thyroid disorders (e.g., Hashimoto's disease). It is critical that individuals be carefully screened for thyroid peroxidase antibodies, antithyroglobulin antibodies and autoimmune thyroid issues prior to any iodine supplementation. **If you happen to be positive for Hashimoto's disease, then it's imperative that you avoid iodine supplementation altogether.** Small amounts of naturally occurring iodine in foods are okay in these cases; just don't supplement. Note that **80 percent or more of cases of low-functioning thyroid are autoimmune related in nature,** whether diagnosed or undiagnosed. And 100 percent of cases of hyperfunctioning thyroids are autoimmune in nature. If in doubt, then test, and avoid iodine supplementation until you know the results.

For people who are able to supplement with iodine, certain nutrients such as magnesium, selenium, vitamins E, A, and D, and B-complex and C-complex vitamins, together with supplementation of full-spectrum (Celtic) sea salt and essential fatty acids, are essential to iodine absorbing well and its being used properly in the body. The details are beyond the scope of this book but need to be considered. In the meantime, be sure to include seafood, seaweed, or kelp as part of your daily diet, as they are among the only reliable food sources of iodine. Kelp and seafood sources tend to be safe and well tolerated by most people. Additional iodine supplementation (beyond simply food sources) can be essential for many people, and I encourage you to seek out a qualified and knowledgeable natural health care provider to guide you through the process of restoring healthy iodine levels. The difference that appropriate iodine status can make is nothing short of miraculous for people who are deficient (according to Dr. David Brownstein, more than 96 percent of people in the United States), and it is well worth the pursuit.

Important note: Iodine is needed for the proper metabolism and use of dietary cholesterol. Diets higher in cholesterol thereby do use and require slightly more iodine.

ADD/ADHD, Learning Problems, Behavioral or Mood Disorders, and the Omega-3 Fatty Acids Connection

A Purdue University study showed that kids who are low in essential omega-3 fatty acids are significantly more likely to be hyperactive, have learning disorders, and display behavioral problems. Deficiencies in omega-3 fatty acids have also been tied to dyslexia, violence, depression, memory problems, weight gain, cancer, heart disease, eczema, allergies, inflammatory diseases, arthritis, diabetes, and many other conditions.

Over two thousand scientific studies have demonstrated the wide range of problems associated with omega-3 fatty acid deficiencies. The American diet is almost devoid of omega-3 fatty acids except for certain types of fish. In fact, researchers believe that about 60 percent of Americans are deficient in omega-3 fatty acids and that about 20 percent have so little that test methods cannot detect any at all in their blood (Gallagher).

Unfortunately, a significant contributor to the growing trend in these problems, even in very young children, is *prenatal nutrition*. Children are being born with essential fatty acid deficiencies at an alarming rate. Furthermore, no infant formula supplies adequate EPA or DHA, fats that are critical to the development of the infant nervous system. Worse yet, soy infant formulas containing phytic acid, trypsin inhibitors, and hemagglutinins—not to mention phytoestrogens impacting normal hormonal development—contribute to mineral deficiencies, impacting normal growth and neurological development.

When what little EPA and DHA that expectant mothers may have is drained away during pregnancy, postpartum depression is the result. *Expectant mothers have a dramatically increased requirement for EPA and DHA* and should supplement these fats in the form of molecularly distilled sources of fish oil as well as with a little cod-liver oil to supply critical and commonly deficient fat-soluble nutrients. (Vitamin A is only potentially deleterious during pregnancy in its synthetic forms.)

Trans fats, excessive amounts of carbohydrates, processed foods, and too many omega-6 fatty acids in children's diets serve only to severely exacerbate the situation and compound learning and behavioral problems. Diets moderately high in quality (read: q-u-a-l-i-t-y) animal-source protein (not fast-food burgers and feedlot meat) and sources of omega-3 fatty acids (from cold-water fish, fish oils, and grass-fed meats) are unquestionably vital to a developing young mind and body—and, indeed, to healthy cognitive and physiological functioning at any age.

Memory—*Husker Du?*

Among the most critical of faculties allowing us to function effectively day to day is basic memory. Memory problems are one of the most common complaints I see and one of the most challenging issues people struggle with. Memory loss is often the result of a progressive degeneration of the brain due to stress, excess cortisol, food sensitivities, glycation, low-fat and low-cholesterol diets, statin use, or environmental factors, and it is something to be taken very seriously. Certain nutritional deficiencies can also generate or exacerbate this problem.

Perhaps the single most common factor impacting memory function is stress. Our ancestors could never have imagined the degree and sheer volume of chronic stressors on every level most of us experience today. We simply weren't designed for this. Cortisol receptors in the hippocampus (the part of our brain directly over our ears) become oversaturated with this stress hormone and can prompt this part of the brain to start to degenerate. It is no laughing matter when you increasingly forget your words in the middle of a sentence, forget to do everyday things, or forget the name of your best friend.

Deficiencies of important fat-soluble nutrients, B vitamins (particularly methylcobalamin B12), iodine, zinc, essential fatty acids, and other nutrients take their toll and can accelerate the decline. Chronic sugar or starch consumption is perhaps the single best way to accelerate the problem. Food sensitivities (e.g., gluten, casein, and others) can set up a vicious, never-ending inflammatory response that can degenerate the brain at a record pace, even causing brain lesions visible on brain scans. Sufficient restorative sleep is also a major factor in day-to-day brain function.

Pay attention!

Is your memory "not what it used to be"? Please don't ignore the signs. The sooner you take steps to remove antagonistic dietary culprits, replenish depleted nutrients, address sleep issues, and support healthy regeneration of viable brain tissue, the more likely you are to stop and maybe even partly reverse the deterioration of your memory *plus* improve the quality of the functioning of your mind and your experience of life.

So what are some key steps to reclaiming or greatly improving your memory and restoring the health of your brain?

1. Practice stress reduction daily using whatever tools or methods work best for you: meditation, yoga, neurofeedback or biofeedback, heart-rate variability training, proper breathing exercises, massage, walking in fresh air—anything. This is not a luxury. It is a necessity.

2. Get six to eight hours of restful sleep each and every single night in a completely dark room.

3. Keep your brain active doing puzzles or simply learning new things. The more you learn, the better you learn! Advanced Brain Technologies sells an inexpensive and well-researched program known as Brain Builder, which is computer software designed to exercise memory and processing skills. It is superb.

4. Minimize—or better yet, eliminate—sugar and starch from your diet.

5. Make sure you have adequate levels of essential fatty acids, such as EPA and DHA (fish oil) and GLA (black currant seed oil), in your diet and avoid low-fat and low-cholesterol regimens like the plague.

6. Make sure you are properly hydrated. Take your body weight (in pounds) and divide by two; this is about the number of ounces of water that your body needs for proper hydration daily. If you drink caffeine, juice, or any other diuretic beverage, you should add more water (12–16 ounces for every 8 ounces of diuretic beverage). Don't exceed a gallon of water (128 ounces) per day.

7. Be sure to test for common food sensitivities—particularly gluten and casein—and eliminate foods containing these substances as completely as possible if they are an issue to prevent further damage to your brain and body. If in doubt, test; see www.enterolab.com or www.cyrexlabs.com.

8. Take a quality phosphorylated or whole food–based B-complex vitamin with meals.

9. Minimize the use of cell phones and cordless phones. Scientific evidence is mounting almost exponentially showing evidence of significant brain damage and increased risk for brain lesions and cancers from such use. If you have to use a cell phone, always use

the speakerphone option and keep it at least six inches from your head. Headsets (including Bluetooth) can actually make the damage worse. Air-tube headsets and ferrite beads both work well to help minimize exposure during use.

10. Supplement additionally with *sublingual* vitamin B₁₂ in the form of methylcobalamin. It is a key methyl donor in the brain and essential to nervous system health and functioning. Many find it quite mentally energizing. There are some quality vitamin B₁₂ oral sprays using cyanocobalamin that work well too. Vitamin B₁₂ is notoriously (and dangerously) deficient in vegetarians and vegans, but increasingly, many meat eaters are also developing vitamin B₁₂ deficiencies due to digestive impairment or loss of intrinsic factor. Long-term deficiency can result in irreversible neurological damage, anemia, memory issues, serious mood and cognitive dysfunction, and even dementia-like symptoms. Supplementation is always the safest insurance.

11. Omega-3 fish oil is standard issue for better brain function and cognition, overall. The most abundant fatty acid in the human brain is DHA, but if it isn't in your diet, it isn't in your brain either! This one is critical and supplementation should be considered for optimal brain function.

12. Supplementing with other methyl donors may also be useful, such as S-adenosyl methionine (SAMe), dimethylglycine (DMG), trimethylglycine (TMG), betaine, choline, B₆, and folic acid.

13. Use phosphatidyl serine to help reverse mild brain degeneration and also to help produce more choline endogenously. Research studies showing significant improvement typically used 800 to 2,000 mg of phosphatidyl serine per day. Phosphatidyl serine also has been shown to improve memory, focus, and concentration. In the research studies, phosphatidyl serine was conjugated with DHA (from fish oils) to optimize its use, which most available oral phosphatidyl serine supplements are not. Transdermal phosphatidyl serine delivery creams (such as AdrenaCalm by Apex Energetics) may be much more practical and cost effective than oral preparations and seem to yield very positive results.

14. Precursors to acetylcholine, an important memory and cognition neurotransmitter, can also be extremely useful to supplement with. The best sources are L-alpha glycerophosphorylcholine (or

alpha-GPC) and dimethylaminoethanol (or DMAE). The effects are typically quite noticeable.

15. L-carnosine may be the single best protectant against glycation of brain tissue, as well as being a potent antioxidant. It has also shown significant benefits in people with autism. Found mainly in meat, L-carnosine tends to be deficient in vegetarian diets.

16. The glutathione precursors L-cysteine or N-acetyl cysteine (NAC), S-adenosyl methionine (SAMe), and transdermal glutathione creams (such as OxiCell and Super OxiCell by Apex Energetics) may improve levels of this critical antioxidant and anti-inflammatory substance.

17. Benfotiamine is a fat-soluble source of vitamin B_1 that provides additional protection against glycation reactions while guarding cells against the toxic effects of chronic glucose exposure. Even people with normal glucose levels encounter damaging sugar reactions over a lifetime and may benefit from some supplementation.

18. Vinpocetine is a phytonutrient that has been shown to improve memory, concentration, cognition, and cerebral circulation and has other protective effects as well.

19. Huperzine-A is a plant-based sesquiterpene alkaloid compound that helps to increase levels of acetylcholine in the brain. It functions as an acetylcholinesterase inhibitor and N-methyl-D-aspartic acid (also called NMDA) receptor antagonist (protecting the brain against glutamate- or MSG-induced damage) and has been used as a potentially effective treatment for people with Alzheimer's disease.

There are other potentially helpful supplements and techniques for improving memory, but the above list covers some of the more-important and better-researched approaches. **Please don't feel as though you have to supplement with all of this,** but do consider following at least the basic dietary and lifestyle suggestions. They go a long way toward making a real difference!

Mineral Deficiencies and Learning, Emotional, and Behavioral Disorders

The second-most common of all modern nutritional deficiencies involves **trace elements.** Needed in only the minutest quantities in the human body, trace elements are vital to the health of our brain and nervous system as well as every other organ and function. Modern, conventional agricultural practices have succeeded in depleting our soils of trace elements, and the use of pesticides can block their uptake in many plants. High regional rainfall amounts can also dramatically affect soil composition and result in mineral-deficient soils in many areas.

More than seventy trace elements have been identified, though comparatively few are as yet recognized as essential for health. Getting them in broad-spectrum form ensures that you aren't missing anything that science just hasn't gotten around to discovering the value of yet. Among the few reliable sources of broad-spectrum trace elements needed for optimal health are ocean-source seafoods, unrefined and mineral-rich Celtic or Himalayan sea salt (vastly more flavorful and healthful than conventional, refined table salt), and supplements such as ConcenTrace Trace Mineral Drops by Trace Minerals Research, which is relatively inexpensive, of high quality, and widely available.

Please avoid the use of what are called colloidal minerals, popularized some years ago by a veterinarian named Dr. Joel Wallach. They contain often dangerous levels of aluminum and other toxic heavy metals and should always be avoided (Schauss 1997). They are also quite expensive. Note that this is not referring to colloidal silver (used as an antimicrobial agent), which falls into a different category.

The consumption of organic, biodynamically grown vegetables is also very helpful, though the mineral composition of these foods *is wholly dependent on the composition of the soil in which they were grown.* Minerals are, in fact, best absorbed and used from animal or seafood sources through ionization by hydrochloric acid and natural amino-acid chelation. *Adequate levels of hydrochloric acid, in addition to dietary fat and fat-soluble nutrients, are needed to facilitate their absorption.*

Among the trace minerals, zinc deficiency is one most commonly associated with learning disabilities, ADD/ADHD, cognitive dysfunction, emotional lability, delinquent behaviors, and eating disorders. Zinc is also critical for immunity and healthy digestive function; it is found predominantly in animal-source foods and is commonly deficient in people who have depression. Consuming significant amounts of soy, in particular, as well as large amounts of grains or legumes (due to their phytic acid), is known to cause zinc deficiencies.

Among other common causes of zinc deficiency are inadequate protein intake from meat and seafood, which possess the richest natural sources, inadequate hydrochloric acid production, chronic stress, eating disorders, chronic infection, and a little-known genetic metabolic condition known as pyroluria (see appendix F). Supplementation with zinc sulfate in solution or ultra-bioavailable ionic zinc may be necessary, along with increased consumption of zinc-rich foods to remediate deficiency states; in tandem with other cofactors and nutrients, this can significantly improve ADD/ADHD symptoms. Tablets and capsules of zinc are less efficiently absorbed by those people who are most deficient. Also, be careful not to oversupplement with copper by taking zinc supplements that have added copper in them. If you are zinc deficient, it is probably better to take zinc as an isolated supplement. A simple, quick, and inexpensive *zinc tally test* (a taste test using a zinc sulfate solution), offered by most natural health care providers, can quickly, inexpensively, and fairly reliably determine the presence of zinc deficiency.

Note, too, that zinc deficiency (like any other mineral deficiency) essentially creates a vacuum that also attracts structurally similar but highly toxic elements. In the case of zinc deficiency, this means cadmium (part of all carcinogenic processes) and mercury, which seek to replace zinc at its vacant receptor sites—a very real problem. **One of the best preventives of heavy metal toxicity is healthy mineral sufficiency!**

Zinc and copper are two minerals that work together but require certain ratios to work optimally in the human body. Zinc needs to be in about an 8:1 or 12:1 ratio with copper for optimal neurological and physiological functioning. When the diet becomes deficient in zinc, or when the body loses large amounts of zinc to stress, which can *triple* its rate of excretion from the body, or in the case of diets high in phytic acid (found in soy, other legumes, and grain products), the ratio moves closer to 1:1. This can result in copper toxicity, which manifests as the aforementioned zinc deficiency symptoms such as learning disabilities, ADD/ADHD, cognitive dysfunction, emotional lability, and delinquent behaviors (Schauss 1997).

Zinc supplementation may be necessary in some cases where stress, deficiency, or dietary inhibitors (i.e., phytic acid in grains, legumes, and soy) have been prevalent for extended periods of time. Zinc monomethionine is available in a pill form that is preferable to many other pill forms and is commonly and inexpensively found in health food stores, though liquid ionic forms and zinc sulfate in liquid solution are far superior for absorption and bioavailability. Liquid ionic forms (with no added copper) are best used in markedly deficient states. Safe doses for zinc are 50 mg for highly bioavailable forms and 100 mg for low bioavailable forms in average individuals. Ionic zinc tends to be effective at even lower daily doses. Individual needs may vary widely. Although the RDAs for this nutrient are much lower—only 15 mg for men aged eleven and older and 12 mg for nonpregnant and nonlactating women, for instance—much higher doses may be needed for a time to treat deficiency or specific conditions. People with pyroluria (see appendix F) may require much higher than average levels of zinc supplementation. The average Paleolithic daily intake was probably close to about 50 mg. *Note:* Zinc toxicity is rare in humans. Individuals on vegetarian, vegan, or high soy-food diets may be especially vulnerable to zinc deficiency.

Sources in Food

The best dietary sources of zinc are foods of animal origin. Excellent sources include oysters, herring, meat, and egg yolks. Adding as little as 3 ounces of extra-lean beef daily (again, please, from organic, solely grass-fed, and free-range sources) can significantly improve zinc status, as long as there is sufficient hydrochloric acid to digest and ionize it. Zinc in commonly cited natural sources such as pumpkin seeds tends to have poor bioavailability because of the presence of phytic acid and the need for proper ionization (the presence of hydrochloric acid); soaking and sprouting these seeds can improve their digestibility, lower the amount of phytic acid, and improve zinc availability somewhat. Note again that it is possible to induce zinc deficiency through a diet rich in grains and legumes and particularly soy. Diets high in processed foods, particularly sugar, contribute significantly to deficiency. Zinc levels are also suppressed through acute and chronic infections, pernicious anemia, alcoholism, renal disease, cardiovascular disease, some malignancies, protein calorie malnutrition, and stress. Stress alone can more than triple one's rate of zinc excretion.

Iron and other mineral deficiencies are especially common worldwide where cereal grains make up a major portion of the diet and with vegetarian or vegan diets in general. Digestive impairment, autoimmune issues, and gluten sensitivities are all conditions where iron deficiency (and clinical or subclinical anemia) may be strongly suspect. In the past several years, researchers have found that iron deficiency is associated with often irreversible impairment of a child's learning ability, IQ, and behavior.

Although significant levels of *nonheme* iron exist in foods such as spinach and some legumes, it is poorly absorbed and used (roughly 1–5 percent). Vitamin C helps improve iron use from these foods somewhat. In contrast, red meat contains *heme* iron—the source most readily used by the human body. Iron from meat sources, particularly red meat, is not less than 20 percent bioavailable. The presence of heme iron in a meal also improves the absorbability from nonheme iron sources. The next-best sources are poultry and fish. It is always better to replenish iron via diet rather than supplementation as various toxicities and side effects are common with supplemental sources, particularly those such as the commonly prescribed ferrous sulfate.

Often simply improving hydrochloric acid production can be the single factor that makes a marked difference in mineral status. If you have to supplement with iron, please make it an organically derived, food-based, or amino acid–chelated form. Please avoid ferrous sulfate.

It is important to note that excesses of iron are also a problem for some people and may pose a greater threat than any other form of what is commonly termed *heavy-metal toxicity*. Iron can be a powerful free-radical producer and carcinogen. The most common sources of excess iron are cast-iron cookware, iron supplements, distilled alcohol, and baked goods from enriched flours—all of which are best avoided by everyone.

Also, however (and this is important), it is possible to have what appears to be an excessively high level of *serum* iron and even elevated ferritin while experiencing actual *intracellular* deficiencies, according to Dietrich Klinghardt, M.D., Ph.D. (Klinghardt 2008). This is most common where chronic infections (e.g., viral, bacterial, parasitic) are present, and these should be ruled out. The body will use iron and copper as oxidizing agents against viruses and other microbial agents. The elevated serum levels of these minerals reflect spent ammunition. Addressing the infection by taking high doses of C-complex vitamins or other reducing agents to help regenerate iron and support proper immune function, according to Klinghardt, can turn this situation around. If excess iron toxicity is truly determined to be the case, however, the best approach is simply to get rid of your excess iron-laden blood by donating it. This is faster, cheaper, and usually more effective than chelation methods.

Among the symptoms of iron deficiency and anemia are listlessness, pallor, fatigue, apathy, impaired IQ and cognitive function, and various behavioral disorders.

It's important to note that nothing else in your mental or physical health can possibly improve when any form of anemia is involved (whether it's related to deficiencies of iron, vitamins B12 or B6, or other nutrients) until that issue is resolved. **Anemia, when present, should be considered a first-order priority when addressing any health issues.** It's also important to point out that not all cases of anemia—even iron anemia—are the result of an actual iron deficiency! It is possible to have even excessive levels of serum iron and still be anemic when there is poor conversion to hemoglobin. Both sufficient hydrochloric acid production and amounts of vitamin B6 are essential for this conversion to take place. Improving digestion is always the most important place to start.

Although iron is commonly found in leafy greens such as spinach and in some legumes, it is very poorly absorbed from these sources. Red meat is the best available source, followed by poultry and fish. Deficiencies early in a person's development can often lead to irreversible damage to IQ, cognition, and immune function. Dietary replenishment is vastly preferable to supplemental approaches because of potential toxicities and side effects of commonly prescribed supplement forms, but improving digestion should usually come first.

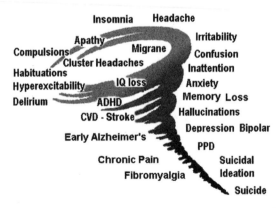

Fig. 26.1. Mental illnesses associated with increasingly severe neuronal magnesium deficiency

Magnesium insufficiency or deficiency is virtually epidemic and can be ill afforded by a society living with so many social, dietary, and environmental stressors. Sympathetic nervous system dominance was something we were designed to be engaged in during an emergency situation such as, say, being chased by a saber-toothed tiger. Today, the majority of Americans are being "chased by saber-toothed tigers" 24/7. We were designed to function in a dominantly parasympathetic state—a rarity today, indeed. Magnesium is critically important to the functioning of a healthy parasympathetic nervous system and of 325 or more enzymes in the body, and it is readily lost with the consumption of high-sugar and high-starch foods.

Magnesium has been consistently depleted in our soils. It has been further depleted in plants by the use of potassium- and phosphorus-laden fertilizers that alter the plants' ability to up-take magnesium. Water from deep wells supplies additional magnesium not found in food, but surface water, our common source, lacks magnesium. Food processing removes magnesium. Broiling, steaming, and boiling remove magnesium into the water or drippings. High-carbohydrate and excessively high-fat diets increase the need for magnesium, as does physical or mental stress. Diuretic medications and insulin further deplete total body levels of magnesium. As we age, magnesium uptake may be impaired. Dieting reduces the intake of already low levels of magnesium. Magnesium protects the cells from the adverse effects of aluminum, mercury, lead, cadmium, beryllium, and nickel. Evidence is mounting that low levels of magnesium contribute to the heavy-metal deposition in the brain that precedes Parkinson's disease, multiple sclerosis, and Alzheimer's disease. It is probable that low total body levels of magnesium contribute to heavy-metal toxicity in children and are one of the causes in the development of learning disorders (Sullivan at www.krispin.com/magnes.html).

Magnesium is one of the more overlooked and among the most depleted minerals in the modern diet. It is readily depleted by high-carbohydrate diets, and its deficiency can lead to high blood pressure, anxiety disorders, extreme and chronic muscle tension, impaired liver and brain function, cancer, and heart disease. Liver detoxification enzymes are magnesium dependent, and magnesium can help offset the toxicity of many ingested substances.

Optimal dosages for adults and children can vary considerably relative to dietary habits and whatever physical or mental demands, symptoms, or issues an individual has. On average, 2.5 to 4.5 mg of magnesium *per pound* of ideal body weight is likely sufficient for the average healthy individual. For best absorption, smaller doses at a time (100–200 mg), two or three times a day, are more optimal. Superior bioavailability can be found in forms such as ionic magnesium, magnesium glycinate, and transdermal magnesium sources such as "magnesium oil" and Epsom salt dissolved in bathwater. Add more supplemental magnesium if any items from the following list of disorders resulting from magnesium deficiency apply to you, since more may temporarily be needed to replenish a deficiency, or if you are particularly active or under extra stress. Cut back on supplementation if stools become too soft or loose. Ionic forms are better at avoiding this problem, as they are better at absorbing intracellularly, where it is most needed, and are less likely to be readily excreted by the colon.

As it stands, most individuals can likely benefit from some magnesium supplementation. Just remember that no nutrient functions in isolation in the body and be sure to eat foods that provide adequate minerals (including calcium) from other sources.

The following disorders are commonly associated with magnesium deficiency. (Other conditions are also associated with chronic and acute low-magnesium intake, and further research is continuing to confirm these relationships.)

- ADD/ADHD
- Alzheimer's disease
- angina
- anxiety disorders
- arrhythmia
- arthritis—rheumatoid and osteoarthritis
- asthma
- autism
- autoimmune disorders—all types
- cavities
- cerebral palsy—in children from magnesium-deficient mothers
- chronic fatigue syndrome
- congestive heart disease
- constipation
- crooked teeth or narrow jaw—in children from magnesium-deficient mothers
- depression
- diabetes—types 1 and 2
- eating disorders—bulimia and anorexia
- fibromyalgia

- gut disorders—including peptic ulcer, Crohn's disease, colitis, and food allergy
- heart disease—arteriosclerosis, high cholesterol, and high triglyceride levels
- heart disease—in infants from magnesium-deficient mothers
- high blood pressure
- hypoglycemia
- impaired athletic performance
- infantile seizure—in children from magnesium-deficient mothers
- insomnia
- kidney stones
- Lou Gehrig's disease (ALS)
- migraines—including cluster type
- mitral valve prolapse
- multiple sclerosis
- muscle cramps
- muscle weakness and fatigue
- myopia—in children from magnesium-deficient mothers
- obesity—especially obesity associated with high-carbohydrate diets
- osteoporosis (in such cases, just adding magnesium reversed bone loss)
- Parkinson's disease
- PMS—including menstrual pain and irregularities
- primary pulmonary hypertension
- Raynaud's syndrome
- sudden infant death syndrome (SIDS)
- stroke
- Syndrome X—insulin resistance
- thyroid disorders—low, high, and autoimmune (low magnesium levels reduce production of the thyroid hormone T4)

Unfortunately, serum blood tests are an unreliable tool for measuring magnesium levels, as they do not measure intracellular magnesium, where it is most important. Serum levels usually do not become low (below about 2.0 mg/dL), however, until intracellular levels have been largely depleted. **Iodine deficiency** is a broadly rampant issue and one that can impact **every aspect** of endocrine, cognitive, mood, and immune functions. It is easily the most underrecognized and widely impacting trace mineral deficiency problem today, an issue recently brought to light by two independent medical doctors: Guy Abraham and David Brownstein.

Although *iodine deficiency* isn't one of the first things that comes to mind for most people in cases of learning disabilities or mood and cognitive dysfunction, this mineral is so widely deficient (and so widely misunderstood) in the American population that it likely impacts most known health problems today and cannot be ignored as a timely and critical issue.

The thyroid hormones T3 and T4 are made up of the amino acid L-tyrosine combined with either three or four molecules of iodine, respectively. Thyroid problems are growing widely and can lead to all manner of brain dysregulation and learning, memory, and mood disorders. Care must be taken, however, to rule out autoimmune thyroid issues (e.g., Hashimoto's disease) prior to iodine supplementation. Cases of Hashimoto's disease need to be clearly identified and addressed more cautiously. Iodine is a major cofactor in the production of thyroid peroxidase; this is the very substance that a person with autoimmune thyroid problems is producing antibodies against (thyroid peroxidase antibodies), and its production will subsequently serve to accelerate destruction of the thyroid. *Not* good. There is currently some controversy and mixed information over this, but unfortunately the literature is quite clear with respect to the problematic nature of iodine supplementation for individuals having Hashimoto's disease. The risk of significantly accelerating the onset of a thyroid immune attack and often also inducing thyroid hyperactivity symptoms is very real. Even when iodine deficiency is suspected in autoimmune thyroid disorders, the problems and risks associated with iodine supplementation likely outweigh any potential benefits. Unfortunately, in these populations, adding supplemental iodine is simply not a good idea. Small amounts of naturally occurring iodine in seafood are likely okay.

Iodine requires cofactors such as B-complex and C-complex vitamins, magnesium, E-complex vitamins and selenium, broad-spectrum trace elements (using something like Celtic sea salt), and essential fatty acids in order to be properly absorbed into the tissues and properly used. It is important that tissue levels of these nutrient cofactors be healthy prior to iodine supplementation in individuals with nonautoimmune (non-Hashimoto's) thyroid disease. Failure to ensure this may result in uncomfortable reactions.

Although iodine is commonly recognized as needed for healthy thyroid functioning, many people are not aware that iodine is greatly needed for the normal functioning of each and every cell as well as the normal manufacturing of all hormones and the functioning of the entire endocrine system (also for improving the sensitivity of hormone receptors), broadly impacting many aspects of health. Every organ and all tissues contain and must have iodine. The brain is no exception.

The therapeutic actions of iodine include antibacterial, antiviral, antiparasitic, and anticancer effects, elevating pH values, and serving as a mucolytic agent (breaking up mucus in the body). Conditions that can be successfully improved or treated with iodine are:

- ADD/ADHD
- atherosclerosis
- brain fog
- breast diseases
- deafness
- Dupuytren's contracture
- excess mucus production
- fatigue
- fibrocystic breasts
- goiter
- headaches and migraines
- hemorrhoids
- hypertension
- infections
- keloids
- liver diseases
- memory problems
- ovarian disease
- parotid duct stones
- Peyronie's disease
- prostate disorders
- sebaceous cysts
- senility
- thyroid disorders
- vaginal infections

Apart from iodine-poor soils and reduced iodine in the food supply, one major reason for rampant iodine deficiencies involves toxic levels of other halogens in our environment and our water and food supplies. First on the list of offenders are bromine/bromide, included in *all* baked goods (as an anticaking agent), soft drinks, sports drinks, medications, and highly processed vegetable oils; in *many* pools and spas as a disinfectant; in *most* household items (including flame retardants in everything from carpets and furniture and car upholstery to electronics); and in pesticides. Bromide/bromine toxicity is everywhere and affects nearly everyone. Fluoride in municipal water supplies is also a major problem, as is chlorination. All these substances serve to displace iodine in the body and all its tissues, are markedly toxic, and often require large doses of iodine to reverse the problem.

Taking excessive amounts of iodine (or too much too quickly) can lead to uncomfortable detox symptoms (sometimes referred to as Herxheimer reactions) as these halogens are displaced. Therefore, it is important to approach iodine supplementation carefully, knowledgeably, and systematically, preferably under the guidance of a knowledgeable health care practitioner. Iodine's cofactors (previously listed) are essential to successful iodine supplementation.

Good dietary sources of iodine include all seafood, kelp, and other seaweeds. Iodized salt supplies only *iodide* and is not sufficient to supply all tissues with needed complete iodine. Only about 10 percent of this form of iodine in iodized salt is actually bioavailable. Unrefined, full-spectrum sea salt that is not iodized is a fairly poor source of iodine, incidentally, though it is very helpful with the body's use of iodine. Among the best supplemental sources of higher-potency iodine are Iodoral (combines elemental iodine and iodide, the two forms needed by the body) and Lugol's solution (mostly available by prescription and tastes awful). Kelp supplements can provide smaller amounts of naturally occurring complete iodine that are well tolerated and easily absorbed, though may be inadequate to reverse severe deficiency states or bromide/bromine or fluoride/fluorine and chlorine toxicity. Detoxification of undesirable halogens (along with other compounds and heavy metals) for those with autoimmune thyroid issues may be more safely accomplished with the use of sodium alginate or modified citrus pectin as gentle oral chelating agents.

It can take three to six months of diligent iodine supplementation to reach full iodine sufficiency throughout the body (longer in some people who have more-severe health challenges), according to Brownstein, and maintenance levels of iodine supplementation may be required long term for many people. For more information concerning iodine's role and the associated risks in cases of autoimmune thyroid disorders and Hashimoto's disease (and the ultimate source of information and resources for these populations), read *Why Do I Still Have Thyroid Symptoms When All My Lab Tests Are Normal?* by Datis Kharrazian, D.H.Sc., D.C., M.S., or go to the website www.thyroidbook.com.

Other Nutrients That May Help Alleviate ADD/ADHD Symptoms

L-tyrosine, an amino acid, together with vitamin B$_6$, is an important precursor to both norepinephrine and dopamine. These neurotransmitters are largely associated with positive mood and the brain's capacity to focus and remain alert. Depletion of these important catecholamines is commonly found in people with attentional disorders and some forms of depression. The effect of methylphenidate and other stimulants, to some degree, is to force a release of these neurotransmitters, which can ultimately be depleting (and cause other problems). Other popular drugs such as Strattera work by inhibiting the reuptake of these neurotransmitters. Supplementation with L-tyrosine can be a drug-free, natural alternative to these potentially damaging artificial substances. Adequate B vitamins (B$_6$ in particular) are also needed for the proper metabolic conversions. Poor protein intake, excess carbohydrate intake, and poor digestion can result in amino acid deficiencies and poor neurotransmitter function. Chronic sugar or starch consumption can block healthy functioning of these and other neurotransmitters and also cause their depletion. Dosages used in studies ranged from **up to** 5,000 mg of L-tyrosine per day on an empty stomach for children to **up to** 10,000 mg per day for adults (in divided doses). The needed dosages will vary widely, and care should be given to appropriately determining individual requirements. This amino acid can also be a godsend to people who are addicted to stimulant drugs (including caffeine) and can rapidly facilitate relief from these addictions, in tandem with improved diet and additional nutrients. It is important to start with the lowest dose and increase it every half hour on an empty stomach until the desired effect is reached to arrive at the individually appropriate dosage. Do not oversupplement! Be cautious in cases where one may be in active stress response or stress overload, as L-tyrosine can exacerbate the overproduction of adrenaline and even (seemingly paradoxically) lead to suppression of thyroid function as a result.

L-alpha-glycerophosphorylcholine (better known as alpha-GPC) and **dimethylaminoethanol** (DMAE) serve as important precursors to acetylcholine; they are essential to your brain's memory and learning capacity. These substances can safely stimulate and nourish the brain in a nonaddictive manner. Sardines, anchovies, and other fish are richly abundant in DMAE. It can also inhibit and help rid the body (skin and organs, including the brain) of *lipofuscin,* a pigment in the skin and brain that is normally associated with aging. (It causes what are sometimes referred to as age spots.) Dosages of both alpha-GPC (600–1,200 mg per day) and DMAE (50–500 mg per day) can help people with a wide variety of cognitive and behavioral problems as well as support healthy mood function and sleep. In one study using DMAE, hyperactive children showed improvement in just ten weeks. In another study, children with learning disabilities did better in concentration and skill tests, all without adverse side effects such as increases in heart rate and blood pressure, agitation, and unhealthy appetite suppression. Alpha-GPC is well tolerated and widely accepted to be safe.

Acetyl L-carnitine is very structurally similar to acetylcholine. It has a variety of benefits to the brain, including prevention of glycation (especially in tandem with R-lipoic acid), prevention of degenerative processes including Alzheimer's disease, and improvements in cognitive function.

L-tryptophan or **5-hydroxytryptophan** (5-HTP) can be helpful in cases of hyperactivity. For a young child, 25 mg of 5-HTP may be a good starting dose, to be incrementally increased as needed, or 250 mg of L-tryptophan on an empty stomach (not both). If sleep is also an issue, L-tryptophan may be the better choice, as 5-HTP can generate increased cortisol, which can disrupt sleep. Note that sugar consumption can disrupt the therapeutic effect.

Vinpocetine (10–20 mg, three or four times a day), a supplemental phytonutrient, can significantly improve cerebral circulation and cognitive functioning. It has effects on blood vessels in the brain, blood flow in the brain, and even brain cells themselves. Many people report improved concentration ability. Vinpocetine can be of value in enhancing the delivery of oxygen and nutrients to the brain as well as possibly in preventing the damage that occurs if nutrient delivery is impaired. According to some research, it may also help to prevent the neurotoxic effects implicated in Alzheimer's disease. It also has antioxidant properties and has been shown to improve memory.

27

Relief from Anxiety and Depression in Our Uncertain World

■ ■ ■ ■ ■ ■ ■ ■ ■ ■ ■ ■

Anxiety and depression are easily the most prevalent psychological disorders today and commonly coexist in people who are afflicted. They are epidemic. Major depression alone is expected to be the second-leading cause of disability by 2020 *worldwide*—second only to ischemic heart disease, according to the Institute of Functional Medicine. In the United States, one-quarter of the population is at risk for major depression.

I personally suffered from intractable depression and chronic dysthymia for thirty-five or more years before I discovered neurofeedback. Along with depression, I also suffered from anxiety and panic attacks that altogether defined my entire existence for far too long. The symptoms robbed me of my full experience of life and continually weighed like a dark cloud over every pursuit. I used to liken it to swimming with ankle weights on; I would periodically get up a head of steam and fight my way to the surface into the fresh air and sunlight, where I could drink in the air and make some headway in my life, only to eventually be weighed back down into the black, smothering depths of despair and futility. As time went on, these bouts became more frequent, insidious, prolonged, and severe. It almost came to a point where I could not see any reason to fight my way back to the surface any longer. In some ways, I really just didn't want to be here on the planet anymore.

Today, it's hard to imagine having ever been there. For the last fifteen years or more now, this has been a total nonissue for me. I can remember well what it was like and feel deep empathy for others who are similarly suffering. Let's just say, "I get it."

A common misconception about depression is that it is somehow a lazy person's disorder and that all people have to do is simply pull themselves up by their own bootstraps and get it together. Depression is in actuality a state of "chronic efforting." It's a state of spinning one's wheels in the freshly fallen snow (I'm originally from Minnesota; snow metaphors work for me). Your wheels spin and spin until smoke starts coming from the transmission. Eventually you run out of gas and wear down the engine. For too many people, the solution is simply to get more gas when what you really need is to stop, let the tires cool, then ease gently out of the ditch. (There's your crash course in Minnesota Winter Driving 101.)

For the majority of the people I see, depression is really a state of "anxiety to exhaustion." It is a state of learned helplessness.

Although the answer for me was ultimately neurofeedback—for which I will be eternally grateful and devoted—knowing what I know today about diet would, I believe, have made a major difference in that equation for me much sooner.

Make no mistake: insulin and leptin are major players in this equation. Both hormones, when elevated, stimulate sympathetic overarousal and can easily provoke agitative and exhausting anxiety states. Advanced glycation processes additionally degenerate the brain, damaging the brain's natural inhibitory capacity and sending it into chronic sympathetic overdrive. Overproduction of catabolic cortisol further serves to degenerate living brain tissue at the temporal lobes, damaging the brain's capacity to effectively mitigate the stress response. Proper signaling to the adrenals becomes lost. The brain becomes a wild horse with no reins, running in unbridled and unpredictable fury around the clock. Deficiencies of amino acids (due to digestive problems or protein-poor diets), iodine, zinc, magnesium, B-complex vitamins, essential fatty acids, and other substances fuel the problem. Food sensitivities lead to chronic states of inflammation and overarousal.

Add this to acute—or even average—life stressors, and the effect can be quite punctuated and even intolerable. Fluctuations in blood sugar levels further destabilize the system and mood, adding to cortisol problems. Elevated stress hormones, as a result of the insulin and leptin surges, stimulate even more insulin, which, in turn, causes the body to lose magnesium, which is necessary for relaxed, parasympathetic functioning. In short, it's a vicious cycle.

Depression has also been found in 67 percent of patients with untreated celiac disease (Addolorato et al. 2004). The same study found that high levels of anxiety are also exceedingly common in such patients (73 percent). Gluten sensitivity (or the possibility of it) cannot be ignored here as a contributing factor or underlying culprit. In an article in the journal *Alimentary Pharmacology & Therapeutics,* the authors stated, "Depression is reported to be a feature of celiac disease and is ranked as its most common neuropsychiatric disturbance" (Hallert et al. 2002). Food sensitivities, in general, always need to be considered wherever depression or anxiety is an issue. Small intestinal bacterial overgrowth (SIBO) should also be ruled out (see www.SIBOinfo.com).

Chronic adrenal dysregulation in women can lead to deficiencies of estrogen at menopause. This diminished estrogen in women lowers serotonin receptor activity, leading to commonly reported depression issues in postmenopausal women. Abnormally diminished estrogen also results in cerebral inflammation and subsequent brain degeneration. In men, dysglycemia and concomitant adrenal dysregulation can cause similarly diminished testosterone levels, which, in turn, depress dopamine function.

Furthermore (as you may recall), our rate of zinc excretion goes up several-fold under stress, and our requirement for B vitamins, which are essential for healthy nervous system functioning, rises sharply, and they are depleted rapidly by stress and chronic carbohydrate consumption. Sympathetic overarousal also shuts down digestion and hydrochloric acid production (further compromised by dietary carbohydrates), additionally blocking the absorption of important minerals and preventing the proper digestion of protein into the amino acids that are needed for neurotransmitter production. We rapidly lose electrolytes under stress, and our body's bioelectrical system suffers, its neurological timing mechanisms suffer, and the system struggles for equilibrium. Also, essential fatty acids get used up rapidly battling elevations in inflammatory cytokines induced by leptin surges, which rapidly destroy mitochondria and decrease energy levels, and our need for omega-3 fatty acids climbs.

We're drained of our reserves. The brain suffers. Energy plummets.

We see the entire world around us through this chaotic biochemical lens. Life looks bleak, if not overwhelming. For some people, this is entirely identifiable as a state of chronic anxiety. For others, it spirals and descends into depression or some combined state of misery.

Are you seeing the common thread here?

Food sensitivities, EMF pollution, and everyday stressors add another layer to the draining mix. Adrenals move progressively toward exhaustion; the thyroid suffers. One seeks alcohol or carbohydrate-rich snacks to help stimulate struggling serotonin levels, while actually further depleting them or dissociating one from everyday reality. And so, the cycle self-perpetuates.

Life sucks.

Author, scholar, CIA analyst, and professor emeritus Chalmers Ashby Johnson once said about the U.S. military-industrial complex, "I guarantee you when war becomes profitable, you are going to see more of it." In exactly the same manner, as physical and mental illness has become extremely profitable, we are seeing and will continue to see more of it. In 1985, the total annual sales for all antidepressants in the United States was approximately $240 million; today, it is in excess of $12 *billion*. Between 1987 and 1997, the percentage of Americans in outpatient treatment for depression more than tripled. For those in both outpatient and inpatient treatment, the percentage who are on prescribed medication nearly doubled.

Depression is not a Prozac deficiency. Anxiety is not a deficiency of any pharmaceutical anxiolytic agent. Personal issues certainly cloud the equation, but psychotherapy is ill suited to get at the *physiological* underpinnings of depression or anxiety. Both disorders are commonly the product of a vicious cycle that becomes self-perpetuating and colors the lens through which life is experienced. It is a substantially tainted lens. Legitimate life issues become entangled, exacerbated, and confused by what can only be termed *physiological dysregulation*. Improved diet, improved digestion, and nutrient repletion are everything to these populations.

Neurofeedback can sometimes dramatically help restore healthy timing and better self-regulation, but it is diet that ultimately corrects the underlying biochemistry. The brain simply needs certain raw materials to work with; it also needs to be able to get other things that don't belong there out of the way.

Although all this might sound very complex, the basic foundational formula and dietary approach (presented all along in this book) is actually quite simple. **Most supplements are optional.**

Nutrients to Support Depression and Anxiety

- Very low carbohydrates, moderate protein, and sufficient fat intake as needed to satisfy appetite, including supplementation with omega-3 fatty acids and GLA (black currant seed oil). Eat as many fibrous vegetables and greens (raw and lightly cooked) as desired for bulk and antioxidant content.
- Test for gluten sensitivity and/or simply avoid all gluten-containing foods.
- Adequate hydration.
- B-complex vitamin supplementation.
- Trace Mineral Drops or use of full-spectrum (Celtic or Himalayan) sea salt.
- Magnesium (600–800 mg per day): Magnesium glycinate is a highly bioavailable form. Liquid ionic forms may be better used by people with impaired digestion and can also reach intracellular levels more effectively. Liquid ionic magnesium can also be effective at much smaller doses.
- Zinc (either ionic form or amino acid chelated).
- L-tryptophan (comes in 500 mg caps): May be useful for both anxiety and depression symptoms and is a direct precursor to serotonin. A widely available metabolite, 5-HTP, can also be helpful but can additionally raise cortisol levels, which may not be desirable for some people, especially if sleep is an issue. A commonly recommended approach to taking L-tryptophan involves starting with one capsule of L-tryptophan on an empty stomach, noticing how one is feeling, and if no enhanced sense of well-being is noticed after twenty to thirty minutes, another capsule is taken, and so on. When a positive shift is experienced, that is considered the effective dosage. Do not take L-tryptophan if you are also taking antidepressants unless you are under careful, qualified medical supervision.
- For anxiety coupled with mind racing and physical tension, theanine, an amino acid, can be wonderful. Again, one widely used protocol involves starting with a low dose (on an empty stomach) and working up in dosage the same way as with L-tryptophan, taking only what is needed to achieve better relaxation (for many, this is somewhere between roughly 200 and 400 mg per day). Theanine is found in green and black tea, and it can serve to enhance the

activity of the body's primary inhibitory or calming neurotransmitter, GABA, which can also be used supplementally. Theanine also has known positive effects on serotonin and dopamine levels. Smaller doses can be mildly stimulating, while larger doses tend to be quite calming. It has also been shown to lower high blood pressure. It readily crosses the blood–brain barrier and can be significantly neuroprotective, especially for people with impaired cerebral circulation.

- GABA is both an amino acid and an inhibitory or calming neurotransmitter. It can be successfully used for issues concerning anxiety, racing thoughts, and physical tension. Though oral GABA cannot normally cross the healthy, intact blood–brain barrier, wide-ranging benefit is often reported with GABA supplementation. Be warned, however, that if GABA supplementation helps you, the bigger problem may actually be a leaky blood–brain barrier.

- Taurine is another amino acid that is very useful for anxiety-related issues and instabilities. Taurine is the end product of sulfur metabolism and is an antioxidant. It is a constituent of healthy bile and can help support biliary function as well. Taurine has its highest concentrations in electrically conductive tissue such as the brain, the heart, and the nervous system. It greatly helps curb excitatory activity and nervousness without being sedating, and it functions as an inhibitory neurotransmitter. Also, high concentrations of taurine occur naturally within the retina of the eye. There is no known toxicity. Taurine typically comes in 500 to 1,000 mg capsules and can be taken in a similar fashion as the other amino acids. Usually 1,000 to 2,000 mg does the trick, but some people need more or less. Very high doses, in excess of 5,000 mg, can result in a diuretic effect (but one that spares electrolytes). Taurine tends to be very safe and is well tolerated by most people.

- L-tyrosine is a precursor to norepinephrine and dopamine, two neurotransmitters commonly associated with some forms of depression. L-tyrosine comes in 500 mg capsules and is typically taken the same way as the other amino acids. It has a stimulant effect and may be inappropriate for people in active or acute stress response (it can worsen or cause agitation). Also, don't use L-tyrosine if you have malignant melanoma (it is a precursor to melanin). Don't use it if anxiety is a significant part of the problem for you.

- DL-phenylalanine (also known as DLPA) is yet another amino acid precursor to L-tyrosine, norepinephrine, and dopamine, and it also helps to enhance the activity of beta-endorphins. The same restrictions apply as to L-tyrosine. The D-fraction may be especially useful when there is pain or a tendency toward "addiction to pleasure-seeking stimuli," as it helps specifically enhance the function of endorphins by functioning as an endorphinase inhibitor.
- Light boxes: Light, after all, is decidedly a nutrient! When seasonal affective disorder issues are present, these light boxes, which emit up to 10,000 lux, can be extremely useful and transformative of mood and circadian rhythms. Use for fifteen to thirty minutes in the morning to shut down undesirable, chronic, inappropriate melatonin production. This can help lessen fatigue or depression during the day and can significantly enhance serotonin production. If staying asleep at night is a significant problem, using the light box later in the afternoon or early evening (at least two hours before bedtime) can improve sleep quality, too. Spending some time outdoors at around noontime daily (an hour or so if possible) is another natural means of getting adequate "light nutrition." Avoid sunscreens or even sunglasses if possible. Being in the shade is okay.
- Vitamin D deficiency has also been identified in people with seasonal affective disorder and other forms of mood dysregulation, and supplementation should be considered. Read chapter 9 for information on vitamin D supplementation and dosage guidelines.

In addition, when using nutrients to assist with depression and anxiety, please note the following related points:

- Among amino acids, competition with each other for metabolic transport sites across the blood–brain barrier tends to make supplementation of amino acids most effective when specifically desired amino acids are taken in isolation from one another, on an empty stomach, and in the absence of dietary protein.
- Transport of amino acids across the blood–brain barrier is blocked by elevated glucose levels.
- Most amino acids require the presence of cofactors and accessory

nutrients to make their proper conversions into neurotransmitters. Vitamin B$_6$ (also known as *pyridoxine;* the bioactive form is known as *pyridoxal-5-phosphate,* or P-5-P) is most often needed, and it is depleted by all antidepressant medications. Other commonly needed nutrients for proper neurotransmitter conversions include iron for both serotonin and dopamine, and folic acid, which is commonly deficient. Always be sure you are supplementing with B-complex vitamins at mealtime and that you are not anemic.

- The symptoms that you have experienced are probably the best indicators of which amino acid is likely to work best for you. Although urinary neurotransmitter testing has gained some popularity, the approach is deeply flawed, inaccurate, and very expensive. It is far better to rely on symptoms as the most accurate (and affordable) available indicators of neurotransmitter deficiency.
- Amino acids tend to be self-weaning over time and are far safer and faster acting than nearly all prescribed medications used to treat the same symptoms. In most cases, the effects are readily experienced within minutes to hours, rather than days or weeks. Long term, a better diet and improved digestion are likely to be your best insurance for sustained mental health.

The following lists cover the common symptoms that are associated with various neurotransmitter deficiencies and the amino acids that are most effective in replenishing your brain's supply.

Serotonin deficiency symptoms (may respond to L-tryptophan or 5-HTP):

- depression
- worry and anxiety
- negative thinking
- seasonal affective disorder (SAD) symptoms
- anger or aggressiveness
- poor sleep patterns
- shyness or fearfulness
- loss of pleasure in things you used to enjoy
- cravings for carbohydrates

Note: Iron is needed for the conversion of L-tryptophan to serotonin. Anemia can make this conversion very difficult in some people, so it is important to rule out even "subclinical" anemia.

Dopamine deficiency symptoms (may respond to L-tyrosine or L-phenylalanine):

- depression
- lack of physical or mental energy
- low libido
- poor self-esteem
- poor motivation or enthusiasm
- distractibility
- "short fuse"
- cravings for stimulants and carbohydrates

Note: Iron or folic acid is needed for the conversion of L-tyrosine to L-dopa. Anemia may make this conversion very difficult in some people, so it is important to rule out anemia.

GABA deficiency symptoms (may respond to GABA, theanine, or taurine):

- racing thoughts
- inability to relax or loosen up
- poor sleep
- feelings of anxiety or panic for no reason
- feelings of impending doom
- cravings for alcohol, food, nicotine, or drugs to calm yourself

Endorphin deficiency symptoms (may respond to DL-phenylalanine or particularly D-phenylalanine):

- extreme sensitivity to emotional or physical pain
- crying or tearing up too easily
- avoidance of painful issues
- chronic issues with physical or emotional pain
- cravings for comfort foods or "numbing" indulgences

Precautions

Avoid taking the following amino acids:

- L-tyrosine, L-phenylalanine, or DL-phenylalanine: *if* you are prone to migraines, are on antidepressants, have high blood pressure, or have bipolar disorder or manic depression
- L-glutamine: *if* you knowingly have cancer
- L-tryptophan or 5-HTP: *if* you have a carcinoid tumor
- GABA or taurine: *if* you have very low blood pressure

So How Does Exercise Fit In to This Equation?

Studies show that simply walking longer distances for exercise three times a week can improve measurements of focus and attention for older adults. Some research even indicates that gray-matter volume within several brain regions, including the frontal and temporal cortexes, is larger in people (women, in particular) who regularly exert themselves aerobically. Exercise has been shown to have an effect on mood that is equal, if not superior, to the effect of taking selective serotonin reuptake inhibitor (SSRI) medications (antidepressants).

Animal studies show that exercise increases the expression of the neurotransmitter receptors involved in learning and "brain plasticity" (the ability of the brain to function more flexibly) and enables animals' brains to generate new neurons. It can also improve oxygenation and circulation to all tissues, including the brain. Clearly, exercise is a decidedly helpful thing.

Emotion is created by motion.
TONY ROBBINS, *PERSONAL POWER*, 1993

By moving our bodies, we engage a greater and more flexible capacity for emotion. More than one hundred studies done regarding the impact of exercise on anxiety and depression have shown a consistent and significantly positive benefit, roughly equal to that of most traditional therapies. In addition, other variables positively affected by exercise include generally improved mood, enhanced self-esteem, improved ability to recover from psychosocial stressors, and more-restful sleep. Recent studies have found that exercise boosts activity in the brain's frontal lobes and the hippocampus. Animal studies have found that exercise effectively increases levels of serotonin, dopamine, and norepinephrine—all associated with enhanced mood function.

Exercise has also been found to increase levels of brain-derived neurotrophic factor (BDNF), which is thought to help improve mood and also help brain cells survive longer. This, in turn, points to the role of exercise in helping to prevent dementia or benefiting people who have it; it's about a lot more than just enhanced endorphin production or "runner's high." Everyone should find a way to engage in something physical, preferably doing something he or she enjoys.

In the largely sedentary society in which we live, we need to remember to get outdoors into the fresh air and sunshine and move our bodies in ways they were designed to move. Adding oxygen and circulation to the equation can only provide positive benefits in the quest for mental health.

Consider, too, that any emotional state you can think of also corresponds to a certain type of body language. When you feel depressed, your body moves slower, your eyes tend to be more downcast, your shoulders roll forward, and you have a slackened facial expression—you can spot 'em a mile away. Conversely, happy people stand more erect, with their eyes more forward or cast upward (less inwardly directed), with a more brisk and open freedom of movement and something called a smile. It's easy to spot this, too, and studies also show that replicating the postures and expressions of emotional states tend to consistently replicate the states themselves. In other words, if you feel depressed and decide to artificially adopt the posture and facial expression of a happy person, it will virtually become impossible for you to maintain that depressive state as long as you do so. Mood is as much about body language as it is about inward states. Adopting the posture, facial expression, and movements of whatever state you want to have can have a remarkable effect—and when sustained for prolonged periods of time can have an even transformative effect. What the heck, right? It can't hurt to try!

28

What about Food Allergies and Sensitivities?

■ ■ ■ ■ ■ ■ ■ ■ ■ ■ ■

Food allergies and sensitivities are an extensive and complex subject and an extremely common problem among people with learning disabilities and other behavioral, physiological, emotional, and neurological problems. Frequently, symptoms can easily resemble those of nutrient deficiencies and heavy-metal toxicities as well as traumatically generated psychological disorders. Doris J. Rapp, M.D., lists the following nervous system symptoms as possible signs of food allergies or sensitivities.

- hyperactivity: wild, unrestrained
- talkative behavior: explosive, stuttering, constant
- inattention: disruptive, impulsive
- short attention span
- restless legs, finger tapping
- clumsiness: uncoordinated, tremors
- insomnia or nightmares
- nervousness: irritable, upset, short-tempered
- high-strung, excitable, or agitated behavior
- moodiness or depressed behavior: tired, weak, weary, exhausted, or listless
- easily moved to tears or easily hurt
- high sensitivity to odor, light, sound, pain, or cold

Sound like anyone you know?

Other medical symptoms related to food allergies or sensitivities are the following.

- nose: year-round stuffiness, watery nose, sneezing, nose rubbing
- aches: in the head, back, neck, muscles, or joints ("growing pains" or aches unrelated to exercise)
- belly problems: bellyaches, nausea, upset stomach, bloating, bad breath, gassy stomach, belching
- bladder problems: wetting pants in daytime or in bed, need to rush to urinate, burning or pain with urination
- face: pale color, dark eye circles, puffiness below eyes
- glands: swelling of lymph nodes of neck
- ear problems: repeated formation of fluid behind eardrums, ringing ears, dizziness
- excessive perspiration
- low-grade fever
- chronic inflammation anywhere in the body
- proneness to allergies
- resistant to weight loss (even with exercise and a low-calorie diet)

Elimination diets are the most inexpensive and accurate method to determine whether food allergies or sensitivities are to blame for such symptoms, but they require patience, extra vigilance, and disciplined effort. They work by eliminating suspected culprits—the most common are gluten, soy, corn, peanuts, chicken eggs, and dairy (casein)—for a period of time (no less than two weeks; a month or more is better, and for accurately determining gluten sensitivities, this can take six months or more). Then, in reintroducing each of these, one at a time every seventy-two hours, a determination of sensitivity can usually be made. The effects become obvious, either immediately or within those seventy-two hours. I do *not*, however, recommend any experimental reintroduction step with gluten-containing foods, since the potential detriments of gluten sensitivity reactions are so potentially destructive and so prolonged in their effect.

Oftentimes, the food an individual craves most is to blame and can be a strong hint indicating where to start. Some health care professionals offer other, varying forms of testing in this area, though most testing is expensive and limited in accuracy.

The most current and cutting-edge means of testing for food sensitivities involves a series of proprietary testing arrays through Cyrex Labs (www.cyrexlabs.com). Its tests must be ordered through a qualified, licensed health care provider. Cyrex Labs tests have an unprecedented accuracy rate in identifying gluten sensitivity and are also able to identify an expanded array of cross-reactive compounds not typically tested for by other labs. One additional array is also able to accurately identify the locations in the body where gluten is doing the most damage—something vital to know so that compensatory and supportive steps can be taken to safeguard the affected tissues. A highly accredited company called EnteroLab (www.enterolab.com) has a proprietary stool antigen test that is easily six times more accurate than any conventional blood test for identifying certain basic sensitivities. Blood tests for food sensitivities are typically (with the exception of those offered by Cyrex Labs) no more that 30 percent accurate. False negatives through blood tests are the **rule**, not the exception. Anyone can order a test kit by contacting the company, without a prescription. Enterolab also tests for an additional genetic marker that shows an inherent tendency toward gluten sensitivity and celiac disease, which is a major plus in helping to get around the issue of false-negatives (an extremely common problem in food-sensitivity testing). The Enterolab website is also an invaluable source of accurate information. Insurance reimbursement for either the EnteroLab or Cyrex Labs testing may be possible. The prevalence of gluten and casein sensitivities alone makes these testing methods indispensable for almost everyone, particularly when unexplained health issues of any kind are present.

Whenever food allergies or sensitivities are a problem, digestion can be a core cause, though repairing digestion may not necessarily fix all food sensitivities. Gluten sensitivity, in particular, should be considered permanent. To be deluded into believing otherwise poses a potent and potentially lethal risk that's simply not worth it. Once gluten sensitivity damage is healed, however, it may be possible to cautiously reintroduce other nongluten related foods in a limited way once again.

Essentially, the problem begins when undigested food particles pass inappropriately through a compromised intestinal wall (via leaky gut syndrome) and become antigens—targets for your immune system. With a healthy gut, this should not happen. Reestablishing gut and digestive system health and integrity is critical for long-term recovery.

Digestive issues are critical to consider when learning, attentional, autoimmune, cognitive, or emotional and behavioral problems exist. Restoring normal digestion and healthy gastrointestinal flora should be among the first steps taken toward improving these conditions.

Some food allergies and sensitivities can be cyclic in nature and respond to several months' abstinence, after which one can reincorporate certain offending foods in a limited way. Other sensitivities (such as gluten and possibly casein) may well require permanent and total abstinence. Where autoimmune conditions and autism (which can be categorized as an autoimmune brain disorder) are concerned, sensitivities to gluten and casein should be assumed, and these foods should be completely and permanently eliminated. For many people, the results of successful, long-term elimination can be dramatic. Even when elimination of substances such as gluten and casein does not result in automatic remediation of certain issues, however, at the very least one key obstacle toward improvement has been removed. **Please don't just assume it doesn't matter!** Elimination of gluten may only be the first step for many, and this needs to be followed up with testing for possible cross-reactive compounds, as well as actively addressing the accompanying chronic states of systemic inflammation and then systematically taking steps to heal the damage, which may *not* happen on its own. Healing the gut is a process that must be approached actively and systematically.

Exploring the possibility of food sensitivities or allergies is a potentially very worthwhile consideration when dealing with a seemingly inexplicable array of symptoms. Two very informative books on the subject are *Is This Your Child?* and *Allergies and the Hyperactive Child,* both by Doris J. Rapp, M.D. Another, more recently published and superb book on this subject that is highly recommended is *Gut and Psychology Syndrome: Natural Treatment for Autism, Dyspraxia, Dyslexia, ADD/ADHD, Depression and Schizophrenia* by Natasha Campbell-McBride, M.D., MMedSci (neurology), MMedSci (nutrition). A website that contains quite a bit of information on gluten-free and casein-free diets is www.gfcfdiet.com. Also see www.celiac.com for a complete list of foods that contain gluten as well as information on often surprising and hidden sources of gluten. You can locate a gluten sensitivity center near you for any qualified assistance and information you might require at www .conquergluten.com.

Once a food to which one is sensitive has been removed, a regimen of supplementation for no less than a year and preferably two can help restore gastrointestinal mucosal integrity, calm the inflammatory cycle, and improve immunologic function. A list of the principle supplements for accomplishing this follows.

- L-glutamine: primary source of fuel for enterocytes; helps to fuel the regeneration of a damaged small intestine.
- Probiotics (various strains): help to restore normal gut health and immune response.
- Grass-fed bovine colostrum: functions to reduce inflammation, protects against irritation from toxins, checks any potential infection while promoting epithelial growth and repair (helping to reduce excess permeability and leaky gut), can help promote recolonization by friendly gut flora, and is a very potent immune system modulator.
- Proline-rich polypeptides (also known as colostrinin): are composed of a group of related polypeptides derived from bovine colostrum that have the unique ability to stabilize and modulate both immune and cytokine (inflammatory) processes in the body. Pure bovine proline-rich polypeptides are available in oral sprays that can greatly enhance the effectiveness of restorative therapies.
- Vitamin D$_3$: helps support healthy immune function, mitigates inflammation, and can help restore normal intestinal permeability.
- Omega-3 fish oil or krill oil (supplement for EPA, in particular): helps promote production of anti-inflammatory prostaglandins.
- Curcumin (found in turmeric): has a powerful anti-inflammatory effect.

When one finds learning disabilities, ADD/ADHD, unexplained violent behavior, mood swings, and seeming psychiatric disorders, additional issues to consider include heavy-metal toxicity and food-additive or salicylate reactions (for more information, search for "Feingold diet" on the Internet). Visual- or auditory-processing deficits can also manifest in many people with learning disabilities. Seek appropriate professional assistance for diagnosis and treatment.

29

The Impact of Modern Dietary and Environmental Stress on the Brain

■ ■ ■ ■ ■ ■ ■ ■ ■ ■ ■ ■

This subject could be a whole book unto itself. Our primal mind has no defense against the stressful world it now faces, and we are paying a terrifying price for it. We are bombarded from all sides by a chemical (e.g., pollutant, excitotoxin), societal, media, and EMF onslaught—as well as our dietary self-induced tidal waves of insulin and leptin. All of this is relentlessly generating damaging excitatory activity in our brains. It is unprecedented in our history. The toll this takes is insidious as well as profound, and it must be appreciated if steps are to be taken to mitigate its effects.

The richest repository of cortisol receptors in the brain lies in the hippocampus, which exists as part of the temporal lobes (right above both ears). The hippocampus is a part of the brain's limbic system. It serves a role in the formation of new memories and the retrieval of older memories as well as in spatial navigation and the regulation of affect (emotion). It is typically the first area of the brain affected in Alzheimer's disease and other forms of degeneration. The hippocampus is the part of the brain most responsible for mitigating stress response, as evidenced by its preponderance of receptors for cortisol (our major stress hormone)—more than there are in any other areas of the brain.

Unfortunately, we were never designed to be bombarded with stress (or marinated in cortisol) 24/7; this delicate and sensitive part of the brain can become significantly damaged from excessive and chronic exposure to stress hormones and excitatory activity. Its cells wither, degenerate over time, and die off, creating impaired memory function and even psychological disturbances ranging from anxiety to paranoia and emotional instability. Modern imaging studies increasingly show a common trend in the general population toward obvious signs of shrinkage and "Swiss cheese"–looking temporal lobe degeneration. It's a horrifying trend. This is now being referred to clinically as a "normal variant of aging" by radiologists. The fact that it is so very common, however, hardly makes it "normal."

This dangerous trend underscores the need for stress reduction as a mandatory practice for everyone. Neurofeedback can be an especially powerful mitigator of chronic stress and can also be used to teach the brain vastly improved self-regulation of its stress-related circuitry. In my neurofeedback practice, every client gets some form of temporal lobe training to help calm the damaging excitatory activity there that is typical for most people in today's environment. Neurofeedback often dramatically improves self-regulation of stress-related circuitry. Other methods of biofeedback can also be extremely useful for stress reduction, especially heart-rate variability training (www.HeartMath.com) and *capnotherapy*, or "breath training" (www.betterphysiology.com).

This bombardment of stress also underscores the potential benefits of antiglycating nutrients such as L-carnosine, acetyl L-carnitine, benfotiamine (a fat-soluble source of vitamin B_1), and pyradoxamine (a fat-soluble source of vitamin B_6); supplemental adaptogens such as eleuthero-ginseng, ashwagandha, maca, holy basil, rhodiola, schisandra, and others; and regenerating, cortisol-attenuating, and protective nutrient substances such as (particularly) phosphatidyl serine, vitamin B_{12} (and other methyl donors), and CoQ10 (ubiquinol). Overall, insulin levels also need to be lowered.

Most of all, the impact of stress on the vulnerable brain may be the best argument yet for minimizing the excitatory effects of excess insulin and leptin and the oxidizing and glycating effects of dietary sugar and starch.

Another point worthy of ample consideration is the impact of chronic excitatory activity on our frontal lobes—our "executive brain."

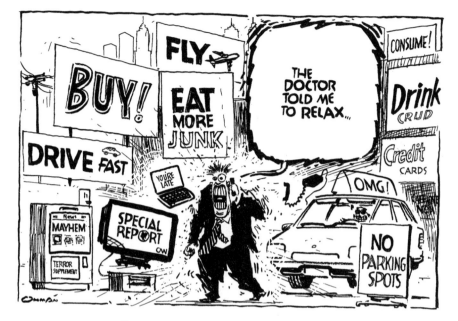

Fig. 29.1. The assault of our modern world

This is the part of the brain that, in many ways, makes us most human. It controls many aspects of short-term memory, inhibitory activity, consequential thinking, focus, planning, and affect regulation or emotion. This part of the brain is usually not fully developed until we are in our early twenties—as reflected in the sometimes erratic and irresponsible tendencies of juveniles. As mature adults, however, this part of our brain allows us to better consider our environment, effectively use our short-term memory, properly focus and process our thoughts, plan our actions thoughtfully, and control erratic impulses.

What we are really talking about when we talk about overarousal, excess sympathetic nervous system activity, or excitatory activity is basically a fight-or-flight state. As mentioned before, this part of our nervous systems was designed to kick in only under threatening extremes, such as, say, being chased by a saber-toothed tiger. Unfortunately, we live in a society today where many of us are being chased by saber-toothed tigers 24/7. Many people have a nervous system that functions habitually in this way. These people often end up seeking neurofeedback (if they're lucky), medications or other drugs, or alcohol to manage this constant hellish hijacking of their brain. Many constantly feel like prisoners of their own nervous systems.

What is the impact when everyone functions in this way, not only on us, individually, but on our society as a whole? The sociological implications are certainly chilling, to say the least.

In a fight-or-flight state, the frontal lobes, our executive functioning, as described above, and even our "humanness" basically shut down. We become either purely instinctive animals or machinelike. Our judgment is affected. We lack any meaningful consideration of the future or past. We're stuck in survival mode only. We *react*, as opposed to *respond*, to the world around us, and we become impulsive and unfocused, and we fail to adequately contemplate the consequences of our actions. It's adolescence run amok. It's a recipe for societal degeneration and chaos, *and all this has become a mainstream hallmark of the society in which we live.*

The ravages of exposure to insulin, leptin, excitotoxins, and chronic EMFs are deteriorating more than just our minds; they are deteriorating our entire society.

Summing It Up

Suffice it to say that consuming a diet closely paralleling that of our ancient human ancestors is the best general insurance we have to avoid dietary deficiency, mental illness, and cognitive decline. Although not necessarily sufficient all by itself to address all modern-day needs and conditions, it is nonetheless our best available foundational blueprint for the optimal functioning of our minds, emotions, immune systems, and overall physiology.

Optimizing nutrient ratios by the elimination of simple sugars and starches, moderating protein intake, and ensuring the adequate intake of healthy fat to satisfy the appetite can additionally serve to greatly enhance both quantity and quality of life. This modification (based on more-recent advances in human-longevity research) takes these foundational "Paleolithic principles" to a whole new level.

From a physiological perspective, **what we eat ultimately accounts for easily 70 percent of our health and longevity.** The very foods we eat are responsible for controlling, modifying, and regulating our genetic expression. This is huge. The foods and supplements we take into our bodies may be, in part, looked upon as ingested *genetic instruction manuals.* A whole field of study has sprung up around this concept, known as *nutrigenomics* (the study of how different foods and their constituents may interact with specific genes to increase or lessen the risk of common chronic diseases). Supplementation with commonly deficient nutrients, antioxidants, and antiglycating nutrients and engaging in regular exercise can further benefit the equation and slow mental, physical, and emotional decline. What we eat really does help determine—more than any other single factor—our genetic destiny.

Attitude, beliefs, habitual emotions, and stress are less quantifiable but also enormously important. Still, the better we eat, the better the raw materials with which to manufacture hormones, neurotransmitters, and prostaglandins—"the molecules of emotion," to borrow a phrase from Candace Pert, internationally recognized pharmacologist and author. Positive thinking is something that should flow naturally and not be an uphill battle perpetuated by lousy biochemistry emerging from a crappy diet.

> Emotions, after all, are little more than biochemical storms in the body and mind. A healthy diet invariably makes for a better forecast.

Emotions are not, in essence, the result of what happens to you, but rather, how you respond to what happens to you. A balanced biochemistry allows us to respond, rather than react, to the world around us.

The quality this lends to our experience of life cannot be overestimated. It's not really about living forever. It's about being healthy enough to live fully, live healthfully, and live happily. Of course, the longer we are able to do this, the better.

Isn't that really the point of it all—quality of life?

We don't beat the Reaper by living longer. We beat the Reaper by living well . . . and living fully.

RANDY PAUSCH, PH.D., PROFESSOR AT
CARNEGIE MELLON UNIVERSITY; DIED JULY 25, 2008,
AT AGE FORTY-SEVEN, OF PANCREATIC CANCER

PART THREE

PARADISE LOST

Cancer, like insanity, seems to increase with the progress of civilization.

STANISLAS TANCHOU,
MID-NINETEENTH-CENTURY
FRENCH PHYSICIAN

30
Surviving in a Modern World

We live in uniquely perilous times. Our ancestors never would have imagined a world where meals come in cardboard boxes and meat comes from animals that are filled with dangerous chemicals and hormones, fed unnatural foods, and forced to live in torturous, stressful, and unnatural environments. They couldn't conceive of things such as air and water pollution, excitotoxins, heavy-metal contamination (much of this was not an issue prior to mining), EMF pollution, twenty-four-hour daylight (in the form of electricity), ten-hour workdays, the stress of daily rush-hour traffic, pesticides on plant foods, or the depletion of nutrients in the soils where plant foods grow. How could they have even begun to fathom GMOs, corrupt pharmaceutical interests, or corporate-controlled FDA politics?

For us today, the challenges are much different from what our ancestors faced in the day-to-day primitive past. I personally would almost rather deal with being chased by a saber-toothed tiger or a charging cantankerous woolly mammoth than deal with the corruptive influence of the FDA and multinational corporations or face massively contaminated food, water, and air supplies.

Our environment—our food, water, and air supplies—has decidedly, even radically, changed, even though our physiology has not. This is not a happy conundrum. How do we manage in the face of all this? How do we adapt, much less survive, at all? The odds are definitely stacked against us.

Then again, some things, nowadays, are to our advantage. We no

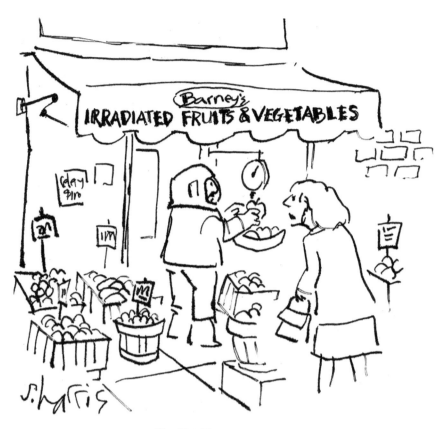

Fig. 30.1. The corner store

longer undergo the same sort of food shortages our ancestors did, we're less vulnerable to fearsome predators (of the four-legged variety), and we have the field of modern scientific research to occasionally give us an edge over nature by helping to reveal her secrets. These advantages, unfortunately, are mostly outweighed by the sheer burdensome toxicity of the environment, the unscrupulous greed and influence of multinational corporations, a compromised food supply, and the deteriorating extremes of our planet.

It's clear that our challenges have changed and that once again our species is being forced to adapt, this time to a radically accelerated state of cataclysmic change to our environment on nearly all levels. The cartoon above seems amusing; however, as of August 21, 2008, the FDA approved the irradiation of all commercially sold spinach and lettuce, without any consumer labeling whatsoever. This effectively destroys all phytonutrients and many heat-labile vitamins (B-complex vitamins and vitamin C) entirely.

Microwaving alone, for instance, destroys 97 percent of all phytonutrients and vitamins in vegetables and other foods, according to a study published in the *Journal of the Science of Food and Agriculture* (Vallejo et al. 2003), and may alter proteins in damaging and mutagenic ways. There may no longer be any cancer-preventive effect from cruciferous vegetables or any other plant food if irradiation of all fruits and vegetables is allowed or otherwise mandated. What's next? How can we possibly survive the accelerating destruction of our food supply through the creation of unnatural "Franken-foods" based on the ongoing and ever-expanding sinister and dangerous GMO technology or the destruction of our environment through industrial pollution and exploitation? And where are these "modern challenges" leading us? These are among the most important questions addressed in this book and in our time.

> The great enemy of truth is very often not the lie—deliberate, contrived, and dishonest—but the myth—persistent, persuasive, and unrealistic. . . . Too often we hold fast to the clichés of our forebears. We subject all facts to a prefabricated set of interpretations. We enjoy the comfort of opinion without the discomfort of thought.
>
> JOHN F. KENNEDY

EMF Pollution: The New Tobacco?

> EMF pollution may be the most significant form of pollution human activity has produced in [the twentieth] century, all the more dangerous because it is invisible and insensible.
>
> ANDREW WEIL, M.D.

EMF pollution affects us all in insidious ways that we've barely begun to recognize. It is known to generate or exacerbate damaging (even mutating) excitatory activity in the brain, and it may well be the single greatest influence on the exponential increase in anxiety-related disorders, autism, and brain cancers.

As a clinical neurofeedback specialist, I have personally observed a radical trend over the last ten to fifteen years toward "high-arousal" disorders and have witnessed an almost exponentially disproportionate shift toward the overarousal spectrum of neurological dysregulation. Doing the work that I do has put me in the unique position of making these observations when they may have been less noticeable for many other people, though I cannot and do not speak for others in my field. After exploring the potential reasons for this, I have concluded that EMF pollution and the exponential increase in cellular towers over just the last ten years, along with cordless phones, Wi-Fi technology, and home electronics, best account—at least in probable part—for this overwhelming, rather sudden, and disturbing shift.

There's no question, too, that current and unprecedented changes in our earth's magnetic fields and ionosphere as well as the influence of solar winds and solar cycles affect the electromagnetic functioning of the brain and body. Dramatic shifts are afoot, and it all influences the way we feel and function (see www.glcoherence.org). These influences are inescapable, and coupled with EMF effects, the human species is being impacted to the core of our body electric in ways we need to understand and address with far greater awareness. Otherwise we become veritable leaves at the mercy of the solar winds and disruptive currents. As EMF is a manmade disruptor in this greater equation, we need to start here and examine this influence more earnestly.

A cursory search using the website at www.antennasearch.com revealed no fewer than sixty-seven cell towers within four miles of my own home. They are everywhere, and they are multiplying. The telecom industry even offers school districts money in exchange for permission to build these damaging, microwave-producing behemoths on school premises, exposing children's vulnerable, developing brains to certain known and unknown EMF dangers.

Dr. Siegfried Othmer, physicist and chief scientist at the EEG Institute in Woodland Hills, California, puts some of this controversial issue into perspective: "Many years ago Russian scientists reported very low-level effects of microwave exposure on rabbits. The findings were met with skepticism by American scientists. After all, there is not sufficient energy there to break molecular bonds, so how could there be a biological effect? Years later there arose the controversy about whether high-tension wires posed a risk to those living nearby. The risk was dismissed for the same reason. But nevertheless there was pressure to undertake a safety study, and a number of those were done. Typically those studies looked at death rates due to leukemia. Now, if one really wanted to know if there was an effect, one would not start by looking at death rates. But this had the advantage of yielding only small numbers, and that sets the stage for endless argument about whether the findings are substantive enough to drive policy. Secondly, it sets an implicit standard that any effect short of one that kills you is really ok. Finally, any such study treats the population as homogeneous with respect to risk. It does not look specifically at people who might be at particular risk."

Othmer went on to say, "Recent neurobiology research has revealed that small voltage fluctuations imposed on neuronal populations can drive them to alter their firing properties. Here we have the operative mechanism whereby 60-cycle electrical fields and cell phones can have physiological effects. The effect can also be optically induced, as we know from children who are sensitive to traditional fluorescent lights. Here the rhythmic light source drives the neuronal populations rhythmically, so that the effect is self-induced, if you will. One can think of the neuronal dance by analogy to people jumping on a trampoline. To a certain extent, they entrain each other. It is more pleasant when everyone jumps together. For an explanation of this effect we cannot look at the molecular level. We cannot even look at the level of the individual neuron. We have to look at group behavior of neurons—because that is in fact how neurons encode behavior. Finally, just as we see in the case of the child who reacts to fluorescent lights by throwing a tantrum, not everyone responds in the same way. A fraction of the population has much more limited tolerance. It is these who need to be considered in any policy debate."

As with the consequences of the use of tobacco, the consequences of EMF exposure are carefully concealed by the industries that generate the dangers, and as such, they may not be fully understood and appreciated for many years (if ever), by which time it may be too late. Unlike cigarettes or secondhand smoke, there is no escape from EMFs; they surround and penetrate us all. All this certainly goes beyond cell phones, however. The radiation these modern technologies generate creates a very real health concern. We get radiation everywhere in our environment today, from microwave ovens to irradiated produce in our grocery stores. We experience considerable cosmic radiation during daytime air travel. There are electromagnetic fields from our computers, our TVs, our radios, our vehicles (*especially* electric and hybrid cars), and even from our alarm clocks and washing machines. In many places around the country, toxic *uranium* is contaminating the drinking water. Any way you look at it, electromagnetic fields and radiation are constant assaults, breaking down our immune systems.

In my own experience working with the functional blood chemistry analysis of many, many individuals over the past several years, one pattern coming up again and again is depressed white blood cell count—in other words, depressed and often highly dysregulated immune function. The logical cause is likely some combination of infectious, biochemical, and bioelectrical influences.

The human body is a bioelectrical system; we are "electric" beings. Our bodies and even our DNA transmit and receive frequencies like *any other antenna*. Our brains are extremely vulnerable to any technology that emits EMFs because the brain immediately starts resonating to the outside signal by a kind of tuning-fork effect.

Andrija Puharich, M.D., a government military researcher in the 1950s, was known for his study of the influence of extremely-low-frequency electromagnetic wave emissions on the mind. Puharich was able to make extremely-low-frequency waves change RNA and DNA, breaking hydrogen bonds to make a person have a higher vibratory rate. In short, we know these technologies impact us in an unnatural and deleterious manner. Puharich discoved that a frequency of 7.83 Hz (the natural frequency generated by Earth's inner ionosphere) made a person "feel good," producing a positive altered state. Other frequencies caused riotious behavior, and still others were able to induce depression—the implication, of course, being that the ability exists to manipulate these frequencies with certain modern frequency-generating technologies. Certain mind tools using the principle of "brainwave entrainment" (such as audiovisual entrainment devices) can manipulate brainwave frequencies to noticeable and decided benefit. The concern lies in the potential of those with, say, less benevolent motives to use similar principles to our individual or collective detriment.

The best we can do is try to minimize the impact of undesirable EMF pollution and interference by taking the following precautions and supporting our innate resilience to stress and overall health:

- Minimize EMF influence by unplugging electrical appliances and Wi-Fi routers when they are not in use, especially in the room where you sleep.

- Seek out nonelectrical alternatives to many home appliances. The Lehman's Non-Electric catalog (www.Lehmans.com) has many alternatives to electricity-dependent household appliances that can also even help reduce your home electric bills.
- Minimize the use of cell phones, and always use their speakerphone option.
- Avoid Bluetooth headsets and all others except air-tube headsets, which are EMF protective.
- Keep away from wireless routers and high-tension power lines. Unplug wireless routers at home while you sleep.
- Minimize or eliminate the use of cordless phones at home and at the office. (Yes, even cordless phones are bad, and likely even worse than cell phones!) Use old-fashioned corded phones at home and at the office instead of EMF-generating cordless varieties. (Corded phones have the added benefit of being able to function during power outages.)
- Finally, take your health and the health of your immune system very seriously. Seemingly harmless dietary indulgences may be costing you more today than you ever realized.

It's time to start taking the threat of EMFs seriously and take whatever steps we can to protect us from and compensate for their insidious biological effects.

What about Detoxification Regimens? Are They a Good Idea?

You betcha! (You can take the girl out of Minnesota . . .)

Detoxification regimens can help purge your body of innumerable toxic metabolites and toxic buildup in your colon, cells, and fat tissue from pesticides, other chemicals, heavy metals, and stress-related compounds. I've got news for you; we *all* have them. Even newborn babies are showing a couple of hundred toxic chemicals systemically when tested. A study released in January 2011 in the journal *Environmental Health Perspectives* revealed that essentially **100 percent of the 268 pregnant women tested were contaminated with highly toxic synthetic chemicals.** The authors stated, "The percent of pregnant women with detectable levels of an individual chemical ranged from 0 to 100 percent. Certain PCBs, organochlorine pesticides, PFCs, phenols, PBDEs, phthalates, polycyclic aromatic hydrocarbons (PAHs) and perchlorate were detected in 99 to 100% of pregnant women" (Woodruff et al. 2011). This is terrifying. Even before birth, no one is safe. The burden this unavoidable contamination places on the human immune system and energy reserves is monumental.

Taking steps to minimize this toxic burden makes good sense, to put it mildly.

Detoxification approaches can range from daily regimens to much more involved programs lasting anywhere from ten days to about a month, usually. Some focus entirely on the colon, and others involve a more systematic detoxification of the entire body. I suggest starting with perhaps a good colon detox with additional support for your other avenues of elimination: your liver, kidneys, and urinary tract, as well as skin and lungs. Once your avenues of elimination are open and well prepared, the rest of the detoxification process tends to go more smoothly and with a lot less discomfort, and a more intensive regimen can be more safely and effectively implemented. Ultimately, one should strive toward *some* form of daily detoxification measures to have any real hope of staying ahead of the game.

Steps to Take toward Detoxification

- Start by eliminating processed and chemically laden foods from your diet once and for all. Go organic, biodynamic, and local with your whole-food choices. We *must* take control of what we can. Don't allow cynicism to seduce or detract you from common sense.
- Get in the habit of drinking roughly half your body weight (in pounds) in ounces of purified water daily. For every diuretic beverage you consume (caffeine, juices, or sodas), include an extra 12–16 ounces of water to compensate for its dehydrating effects.
- Drink quality, unsweetened (or sweetened only with a little stevia) green drinks daily.
- Include a variety of nonstarchy, fibrous vegetables and greens in your daily diet.
- Detox teas of all kinds can be an extremely helpful adjunct. The most powerful variety I know of that is widely available is called FlorEssence (made by Flora, Inc.), found in most health food stores. Take 2 ounces of the concentrate and add a little warm or hot water

to it without sweetening it at all, and sip it on an empty stomach before bedtime. It is a remarkable, powerful, and very gentle product. Although this is a bit expensive for ongoing use, it is a superb adjunct to any detoxification program you may implement.

- Powerful and safe daily detoxing support supplements that I have found helpful include chlorella, cilantro extract, astaxanthin (a potent marine carotenoid), modified citrus pectin (Pecta-Sol), and a very safe and potent detoxifying seaweed extract known as Modifilan.

- Use quality, viable probiotic supplements or living sources of beneficial flora through the consumption of homemade coconut (or, if you aren't casein sensitive, made from raw milk) yogurt or kefir and delicious cultured vegetables. (You can learn to make these at home. It's simple, and you'll save a fortune.)

- Find a quality fiber product such as Garden of Life's Super Seed and begin using it daily in the morning to help cleanse your colon and bind conjugated excess (particularly estrogenic) hormones for safe elimination. You may also want to consider finding a quality colon hydrotherapist who uses a gravity-fed system to help really cleanse and tone the full length of your colon and give it a fresh start. Otherwise, there are colon-cleansing programs out there you can buy online, such as Arise and Shine, that can be very helpful.

- Either buy a far-infrared sauna or find a way to spend regular time in one. These are amazing for detoxifying very readily through your largest organ—your skin—on a downright cellular level. Recent research suggests that exposure of our cells to penetrating infrared light results in improved water structuring and energy production at the cellular level. Far-infrared saunas are a leap forward in detoxification regimens and can greatly relieve your toxic burden over time. I find these far more preferable and beneficial than a conventional sauna, and they are much safer. I use a Sunlight Saunas brand Solo model, though there are many quality far-infrared saunas on the market to choose from.

- Using Epsom salts in your bathwater (a good two cups) can be an inexpensive way to absorb more detoxifying (and calming) magnesium into your system through your skin in a warm, soothing tub of water. Ahhhh . . .

- Consider doing a more comprehensive detoxification program that can help reduce inflammation, support liver and renal function, and help relieve your entire system of years of toxic burden. There are numerous over-the-counter kits that vary significantly in quality. Beware of those designed to be little more than a laxative and diuretic. You also might want to work with a nutritional therapist or health care provider who can walk you through something much more tailored to your individual needs.
- **Detoxify your mind** of toxic fear, negativity, cynicism, and unnecessary negative emotions or thinking by engaging in meditation, biofeedback or neurofeedback using quality audiovisual entrainment tools (see www.MindAlive.com), releasing techniques (see www.sedona.com), positive visualization, and laughter, and by focusing more on feelings of love, appreciation, gratitude, and compassion. Seriously, all "new age" fluff aside, this stuff *works*. The science behind this is crystal clear.

31

What Generation of Pottenger's Cat Are You?

■ ■ ■ ■ ■ ■ ■ ■ ■ ■ ■

Years ago, in the 1930s, a scientist and doctor by the name of Francis Pottenger initiated a series of now famous feeding experiments with cats that spanned more than ten years and several feline generations. His findings transformed many people's view of the role that diet plays in health and reproduction.

Certain groups of these cats were fed quality, fresh, undenatured food and others were fed varying degrees of denatured and processed food, then the effects were observed over several generations. The results from the inferior diets were not so startling for the first-generation animals but markedly and progressively so in subsequent generations. From the second generation on, the cats that were fed processed and denatured diets showed increasing levels of structural deformities, birth defects, stress-driven behaviors, vulnerability to illness, allergies, reduced learning ability, and, finally, major reproductive problems. When Pottenger attempted to reverse the effects in the genetically weakened and vulnerable later-generation animals with greatly improved diet, he found it took fully **four generations** for the cats to return to normal.

The reflections that Pottenger's work casts on the health issues and dietary habits of modern-day society are glaring and inescapable.

The time has come for us to decide just what level of health we choose to have for our children and ourselves. *The choice is truly ours.*

A true state of health cannot be achieved by simply managing a disease process with either supplements or pharmaceuticals. Supplements can, at least, help, but by definition, they are **supplements** to a more fundamentally essential and healthy approach to diet. Also, we must somehow compensate for what we are being bombarded with from all sides.

Overwhelming modern-day circumstances have essentially eliminated our margin for error. The time for innocent indulgence has passed. We can no longer exercise the hubris of pretending we can get away with eating whatever we want, even "in moderation," and somehow avoid the unforgiving consequences simply because we are in denial of them. The consequences of ignorance, for many, will be beyond help. We are too many unhealthy generations of "Pottenger's cats" into the Industrial Revolution and the ravages of a deteriorating food supply, and we are too genetically compromised by all this to indulge in a dietary approach dictated merely by one's superficial tastes (e.g., comfort or junk food) or wishful ideals (e.g., vegetarianism and veganism). Many people no longer have the same resilience of even a generation ago.

With respect to the modern health care crisis, we, as *individuals,* need to take adult responsibility for our own shortsightedness and self-indulgent practices. We basically need to grow up. No one else will ever fix this for us.

There is a real danger in this time of growing economic fear to short-change the quality of the food we eat by leaning on cheap, processed, and starch-based foods as a means of saving money. It is utterly critical that we do not allow ourselves to be seduced by this thinking. Though it makes obvious sense to save money on unnecessary luxuries at such an uncertain economic time, a healthy, quality diet and necessary supplementation should never be viewed as any sort of luxury—**especially** now. If you can't afford to get sick, then you can't afford not to take your preventive health care seriously. More than ever, everyone needs to be encouraged to prioritize quality food and needed supplementation as the ultimate answers to the costly health care crisis. Preventive medicine is **pennies on the dollar** as compared with the cost (on all too many levels) of falling prey to the so-called health care (read: disease management) system. The number one cause of bankruptcy in the United States currently is illness and its associated health care costs.

Our future as a species essentially lies in our past.
Adopting a dietary approach that is consistent with our
foundational primitive physiological requirements is
the first critical step in restoring our health. *It may
well be the underlying key to our very survival.*

How Do We Possibly Adapt to What We Face?

I personally submit that we are now living in a world and in a time where there is no longer any room for error with respect to what we must do to maintain our health and survival. Pottenger's work has shown us that progressive generations with poor dietary habits result in increasingly more vulnerable progeny and that each subsequent generation with unhealthy dietary habits results in impaired resistance to disease, increasingly poor health and vitality, impaired mental and cognitive health, and impaired capacity to reproduce. It is all part of what we are seeing in our epidemic levels of poor health and the overwhelming rates of autism, violence, attentional disorders, childhood (and adult) behavioral problems, mental illness, fertility issues, and birth defects.

Taking control of your health is the single most foundational
means of taking control of your own future. Without our
health and clarity of mind, we have nothing.

We are a few generations of Pottenger's cats, as humans, past the dawn of the Industrial Revolution and the ever-tightening tendrils of the unscrupulous, greed-driven food industry it spawned. We, as a species, have never been more vulnerable. Today, the effects of the increasingly widespread consumption of processed and fast foods are glaringly, if not disturbingly, clear. Add this to an increasingly contaminated environment, nightmarishly dangerous and spreading GMOs, a profit-based (rather than results-based) and broken health care system, and a broken economy on a global scale, along with progressively inferior and deteriorating food and water supplies, and the implications are virtually, if not wholly, cataclysmic. The odds are clearly stacked against us.

How Do We Possibly Overcome This?

Here's how:

First, *we must* take a keen interest in the "machine"—our primal body and mind—that we inhabit. We must strive to understand our own inner workings as much as humanly possible.

When choosing what we eat, we must strive to apply what we know about the selective pressures that shaped our physiology over more than one hundred thousand generations.

We *must not* simply trust others to manage our health for us, especially when others' interests may lie not with our best interests, but instead with profit.

We must avoid the temptation of food as a source of cheap, nutrient-devoid entertainment and instead make conscious, deliberate, and wise choices about what it is we mindfully incorporate into our living matrix.

We must do what our ancestors also did because they had to; we must adapt. We are also forced to take certain compensatory steps our ancestors didn't really need to take. One of the first orders of business in this adaptation is to compensate—as much as is possible—for the toxic, oxidative onslaught from our environment.

Because of this toxic onslaught, *our need for antioxidants and the foods that help us produce them internally has never been greater.* Even though vegetables and greens were mostly an optional source of nutrients in our primitive, ice age past, the time has come to greatly increase their role in our modern diets, both to provide a varied plethora of phytonutrients and antioxidants to our beleaguered, embattled cells and, to some degree, to provide fiber as a means of binding unwanted, conjugated, carcinogenic xenoestrogens and eliminating them from our bodies, preventing their reabsorption. Plant foods are probably more important to us now than ever before.

We must avoid irradiated and chemically treated vegetables as much as possible by buying from local farmers, farmers markets, and co-ops and growing our own. This should be a high priority.

Dietary supplements also have a role to play in supplying us with concentrated sources of key nutrients and both fat- and water-soluble antioxidants. The depletion of nutrients in our soils and other modern factors also make supplementation, to at least some degree, a modern necessity.

Antiglycating supplemental nutrients can also further slow the degenerative ravages of dietary glucose.

I also advocate the use of concentrated, unsweetened, quality "green drinks" (powdered, organic, leafy-green-vegetable and phytonutrient concentrates) as a means of getting more concentrated phytonutrition and providing a detoxifying and alkalinizing nutritional boost to otherwise nutrient-depleted produce from our nutrient-depleted soils. These can also be made using fresh, organic leafy-green produce and either a juicer or a Vita-Mix appliance.

This soil-depletion issue also makes the use of supplement complexes of ionic trace minerals extremely valuable, if not essential, to ensure a complete source of the trace elements that are necessary for innumerable cellular and bioelectrical processes. ConcenTrace Trace Mineral Drops, by Trace Minerals Research, and Himalayan or Celtic sea salt are excellent means of supporting these dietary requirements.

A greatly increased need for quality (pure) hydration is also probable. Although our ancestors likely did not consume "eight full glasses of water per day" or carry around water bottles, the dehydrating tendencies of modern stress and diuretics (e.g., medication, high-carbohydrate diets, gym workouts, caffeine) plus the excessive burden of toxicity in our bodies and in our environment make this a much more sensible modern practice. To find sources of pure, natural water from deep artesian springs near where you live, often at little or no cost, go to www.findaspring.com and search by your location. No healthier water exists. Otherwise, invest in the highest-quality water filtration system you can possibly afford. The least expensive one I have found that is also portable and requires no electricity (making it also ideal for emergency preparedness) is the Berkey Water Filtration System, available through www.directive21.com.

The burden of our overwhelmingly toxic environment and contaminated air, water, and food supplies also leads to a need for active and preferably multiple, varied, and regular practices of detoxification. Engaging in physical movement such as exercise, good hydration, consumption of green drinks, colon hydrotherapy, far-infrared saunas, rebounding (using a mini-trampoline; outstanding exercise for improved lymphatic circulation), and even periodic ten- and twenty-one-day detoxification programs designed by a qualified natural health care provider, certified nutritional therapist, or nutritional therapy practitioner may be necessary and beneficial for many people. The daily use of the aforementioned safe oral detoxification agents can help significantly reduce the body's toxic burden and help free the immune system and the body's energy system for other things.

Minimizing the toxic burden on our tissues and eliminative organs and up-regulating their efficiency are key. Maintaining the up-regulation of our repair and regeneration mode by dietary optimization of carbohydrate, protein, and fat macronutrients as described throughout this book is essential.

Finally, stress management practice today is absolutely mandatory. Fast-paced lifestyles, modern societal pressures, and EMF pollution from cell phones, Wi-Fi routers, and other electrical contamination of our home environment affect us all.

There are any number of stress-management techniques ranging from meditation, biofeedback, and neurofeedback to therapeutic massage that should be incorporated into the lives of *everyone*. This is not about luxury; it is about necessity.

We must accept responsibility for the health and function (and dysfunction) of our own primal bodies and minds, understanding that we ultimately control our own genetic destiny and, to a very significant degree, our own quality *and* quantity of life.

We also need to become activists and to no longer simply and complacently accept the standards for our health and food supplies that are established and maintained by the multinational and monocultural agriculture and food industries; the medical and pharmaceutical corporations; and the other greed- and ignorance-driven corporate interests (or the regulatory agencies such as the FDA that coddle them).

You don't have to be paranoid to pay attention. Be alert. Be aware of what is happening around you and with your food supply. Don't just get angry over injustice; take positive action for yourself and your community. It's important that we don't waste precious energy and time simply pointing fingers at those we deem guilty, but that we work together constructively to improve the conditions that sustain us.

Support the work of the Weston A. Price Foundation and other consumer advocate groups that are striving to make a difference. Vote with your dollars, and support local farmers working hard to do the right thing. Buy locally produced, real grass-fed meats, eggs, and produce. Shop local food co-ops and farmers markets as much as possible rather than larger chain stores, and join community-supported agriculture programs (CSAs) (see appendix G for resources). And if you have the means, then simply grow or raise your own organic food. The more self-reliant we become, the more control we have over our own food supply and the healthier and more affordable our food becomes. Read appendix A, too, for tips on getting started.

The Takeaway Here:
Toward a Journey of Self-Empowerment

Never doubt that a small group of thoughtful committed people can change the world; indeed, it is the only thing that ever has.
MARGARET MEAD, ANTHROPOLOGIST

Despite all we face, it *is* possible to survive—and even thrive—in this modern world. It is possible to avoid the ravages of our nation's health care crisis and corporate manipulations, but only the uniquely informed, vigilant, educated, nutritionally disciplined, and savvy people are the likeliest to do so.

That's a cold, hard reality.

We cannot afford to be ignorant any longer. We cannot afford not to care or to be simply cynical. We cannot afford to blindly depend on a deeply flawed and broken health care (read: disease management) system or government to save us, nor can we depend on the corporate-biased media to accurately inform us. We cannot afford to take *anything* for granted. Mindless indulgences must become a thing of the past. We no longer have any room for error.

We still possess all the potential for physical and mental excellence our primitive ancestors enjoyed, plus we now have the science and the awareness of how to use Mother Nature's agenda and her loopholes to our best advantage. We actually have the capacity and key information that can allow us to live longer and healthier than we ever have before in our long evolutionary history . . .

. . . but only if we have the wisdom to actually use it.

Men occasionally stumble over the truth, but most of them pick themselves up and hurry off as if nothing had happened.
WINSTON CHURCHILL

Where to Start?

■ ■ ■ ■ ■ ■ ■ ■ ■ ■ ■ ■

Although the amount of information covered in this volume may seem a bit overwhelming (to say nothing of paradigm shifting, for some), getting started does not have to be a complicated process. Depending upon just how gung-ho you are willing to be, there are some simple steps you can take to get under way toward improved physical and mental health and well-being.

Step 1: Become very conscious of food and beverage choices. Ask yourself whether what you are eating is something that might have resembled food or nourishment to someone forty thousand or more years ago (in the nutritional heyday before the birth of the food industry). Ask yourself whether what you are eating is more likely to promote your health or constitute a backslide. Live consciously. Do not fear occasional indulgences, just make them occasional and be fully aware of the choices you make. **Read labels carefully!**

Step 2: The closer you can come to eliminating all forms of sugar and starch (including grains, bread, pasta, rice, potatoes, desserts, juices, alcohol, honey, maple syrup, and so on), by far the better. I used to believe it was better to start by cutting the amount of carbs eaten in half, then gradually reducing the carbs further from there, but my clinical experience has overwhelmingly shown that it is far less painful and much more effective to simply eliminate them and get your body used to the idea of using fat, rather than sugar, as its primary source of fuel as soon as possible. Until that time, your body will simply continue to depend on sugar as its primary source of fuel, and you will still be subject to your blood sugar's whims and fluctuations. This actually makes the successful transition to primarily burning fat much harder, and you will likely continue to experience cravings, weight loss resistance, and other issues. Eliminating nearly all carbs (sources of sugar and starch) other than fibrous vegetables and all but very small amounts of fruit (preferably berries) ASAP is the best possible goal. Those with hypoglycemic tendencies will need to use a supplement such as L-glutamine powder or *Gymnema sylvestre* as training wheels to get this issue or temporary cravings under control, while the use of L-carnitine can help more efficiently and rapidly facilitate the body's use of fat as its main source of fuel.

The results of going cold turkey with respect to carbohydrate elimination, combined with moderating protein intake and using fat to satisfy the appetite, can be quite surprisingly and dramatically positive in their effects, and far easier than one would suspect. The liberation from unhealthy cravings and that blood-sugar roller-coaster effect can feel like an almost overnight miracle to some people. Those who have diabetes or alcoholism may need to proceed more cautiously and under the guidance of a knowledgeable health care provider.

Step 3: Eliminate margarine and vegetable shortening as well as any commercial brands of cooking oil *immediately*, if not yesterday. Buy extra-virgin olive oil (organic, if possible), sesame oil, coconut oil, grass-fed tallow and organic or pasture-fed butter (raw butter from a local farm, if available), or ghee. Avoid the use of any other commercial or even organic vegetable oils, as they contain excessive amounts of omega-6 fatty acids and frequently contain trans fats. They are also very prone to rancidity. Rice bran oil, currently being used in many restaurants for high-heat cooking as a means of avoiding trans fats, is probably okay, though of no particular benefit.

Step 4: Substitute Celtic or Himalayan sea salt for refined table salt. It is an excellent full-spectrum source of trace elements (not just refined sodium), and it tastes much better!

Step 5: Get rid of all the sodas, sports beverages, and juices and focus on drinking pure, clean water. Self-serve water dispensers are available at many markets and typically dispense high-quality reverse-osmosis water that has been both carbon-filtered and sterilized using ultraviolet light at a minimal cost per gallon (twenty-five to thirty-five cents). Better yet (and at ultimately far less cost per gallon), install a water purification system in your own home. (Warning: you get what you pay for.)

Step 6: Avoid fast-food restaurants. If you need a meal in a pinch, you could try carrying along some snacks like jerky, pemmican, canned tuna, sardines, or nuts. (See snack list in appendix B.) If this isn't enough, then seek out natural food–type delis for sliced, unprocessed lunch meats and salads (with simple olive oil and vinegar).

Step 7: Begin shopping in more natural, organic, biodynamic-oriented stores and especially farmers markets. Buy locally grown produce. Avoid the center aisles, the prepackaged and nonperishable section, and stick to fresh meats and produce. Check the website www.eatwild .com for the names of local farms carrying grass-fed products (meats, eggs, and dairy), and contact a local chapter of the Weston A. Price Foundation for the largest array of local resources. Frequently, foundation members will pool their purchases in CSAs, allowing for huge savings on meats and produce. It's also a great way to get free helpful advice and moral support (see www.WestonAPrice.org).

Step 8: Begin supplementing with omega-3 oils. Fish oil is vastly preferable to flax oil. More than a teaspoon or a tablespoon may be needed at first. With respect to capsules, the standard fish oil capsule contains around 180 mg of EPA and 120 mg of DHA. The recommended dosage for remediation of especially deficient states is about one capsule for every ten to fifteen pounds of body weight, preferably in two divided doses. Once the symptoms and sense of well-being improve, cut back to smaller amounts, if desired. Flax oil can be additionally beneficial in small amounts but should not constitute the sole source of omega-3 fatty acids in the diet.

Individuals with learning disabilities, mood disorders, or ADD/ADHD and people of Scandinavian, northern European, Native American, or Coastal Irish descent tend to lack the delta-6 desaturase enzyme necessary for proper conversion to the active derivative forms of EPA and DHA, and these people *must* get these nutrients in animal or fish sources.

Step 9: Include 1 or 2 teaspoons for children and at least 1 or 2 tablespoons for adults of high-quality cod-liver oil a day for a superior and reliable source of vitamins A and some D. Getting some full-body exposure to sunlight or additional supplementation with emulsified vitamin D may also be necessary to obtain optimal levels of vitamin D. The body cannot make adequate use of minerals or function optimally without these important fat-soluble nutrients, and diets today tend not to provide adequate levels. Test periodically for adequate levels of vitamin D in the blood.

Step 10: Begin supplementing with a quality vitamin or mineral complex or a multimineral complex. This would preferably be an *amino acid* chelated form that includes particularly those minerals most deficient in soils and, consequently, diets: iodine, magnesium, zinc, selenium, manganese, chromium, boron, and vanadium. The body can do little with vitamins without these and other minerals present, together with numerous trace elements. Trace elements are best supplemented by unrefined Celtic or Himalayan sea salt or by ionic ConcenTrace Trace Mineral Drops, available in most health food stores. Other reliable dietary sources of these trace elements are wild-caught seafood and kelp or seaweed.

Please avoid colloidal minerals (this does not refer to colloidal silver). If stress or immune, mood, or cognitive dysfunction is an issue, adding extra water-soluble nutrients such as B-complex vitamins and vitamin C-complex may be additionally advisable. If ADD/ADHD, depression, anxiety, or immune dysfunction is an issue, additional zinc or magnesium (ionic, in solution or amino acid chelated form) may be important, if not essential.

Step 11: Become physically active, preferably doing something you really enjoy. It should not have to be overly strenuous or time consuming, but it should be something you can see yourself doing consistently. Some form of weight training or other form of anaerobic activity (e.g., kettlebell training, sprinting, power walking) should be considered. No more than an hour or two per week *total,* preferably broken up into roughly three to five separate days, should be sufficient to achieve desired results. Quality of time (that is, intensity) in the gym rather than quantity is key with weights or other forms of anaerobic or resistance training. Weight training, kettlebell training, and other anaerobic challenges give far more bang for the buck than aerobics for weight loss and improved cardiopulmonary health. Anaerobic training enhances growth hormone release (which burns fat and builds muscle) and improves metabolic efficiency via increase in lean tissue mass and increased density of mitochondria (our cell's fat-burning factories). No more than about five minutes of aerobics—strictly as a warm-up—should be done on the same day as a weight-training workout for best results. Do other forms of intense anaerobic-type exercise on the off days, apart from any weight training. Additional time spent walking or cycling daily is fine.

Exercise improves insulin and leptin sensitivity and can improve cardiopulmonary function, but remember that *too much* exercise can work against you.

Step 12: Start exploring some of the references and websites provided here in order to further educate yourself and inspire your progress. Don't take my word for it! Continuing education is hugely reinforcing and utterly key to long-term health.

Step 13: If food allergies or sensitivities are suspected, then spending no less than two weeks to a few months eliminating a suspected food from the diet can be a good way to find out whether it is to blame or not. Gluten-containing grains, soy, corn, peanuts, chicken eggs, and dairy (casein) are the most likely places to start (not surprising, since they are postagricultural foods, containing foreign proteins). Over time, sensitivity to particularly grains (gluten) and dairy (casein) can also precipitate other sensitivities and allergic responses to other things, not to mention autoimmune disorders and worse. Sticking to high-quality protein from a variety of meats and seafood and vegetables and greens for a period of weeks or a few months is a worthwhile first step in finding whether symptoms improve. Further testing by a competent practitioner specializing in this issue may be necessary.

Step 14: Become aware of the pervasive influence of EMF pollution. Take steps to protect yourself from its influence, and do what you can nutritionally and stress reduction–wise to help compensate for unavoidable exposure. Minimize your exposure to cordless phones, Wi-Fi routers, high-tension power lines, and cell phone radiation by taking precautionary measures (such as the use of air-tube-type headsets—not Bluetooth headsets—or speakerphone options) or by eliminating these influences from your home and work environments as much as possible. Your sleep environment is the most important, and unplugging electrical devices in your bedroom at night can greatly improve the quality of rest and regeneration you get from sleep. Get an old-fashioned, wind-up alarm clock. You can explore your own potential exposure to radiation from cell phone towers by going to www.antennasearch.com.

Prepare to be blown away. I discovered sixty-seven cell towers within four miles of my home.

Step 15: Be sure to get a minimum of seven to eight hours of quality sleep every night. Be consistent! Sleep deprivation (less than six hours a night) can lead to insulin resistance and hormonal dysregulation as well as increased risk for cancer. Be sure the room you sleep in is as dark as possible (no night lights) or wear a soft eye mask. Unplug electrical devices in the bedroom and avoid carbohydrates, including alcohol, before bed as these can result in sleep disturbances and nighttime waking. Becoming a fat burner rather than a sugar burner will ultimately remove blood sugar fluctuations from the daytime and nighttime equation and allow for deeper, more restful, and more regenerative sleep.

Step 16: Be sure to hydrate with purified, microstructured (if possible), and contaminant-free water. The rule of thumb here is to calculate half of your body weight in pounds and consume roughly that amount in ounces of pure, fresh, and clean water per day. Don't exceed about a gallon a day, though, unless necessary due to extreme heat, perspiration, or strenuous activity. Too much is as undesirable as too little.

Step 17: Practice stress reduction and detoxification regularly, if not daily. The use of saunas (especially the *far-infrared* type), green drinks, chlorella (to aid in the detoxification of heavy metals), modified citrus pectin (PectaSol), cilantro extract, proper hydration, exercise, skin brushing or rebounding (for enhanced lymphatic drainage), meditation, biofeedback, attitude awareness, and the cultivation of positive and constructive emotional states should all be practiced by everyone. Periodically, a more-intensive detoxification measure such as colon hydrotherapy or a carefully designed twenty-one-day detox program should be considered good, sound preventive medicine. Our bodies and minds need all the help they can get to overcome the burdens of our toxic environment and food supply!

Step 18: Create or find a health or nutritional support group. Joining the Weston A. Price Foundation (www.WestonAPrice.org) or attending foundation potlucks can be fun, educational, and a great source of feedback and support. Regular visits to the *Primal Body, Primal Mind* website (www.PrimalBody-PrimalMind.com) and subscribing to the newsletter can keep you in the loop with new findings, support, and reminders about how to lead a healthier life. Finding friends and family members willing to join in your efforts is essential for long-term success in creating the kind of health you want and deserve. There are too many counterproductive influences in our culture, environment, and media to go it alone.

Step 19: Try (ideally) to incorporate at least 50 percent of your diet as combined animal-source (yes, animal) and vegetable-source foods that are raw or minimally cooked and cultured. The USDA says that meat or fish that has been frozen solid for two weeks is safe from parasitic concerns for raw consumption. Safety guidelines, quality meat and fish sources, and careful preparation here are important, so be careful, but raw and cultured foods have many important benefits that are readily lost to cooking. Marinades made with lemon juice, liquid whey, and vinegars also help minimize risks associated with raw meat or fish. Taking hydrochloric acid tablets with meals containing raw meat or fish can also provide a certain degree of natural protection from food-borne illness. Salads; raw fibrous veggies; microgreens; sprouts; lacto-fermented vegetables; raw-milk yogurt and kefir; raw-milk pastured cheeses, butters, and tartars; raw egg yolks from pastured eggs; carpaccio; sashimi; ceviche; and lox all possess potentially tremendous health benefits. These foods contain vital nutrients, hydrophilic colloids, easily digested undenatured proteins, fresh and nonrancid natural fats and oils, heat-labile C and B vitamins, and enzymes and probiotic cultures that not only improve the digestibility of these foods but also make them immensely beneficial and nourishing in ways cooked foods can never be. This will be a stretch for some, especially where raw protein sources are concerned, but it will be well worth the effort toward gradual incorporation into the diet.

Those people known as raw foodists (typically vegans) have it only partly right. Exclusively raw-vegetable diets really only meet a partial need, and raw veggies, although very cleansing to the system, are less digestible to us (seeing as we lack four stomachs) because of the cellulose-binding aspects of many inherent nutrients. Also, many nutrients in vegetables (e.g., carotenoids) require dietary fat for proper assimilation. Juicing them is not the answer, either. (See chapter 18 for more on juicing.) Although one might initially feel fabulous on such a diet, as detoxifying and therapeutic in the short term as it may be, it cannot be sustainable in the long term for optimal health.

Cleansing is not the same as rebuilding and adequately nourishing.

Sample Menus

■■■■■■■■■■■■

A beautiful new cookbook embracing the principles from *Primal Body, Primal Mind* is now available: *Cuisine for Whole Health: Recipes for a Sustainable Life,* by Pauli Halstead. It can take a lot of guesswork out of meal preparation. Although the book does incorporate some less-than-optimal foods such as rice, quinoa, and honey here and there (which are not essential to any recipe), the recipes are all gluten-free and, for the most part, "primal friendly." They are also incredibly delicious. You can find Halstead's book on www.Amazon.com or at www .CuisineForWholeHealth.com. If you don't want to buy a cookbook, you can go to my website at www.PrimalBody-PrimalMind.com and view a number of wonderful recipes there, or simply choose from the food items listed below. Another exciting new website providing information on how to incorporate low-carb, gluten-free, and related-type eating into your life and your family's life not only painlessly but also **pleasurably** is www .thecookawakening.com. Invaluable individualized coaching and consulting is available. Contact Durga Fuller. You will thank me later.

The following recommendations are given on the assumption that food sources are organic, biodynamic, and free-range or grass-fed wherever possible.

Breakfast

Eggs (if tolerated) should be from ducks or chickens (6–7 g of protein each). Poached eggs can be served with a bit of salmon, if desired. Lox can be enjoyed alone or with cream cheese (again, if tolerated). Stick to no more than about 2 to 3 ounces of meat or fish per meal. Use butter, ghee, avocado, olive oil, or full-fat raw cheese (if tolerated) as needed to satisfy appetite.

Breakfast meats can include freshly ground sausage (many delicious varieties can be found at the meat counter of natural foods–type markets), a small 2-ounce steak, or freshly ground beef or lamb with vegetables of choice (e.g., onions, mushrooms, spinach, broccoli). Breakfast can also be done with a quick stir-fry or evening leftovers. *Who says breakfast has to look like "breakfast"?*

Drink water, tea, or small amounts of organic decaf coffee (in order of preference). Please avoid all juices, even organic ones.

Lunch

Soups or salads with broiled meats or fish and homemade dressing made with extra-virgin olive oil, prepared mustard (read labels carefully), and balsamic or raw apple cider vinegar blended together are *delicious!* Sliced (not processed) meats or full-fat cow, sheep, or goat raw-milk cheeses with veggies, tuna salad (without the pasta), or egg salad (without the potatoes) also work well. Sliced liverwurst or braunschweiger meats (purchased at www.grasslandbeef.com) can also make for a quick, delicious, and satisfying meal, as can a simple and inexpensive tin of sardines packed in olive oil.

Dinner

Consider steak, roasts, pork, lamb chops, fresh ground burgers without the bun, roast chicken, duck, turkey, ground meat (beef, lamb, venison) hash with veggies, ribs, stir-fries, meat loaf (without bread crumbs), broiled or sautéed salmon, halibut, tuna, escolar, mackerel, red snapper (with garlic butter), scallops, Pacific shrimp, stews without potatoes, casseroles without the noodles, hearty soups, or large salads containing meat or seafood. *Again, stick to no more than 2 to 3 ounces of meat or fish per serving, accompanied by various complements.* You'll be shocked by how much money you save and how satisfying this little protein can be. Trust me. I was.

Complements can be mushrooms or onions sautéed with butter or ghee; most any nonstarchy vegetable, such as broccoli, cauliflower, asparagus, snap peas, cabbage, or brussels sprouts; and greens, such as salads and spinach, chard, or kale sautéed with butter, olive oil, or sesame oil.

Kelp noodles can be a wonderful, healthful, carb-free substitute for angel hair pasta or spaghetti. Pine nuts, walnuts, crushed hazelnuts, or slivered almonds can be used as a garnish. M-m-good!

Nutritious Snack Foods
(or Quick, Healthy, Small Meals on the Go)

- Raw nuts (that have preferably first been soaked overnight in salt water, drained, rinsed, and dried in a 150-degree F oven, or better yet a food dehydrator, to eliminate phytates and trypsin inhibitors) are good, including macadamias, almonds, pecans, hazelnuts, Brazil nuts, and walnuts. Pumpkin seeds can be prepared the same way. Organic dry-roasted and salted nuts are also acceptable.
- Nora's Nut Ball Snackers *(oooh la-la!):* See the recipe in the "Dessert" section!
- Hard-cooked or deviled eggs (preferably organic and free-range).
- Sardines packed in olive oil (very rich in zinc and omega-3 fatty acids).
- Tuna packed in olive oil.
- Tuna or chicken salad (without any macaroni).
- Sliced, seasoned avocados.
- A slice or plain spoonful of pâté (no crackers, except maybe the Lydia's Organics brand).
- A plain slice of grass-fed liverwurst or braunschweiger sausage. (See U.S. Wellness Meats, at www.grasslandbeef.com.)
- Olives.
- Kale chips: I swear to you, you will *never* miss popcorn! See the recipe under the heading "Primal Recipes" at my website, www.primalbody-primalmind.com.
- Cream cheese balls, herbed or plain, with an olive center (very tasty!). Credit and kudos to my wonderful, tastefully creative friend Tina Gilbertson!
- Coconut flakes: The Bob's Red Mill and Living Tree Community Foods brands have delicious packaged coconut in larger flakes.
- Green drinks: Try the NanoGreens brand; they taste great! These drinks have incredible antioxidant and phytonutrient content, and they are delicious, gluten-free, and very detoxifying. NuMedica brand also makes a delicious gluten-free, chocolate-flavored green

drink (I know, but it is seriously delicious) and a berry-flavored green drink—both sweetened only with a bit of stevia and extremely rich in phytonutrients and antioxidants.

- Almond or other nut butter, preferably not peanut or cashew butter. (Peanuts are not nuts; they're legumes prone to contamination with aflatoxin, and cashews are starchier, with oils that are potentially irritating.) Dip celery sticks or just a spoon into the jar and eat!

- Plain organic, *whole-fat, homemade, raw-milk* yogurt or kefir with berries—or better yet, coconut yogurt (no lie): Coco-Yo, the world's tastiest and creamiest coconut yogurt, and totally dairy-free, can be ordered from www.HulaKitchen.com. (It makes an outstanding jerky spice, too, that can be mixed with ground meat and dried in a dehydrator for a melt-in-your-mouth experience.)

- Organic full-fat cheese slices (preferably raw-milk based) or a slice of brie (goat or sheep milk) cheese (only if well tolerated).

- Homemade salmon jerky, beef jerky, pemmican (see recipes in *Nourishing Traditions* by Sally Fallon and Mary Enig), or a good homemade-style beef jerky sold at a natural foods–type meat counter.

- Raw veggies and homemade avocado dip or guacamole.

- Thinly sliced turkey or roast beef, either plain or rolled up with raw cheese, cream cheese, avocado slices, or guacamole.

- Raw cultured vegetables.

- Lox or smoked salmon, with or without cream cheese.

- Shrimp cocktail with lemon (preferably from Pacific Northwest, Alaskan, or Mexican Pacific waters, due to potential petroleum and chemical contamination from Gulf waters or radiation from Japan).

Dessert, Anyone (If You Must)?

- Fresh berries of any variety alone, with fresh cream, or blended with coconut milk and a pinch of stevia.

- Sliced fruit (preferably not with protein-containing meals).

Great Healthy Snack Food Recipe

Nora's Nut Ball Snackers

I hope these aren't my only legacy.

The following recipe is for a snack many of my clients have fallen in love with. They are easy to make and utterly delicious. Kids *love* them. They are also very satisfying for both the taste buds and the appetite. Should you find yourself hungry between meals and need a little something, I think you'll agree these are wonderful.

You'll need the following ingredients:

- One regular, 16-oz jar (roughly) of almond butter or any other nut butter that you prefer (other than peanut or cashew butter). Stir surface oil in well!
- 10 oz or more (a very rough approximation) of organic nuts (e.g., almonds, pecans, macadamia nuts, Brazil nuts, pistachios), preferably presoaked and dried. Use a food processor to grind or chop to the desired consistency and chunkiness.
- Handful of organic sesame seeds or chia seeds (great source of mucilaginous fiber to help "keep that train rolling").
- Organic shredded coconut (as much or as little as you like).
- Alcohol-free (glycerin-based) vanilla extract, or crushed or powdered organic vanilla beans.
- One full brick (room temperature) of KerryGold butter (decidedly a key ingredient). You can also try grass-fed ghee. (For an outstanding organic and fully grass-fed ghee, go to www.pureindianfoods .com). Green Pasture (www.greenpasture.org) also makes a butter pecan–flavored butter oil that I have found to be a lovely and nutritious addition to this recipe. If you cannot have butter or want a nut ball that keeps better at room temperature, you can use organic cocoa butter instead. Works great!

You can add any of these optional ingredients.

- Organic coconut flour (Bob's Red Mill makes a good one): Add for additional yummy coconut flavor or better binding.
- Organic coconut butter: You have to taste this stuff to believe it!
- Stevia: For added sweetness, if needed or desired.
- Organic cacao nibs (Dagoba brand has quality ones): Add chocolaty flavor without adding sugar. Also, cacao nibs have roughly twice the antioxidant content of green tea!
- Organic, unsweetened cacao powder can also provide some lovely decadence for people fancying that chocolaty flavor.

- A scoop of Garden of Life–brand Super Seed: A delicious, gluten-free, sprouted and fermented seed-based fiber product with a touch of cinnamon. This is a particularly effective ingredient for turning those nut balls into a regularity-enhancing experience. Plus, it tastes great!
- Whatever floats your boat (and happens to be low carb).

Blend the above ingredients in a bowl thoroughly, then spoon out in little balls onto wax paper on a plate or tray. An alternative and timesaving method is to simply pour the mixture into a pan evenly, then chill and cut into squares or bars (effectively changing the name of this recipe into Nora's Nut Squares or Bars). Refrigerate for a good hour, or until they firm up.

If you want to take the nut balls with you, you might consider placing them in a small portable cooler. You could also individually wrap them in wax paper to secure them (if they can't be refrigerated) so that they don't get all over everything if they melt.

Prepare your taste buds to be seriously dazzled! And kids *love* them.

Protein Content in Foods

■ ■ ■ ■ ■ ■ ■ ■ ■ ■ ■ ■ ■

The source for the information in this appendix is the USDA Nutrient Database for Standard Reference.

For the following sources of complete protein, please note that the amount of protein varies with fat content. More fat equals less protein per serving. The following numbers are approximations.

Protein Content Based on a 3-ounce Serving

- Egg (medium): 6 g
- Fish: 21 g
- Cheese (cheddar): 25 g
- Roast beef: 28 g
- Roast chicken: 25 g
- Other meats (average): 25 g
- Sausage: 12 g
- Ham: 18 g
- Beef burger: 20 g
- Corned beef: 26 g
- Liver: 23 g
- Sirloin steak: 24 g
- Turkey: 25 g
- Shrimp: 18–21 g
- Tuna: 22 g
- Ground beef (regular): 23 g
- Ground beef (lean): 24 g

- Spareribs (lean): 22 g
- Chicken breast: 25 g
- Lobster: 17 g
- Salmon: 22 g
- Feta cheese: 12 g
- Duck (roasted): 24 g
- Whole-milk yogurt (8 oz): 7 g

Protein Content in Incomplete or Plant Sources of Foods

Even though the following foods are sources of incomplete protein, they contribute to the amino acid pool and thus can influence the functioning of the mTOR pathway.

- Nuts (e.g., walnuts, Brazil nuts; ¼ cup): 5 g
- Cashews (¼ cup): 5 g
- Peanuts (¼ cup): 9.5 g
- Peanut butter (2 tbs): 8 g
- Almonds (¼ cup): 7.5 g
- Pine nuts (¼ cup): 7.5 g
- Sunflower seeds (¼ cup): 6.5 g
- Oatmeal (1 cup): 6 g
- Black beans (¼ cup): 4.5 g
- Pinto beans (¼ cup): 3.5 g
- Chickpeas (¼ cup): 4 g
- Tabouli (3 oz): 3 g
- Quinoa (½ cup): 4.5 g
- Lentils (½ cup): 9 g
- Tempeh (½ cup): 20 g
- Brown rice (½ cup): 2.5 g
- Stir-fried vegetables (½ cup): 2 g
- Broccoli (½ cup): 2.5–3 g
- Spinach (½ cup): 2.5 g
- Coconut milk (1 cup): 6 g

An Abbreviated Guide to Supplementation

■ ■ ■ ■ ■ ■ ■ ■ ■ ■ ■ ■

Supplements, to begin with, are merely that: *supplemental* to a solid, foundational diet. Numerous studies of groups of primitive peoples have consistently shown that their diets had a much greater nutrient density and vitamin and mineral content many times what is typically consumed today. (See the table titled "Average Contemporary Hunter-Gatherer Nutrient Intake," in chapter 1.)

Given the mineral depletion of our soils, the difficulty in obtaining adequate levels of essential fats and fat-soluble nutrients from readily available food sources, greater chronic levels of daily stress, and environmental toxins, it stands to reason that some supplementation is desirable, if not necessary, for optimal health. Logically, it is best to obtain supplemental nutrients directly from food sources or complexes whenever possible, as numerous, possibly unidentified, natural cofactors can help facilitate the optimal use of the nutrients in the food. For instance, add extra B-complex vitamins via using nutritional yeast (not brewer's yeast) as a condiment. (It yields a cheesy, nutty flavor.) Just 1 or 2 teaspoons for a child and 1 or 2 tablespoons for an adult per day of high-quality cod-liver oil is a wonderful and important way to add natural vital vitamin A and a little vitamin D as well as small amounts of omega-3 fatty acids to the diet.

Celtic or Himalayan sea salt and ionic ConcenTrace Trace Mineral Drops from Trace Minerals Research can be a wonderfully reliable means of getting adequate trace elements in one's diet that are frequently missing from the soils our food is grown in. A quality food-source multivitamin or mineral complex, too, can be helpful for some people. I generally avoid most popular or generic supermarket and pharmacy brands of vitamins (e.g., One A Day, Centrum). Please read the labels and, more specifically, be aware of the additives commonly found in most commercial supplements. Magnesium stearate and stearic acid are unnecessary additives, and most commercial sources contain trans fats. Studies at the University of Texas Health Science Center and the East Carolina University School of Medicine reveal that these toxic excipients cause a rapid collapse of T-cell membrane function and cell death, therefore suppressing the immune system (Tebbey and Buttke 1990).

According to another study, "When cells were exposed to stearic acids and palmitic acids, there was a dramatic loss of cell viability after 24 hours. Cell death was induced by stearic and palmitic acid" (Ulloth et al. 2003). An article in *Townsend Letter for Doctors and Patients* stated, "Stearic Acid, Magnesium Stearate, Calcium Stearate, Palmitate, and Hydrogenated Vegetable Oils are lubricants which enable manufacturing equipment to run more efficiently but inhibit eventual dissolution of the nutrient. Stearic acid may prevent absorption by individuals with compromised digestive systems. Magnesium stearate and stearic acid also present the problem that delivery of the active ingredient may be considerably further down the intestinal tract than the site originally intended. This may result in the nutrient being delivered away from its optimal absorption site. Not only can this impede absorption, in some cases it might be harmful to the liver" (Czap 1999). The authors of another study remarked, "The addition of palmitate or stearate to cultured cells led to activation of a death program with a morphology resembling that of apoptosis. Palmitates and stearates caused cardiac and other types of cells to undergo programmed cell death" (Sparagna and Hickson-Bick 1999). Not the kind of stuff you'd expect to find in a *health food* supplement. Not all companies use partially hydrogenated sources of magnesium stearate, but it is impossible to tell just looking at the label. My first choice is always a brand that is free of magnesium stearate and other additives.

Another additive of concern is titanium dioxide, which "rapidly damages neurons at low concentrations in complex brain cultures" (Long et al. 2007). Also, titanium dioxide has recently been classified by the International Agency for Research on Cancer as a Group 2B carcinogen that is "possibly carcinogenic to humans" (Canadian Centre for Occupational Health and Safety, 2006). This substance is also widely used in cosmetics and sunblock lotions. In addition, it has been strongly linked to autoimmune conditions (Klinghardt 2008). Just because you find a supplement in a health food store (or pharmacy) does not automatically make it healthy for you. Always read labels, including the "other ingredients."

Supplemental sources that avoid magnesium stearate, stearic acid, and titanium dioxide, although challenging to find, can also improve the bioavailability of vitamins, minerals, and other nutrients and supplements. Additive-free supplements are typically available from health care providers almost exclusively, but there are exceptions. For help, see the resources listed in appendix G.

In some cases, there may be pronounced deficiency states of certain nutrients, as with many people who have ADD/ADHD and other learning disabilities. In these cases, supplement with extra ionic zinc, ionic magnesium, B-complex vitamins, cod-liver oil (to improve mineral absorption and use), and omega-3 fish oil. Initially, more of some nutrients may be needed to make up the deficits.

A list of some supplements worthy of general consideration follows. Not everyone will need all of these, but depending on your state of health and ability to afford quality supplements, some of these may be worthwhile. My focus is with commonly deficient or easily depleted nutrients, antioxidants, and antiglycating substances.

- Omega-3 fish oil caps: Roughly 2,000 mg per day can be adequate for basic health maintenance or cognitive enhancement. When weight problems, mood disorders, or learning disorders are an issue, higher doses are needed to remediate deficiency, starting with one standard capsule for each ten pounds of body weight, preferably in two divided doses (Mercola 2002). Up to 10,000 mg per day may be required in cases of more-serious mood disorders or bipolar disorder (Stoll 1998). In these cases, use liquid preparations rather than capsules.
  Note: Some dietary saturated fat is necessary for both protection and proper use of these delicate essential oils, along with supplemental vitamin D_3 and E-complex vitamins.
- Cod-liver oil: 1 or 2 teaspoons is usually sufficient for children and 1 or 2 tablespoons or more for adults.
- E-complex vitamins: Rich in gamma tocopherols and tocotrienols, together with selenium. Take 400 to 800 IU daily (aids in the pro-

tection and metabolism of delicate essential fatty acids). Use only glycerin-based formulas and avoid all soybean oil–based or canola oil–based formulas.

- Selenium (from selenomethionine): Take 200 to 400 mcg daily (required for optimal use of vitamin E). You can also simply eat more Brazil nuts for a superb source of dietary selenium.
- Whole food–based B-complex vitamins: Take with breakfast and lunch. B vitamins are commonly lost with stress and the use of diuretics as well as with carbohydrate consumption. Taking late in the day may overenergize and possibly interfere with sleep.
- Vitamin B_{12} (as methylcobalamin or as micronized or nanonized cyanocobalamin sprays): Take 1 to 5 mg per day as a sublingual liquid or lozenge. Vitamin B_{12} is needed for healthy brain function, the manufacture of red blood cells, cardiovascular health, and numerous other critical functions. Many people have inadequate or deficient levels and have digestive issues that make the absorption of B_{12} from food difficult. You cannot get too much B_{12}, so it's better to err on the side of supplementation when possible.
- Complexed vitamin C: Be sure the vitamin C you take is complexed with other cofactors (bioflavinoids). Taking ascorbic acid alone can lead to a depletion of other cofactors that ultimately prevents the proper use of ascorbic acid and can actually leave you vitamin-C deficient!
- Ascorbyl palmitate: The fat-soluble form of vitamin C that is able to actually cross cellular membranes and provide antioxidant and antiglycating protection *within* the cell, where nuclear material and mitochondria lie.
- CoQ10: From 50 to 400 mg per day is sufficient for most adults, if affordable (supplies additional protection to essential fatty acids and enhances mitochondrial function). CoQ10 is a potent antioxidant. Ubiquinol is a highly bioavailable form. If you happen to be taking a statin drug, this nutrient (dose on the higher side) is essential for you.
- Black currant seed oil or evening primrose oil (sources of GLA): Follow dosage recommendations on the bottle.

Also refer back to chapter 14 for information on supplements that provide aid with insulin and leptin sensitivity and antiglycation.

Eventually, getting most things from the highest-quality food sources should be the ultimate goal, though for some people that may not always be practical or feasible. Given our modern agricultural practices, modern lifestyles, the prevalence of toxins in our environment, and the occasional difficulty in obtaining the best-quality foods from unadulterated sources, it is realistic to expect to need some ongoing supplementation for optimal health.

It is wise to be mindful that the extra investment in quality food and supplementation now is vastly preferable to a dependence on medications (which only treat symptoms and harbor side effects), surgery, and hospitalization down the road. In the end, the costs of these negative consequences extend far beyond the mere financial toll.

What good is quantity of life without real quality?

Don't spend your money on supplements, though, unless you can afford the best-quality sources. Cheap brands may actually do more harm than good in some cases due to their poor sources and additives.

The Weston A. Price Foundation

■ ■ ■ ■ ■ ■ ■ ■ ■ ■ ■ ■

Dr. Weston A. Price, a prominent dentist and respected scientist in the early 1900s, noticed that between the years 1910 and 1925, children of his dental patients had problems their parents never had. He noticed an emerging pattern of crowded, crooked, or missing teeth and malformed dental arches. (In fact, orthodontia was developed around this time for treating this widespread and newly emerging problem.) Price looked to primitive cultures, long renowned for their splendid, beautiful teeth and physical excellence, and wondered whether there was something present in their native diets that might account for this. He also questioned what effect modernization and the refinement of foods might be having on many primitive societies newly adopting the emerging Western diet.

It was a truly unique era, when air travel had only begun to make far reaches of the globe accessible in a way they never had been before. And yet the tentacles of civilization had not yet reached much of it. Numerous primitive and traditional societies were still thriving in ways they had been for hundreds, thousands, or tens of thousands of years. It was a window of opportunity unlike any other in history. Price saw this and, enviably, took full advantage of it.

Over the next ten years, both Price and his wife traveled over one hundred thousand miles, studying numerous primitive and traditional societies, among them Swiss villagers in remote mountain valleys, South Pacific Islanders, Aborigines, people of remote Celtic isles, African tribes throughout the African continent, American Indians, Inuit, and many others. He noticed that the people of all the primitive and traditional groups he studied typically had all thirty-two teeth, perfectly fitting dental arches, and perfectly formed teeth, and that their teeth had little or no decay as long as they had no access to modern foods. Where cultural and dietary integration to modern lifestyles had begun to occur, he noticed first dental decay and systemic disease, then the emergence of crooked, malformed teeth and dental arches as well as narrowed or malformed facial features in subsequent generations. He also noted a direct correlation between the health of an individual's teeth and gums and the overall health and resistance to disease.

Price sent back to laboratories and analyzed more than ten thousand samples of native foods. Price's analysis revealed that people on native diets consumed more than ten times as much of the many then known vitamins and minerals than did those people eating modern refined foods. Especially significant were the very high levels of fat-soluble, animal-source vitamins A and D in the native diets—frequently ten times the current RDAs. For many other nutrients, the figures were as much as thirty, forty, even *fifty times more* than what is found in modern diets.

Clearly, the implications are staggering. And those people experienced almost none of the many diseases that were then plaguing Western civilization. Price also noted several significant common factors among the diets of each of these unique cultures that he believed accounted for their consistently superior health, superior physical structure, and astonishing freedom from disease. Particularly notable was the central importance of animal-source foods and richly abundant fat-soluble nutrients in all cultures studied. He was unable to find a single vegan primitive society anywhere in the world out of hundreds that he studied, to his own considerable disappointment.

Price published a book, *Nutrition and Physical Degeneration,* in 1939, that chronicled in exhaustively documented scientific detail and photographs the findings of his journeys to the remote corners of the globe in search of the answers to health and disease. This book was required reading for many years in Harvard anthropology classes. It just may be the most important work on diet and health ever written (well, next to this one).

Today, the Weston A. Price Foundation is a nonprofit, tax-exempt charity founded in 1999 to disseminate the research of nutrition pioneer Weston A. Price, D.D.S. The foundation is dedicated to restoring nutrient-dense foods to the American diet through education, research, and activism and supports a number of movements that contribute to this objective, including accurate nutrition instruction, organic and biodynamic farming, pasture feeding of livestock, community-supported farms, honest and informative labeling, prepared parenting, and nurturing therapies. Specific goals of the foundation include establishment of universal access to clean, certified raw milk and a ban on the use of soy formula for infants.

The Price-Pottenger Nutrition Foundation is another organization devoted to this information and is well worth joining as well (www.ppnf.org).

Numerous chapters of the Weston A. Price Foundation are currently active throughout the country and can be found via the foundation's website at www.WestonAPrice.org. Local chapters can be an invaluable source for locating quality grass-fed meats and dairy products as well as biodynamically grown vegetables and free-range eggs. Regular meetings often highlight presentations or potlucks and provide a supportive environment as well as great recipes and tips for individuals and families seeking a healthier way to live. One does not need to be a member in most cases to attend.

APPENDIX F

Pyroluria

■ ■ ■ ■ ■ ■ ■ ■ ■ ■ ■

Pyroluria is a little-known but not entirely uncommon genetic condition affecting roughly 11 percent of the population. People with pyroluria produce excess amounts of a by-product from hemoglobin synthesis called *hydroxyhemoppyrrolin-2-one* (also called OHHPL), an otherwise unimportant waste product. Significantly elevated levels of hydroxyhemoppyrrolin-2-one, however, bind excessively to zinc and vitamin B6, leading to potentially severe deficiencies of these important nutrients. Pyroluria is diagnosed by the presence of elevated kryptopyrroles in the urine.

The diagnosis is widely recognized within the field of orthomolecular medicine and orthomolecular psychiatry but little acknowledged within conventional medical circles. The diagnosis and hypothesis of pyroluria have also been strongly acknowledged and advocated by Carl Pfeiffer, of Emory University, and by staff members at the Princeton Brain-Bio Center, a precursor of the Pfeiffer Treatment Center.

In normal individuals, *kryptopyrroles* are simply waste products created from the production of hemoglobin, and they are typically just excreted and of no significant biological consequence. In people with pyroluria, however, these metabolites cannot be readily excreted, and they then bind relentlessly with zinc and vitamin B6, making these nutrients unavailable to the body to a greater or lesser degree, depending on the severity of the condition. This, of course, is extremely problematic and has all sorts of negative and profound implications for neurotransmitter production, immune functioning, cognitive functioning, digestion, and a few hundred or so other things. The effects can be anywhere from mild to severe. Stress tends to elevate kryptopyrrole levels and their impact in these individuals. If left untreated, this can lead to a wide variety of fairly significant and mounting health problems.

Regular physicians rarely test for kryptopyrrole levels and, in fact, may know little about pyroluria or may even deny the validity of the disorder, as there are no drugs to treat it. Nonetheless, it is becoming increasingly well known and screened for among alternative health care providers, and nutritional management may offer profound relief for many people that is not achievable any other way. Nutritional management of pyroluria, once properly diagnosed, generally involves relatively large doses of zinc and vitamin B6 as well as added GLA supplementation (i.e., black currant seed oil) and diets higher in arachidonic acid and omega-6 fatty acids in general. Omega-3 fatty acids tend to be less well tolerated in this population.

Pyroluria is fairly commonly associated with a number of disorders, such as depression, anxiety spectrum disorders, autism, Tourette's syndrome, bipolar disorder, intractable mood disorders, immune problems, chronic acne, eczema, psoriasis, alcoholism, and others. People with pyroluria also tend, in general, to be fairly stress intolerant.

In formal clinical trials, the following percentages were determined for the occurrence of pyroluria in people with various disorders (see http://kryptopyrrole.com):

- Autism: 50 percent
- Alcoholism: 40 percent
- Schizophrenia: 70 percent
- Depression: 70 percent
- ADD/ADHD: 30 percent

Pyroluria can be readily diagnosed with a simple, inexpensive test that is designed to detect abnormal levels of kryptopyrolles in the urine. Normal results are typically less than 10 mcg/dL of kryptopyrroles. Borderline pyroluria can exist when the results are between 10 and 20 mcg/dL (assess symptoms) and can respond nicely to the aforementioned nutritional support. Anything over 20 mcg/dL, particularly when coupled with typical pyroluria symptoms, is considered full-blown pyroluria.

Although the diagnosis may be considered controversial by conventional medical standards, the clinical effects of proper nutritional support tend to be undeniable and can be quite dramatic. Testing and (when appropriate) nutritional support in symptomatic individuals are well worth exploring.

Pyroluria and borderline pyroluria are readily manageable with high doses of zinc and vitamin B₆ (and some extra GLA)—and that's the really good news. The downside of this is that supplementation must be life-long in order to successfully manage the condition. It is especially important that the zinc be in a *highly* absorbable, readily bioavailable form (not tablets). For these purposes, I tend to recommend ionic forms of pure zinc (not blended with other minerals) in liquid solution (see the related resources listed in appendix G). The results of appropriate supplementation in people with milder cases can be dramatic and profound, though in people with more-severe cases, improvement may be more gradual over three to twelve months.

Testing for this condition is simple, relatively inexpensive, and readily accessible to anyone without a prescription. Call Bio-Center Laboratory in Wichita, Kansas (phone: 316-684-7784 or 1-800-494-7785) or go to its website for more information: www.biocenterlab.org.

Symptoms and Characteristics Commonly Associated with Pyroluria

Testing may be worthwhile if fifteen or more of these symptoms apply to you.

1. Little or no dream recall
2. White spots on fingernails
3. Poor morning appetite or tendency to skip breakfast
4. Morning nausea
5. Pale skin or poor tanning or tendency to burn easily in the sun
6. Sensitivity to bright light
7. Hypersensitivity to loud noises
8. Reading difficulties (e.g., dyslexia)
9. Poor ability to cope with stress
10. Mood swings or temper outbursts
11. Histrionic (dramatic) tendency
12. Argumentative or enjoy arguments

13. New situations or changes in routine (e.g., traveling) particularly stressful
14. Much higher capability and alertness in the evening, compared with mornings
15. Poor short-term memory
16. Abnormal body fat distribution
17. Belong to an all-girl family with look-alike sisters
18. Dry skin
19. Anxiousness
20. Reaching puberty later than normal
21. Difficulty with digestion, dislike of protein, or history of vegetarianism
22. Tendency toward being a loner or avoiding larger groups of people
23. Stretch marks on skin
24. Poor sense of smell or taste
25. Feel very uncomfortable with strangers
26. Frequently experience fatigue
27. Tendency to overreact to tranquilizers, barbiturates, alcohol, or other drugs (in other words, a little produces a powerful response)
28. Tendency toward anemia
29. History of mental illness or alcoholism in family
30. Easily upset by criticism
31. Sweet smell (fruity odor) to breath or sweat when ill or stressed
32. Prone to acne, eczema, or psoriasis
33. Tendency toward feeling anxious and fearful, and carry lifelong inner tension
34. Difficulty recalling past events or people
35. Bouts of depression or nervous exhaustion
36. Prone to frequent colds or infections

Paleo/Traditional Diet Resources and Related Websites

■ ■ ■ ■ ■ ■ ■ ■ ■ ■ ■

Organizations and Laboratories

Ancestral Health Society: The Ancestral Health Society fosters interdisciplinary collaboration among scientists, health professionals, and laypeople who study and communicate about the human ecological niche and modern health from an ancestral perspective.
www.ancestryfoundation.org/AHS.html

The Center for Food Safety: Works to protect human health and the environment by curbing the proliferation of harmful food-production technologies and by promoting organic and other forms of sustainable agriculture. Say no to industrial agriculture and yes to true food!
www.truefoodnow.org

Cholesterol Skeptics: A noncommercial organization of doctors and scientists providing information opposing the prevalent dogma about cholesterol and heart disease.
www.thincs.org

Cyrex Labs: An advanced clinical laboratory offering cutting-edge tests based on the latest scientific advances in immunology, specializing in antibody arrays for complex thyroid, gluten, and other food-associated autoimmunities and related neurodysregulation.
www.cyrexlabs.com

EnteroLab: A fully accredited and registered laboratory specializing in testing for common food sensitivities. Extremely accurate testing and a superb resource for information.
www.enterolab.com

Nutrition and Metabolism Society: The Metabolism Society is a 501(c)3 nonprofit health organization that provides research, information, and education in the application of fundamental science to nutrition. The society is particularly dedicated to the incorporation of biochemical metabolism to problems of obesity, diabetes, and cardiovascular disease.
www.nmsociety.org

Nutritional Therapy Association: A quality introductory source of certified education in nutritional therapy, with an emphasis on physiology, human evolutionary history, and the work of numerous acclaimed nutritional pioneers.
www.NutritionalTherapy.com

Nutritional Toolbox: Advanced nutritional training for health care professionals. Webinars, workshops, seminars, and educational materials.
www.nutritionaltoolbox.com

Price-Pottenger Nutrition Foundation
www.ppnf.org

Weston A. Price Foundation
www.WestonAPrice.org

Products and Supplies

Berkey Water Filteration Systems: A superb-quality, low-cost, portable water-purification system requiring no electricity. Effectively removes viruses, pathogenic bacteria, cysts, and parasites as well as toxic heavy metals and harmful or unwanted chemicals to nondetectable levels.
www.directive21.com

EMF Safety SuperStore: Source of EMF-protective products.
www.lessemf.com

Hula Kitchen: The source for one of my favorite foods, Coco-Yo, a 100 percent dairy- and casein-free, creamy, and delicious coconut yogurt. Hula

Kitchen also makes a wonderful jerky spice (MSG- and gluten-free) that you can mix with any ground meat and then dehydrate for the best, most melt-in-your-mouth jerky you ever tasted! (No more broken teeth!) It also sells quality food dehydrators.
www.hulakitchen.com

Kettlebell Training: Skogg kettlebell training system. For the ultimate kettlebell home-training DVD series, go to **www.Skoggsystem.com**. To see the preview, go to YouTube and type in "Skogg System Promo."

Other kettlebell training information: Books and information plus DVDs about kettlebell training.
www.dragondoor.com

MMI Laboratories, Inc.: Source for liquid ionic zinc and magnesium.
1-888-775-7456 or www.ionicmagnesium.com

Pure Indian Foods: The best source—hands down—for fantastic organic, delicious, fully pasture-fed ghee, suitable for people who love the taste of butter (like me) but cannot tolerate any casein. It also offers herbed and spiced forms of ghee for the more adventurous palate.
www.pureindianfoods.com

Radiant Life: A catalog of quality products, supplements, and foods related to the book *Nourishing Traditions*. Owned and operated by the nicest and most helpful people you'll ever want to meet.
www.radiantlifecatalog.com

RFSafe: Source of EMF-protective products.
www.rfsafe.com

Dr. Ron F. Schmid: A source of quality additive-free supplements available to everyone. Highly recommended. Tell Dr. Ron that Nora sent you!
www.drrons.com

U.S. Wellness Meats: Online mail-order source of superb, organic grass-fed meats.
www.grasslandbeef.com

Websites and Links

Beyond Vegetarianism: An investigative website containing some excellent scientific research relating to Paleo diets.
www.beyondveg.com

A Campaign for Real Milk: Information regarding unpasteurized and unhomogenized (raw) milk products and available sources.
www.realmilk.com

Celiac.com: Website offers a complete list of foods that contain gluten as well as often surprising and hidden sources of gluten.
www.celiac.com

"Cereal Grains: Humanity's Double-Edged Sword" by Loren Cordain, Ph.D.: A scientific paper on the history and health risks of grains, with 342 scientific references.
www.direct-ms.org/pdf/EvolutionPaleolithic/Cereal%20Sword.pdf

"The China Study: Fact or Fallacy?" by Denise Minger: Her meticulous analysis of The China Study should more rightfully be termed a research analysis masterpiece.
http://rawfoodsos.com/2010/07/07/the-china-study-fact-or-fallac

Eat Wild: An entire website devoted to extolling the many benefits of pasture-fed compared with grain-fed meat—very educational. Also lists a nationwide directory of places where quality range-fed meat, poultry, and eggs can be purchased. An invaluable resource.
www.eatwild.com

The Gluten Free/Casein Free Diet Intervention website: Addresses issues of learning disabilities, ADD/ADHD, autism, and other health issues as related to grain and commercial dairy products in the diet.
www.gfcfdiet.com

Green Pasture: A superb source for high-vitamin cod-liver oil and quality high-vitamin butter oil.
www.greenpasture.org

Identifying hidden sources of MSG: www.truthinlabeling.org/hiddensources.html
www.truthinlabeling.org/addendum.html

The Institute for Responsible Technology: Your source for thorough, clear, and *hugely* important information about GMOs. *Please* spend time on this website!
www.responsibletechnology.org/GMFree/Home/index.cfm

Dr. Joseph Mercola Website: Great resource filled with hundreds of diet- and health-related articles, many elaborating on the topics of low-carbohydrate diets, Paleo diets, soy dangers, and more. Free subscription to e-newsletter available. Very worthwhile.
www.Mercola.com

Microwave News: Definitive source of research information and news concerning the effects of EMFs.
www.microwavenews.com

Native foods: Explore Dr. Weston A. Price's research, information related to the book *Nourishing Traditions,* and how to integrate this information into your daily life through connection with an online forum.
www.onelist.com/community/native-nutrition

Paleolithic Diet Nutrition Page
www.PaleoDiet.com

Primal Body, Primal Mind: A cutting-edge educational and informational resource.
www.PrimalBody-PrimalMind.com

ThyroidBook.com: The definitive resource guide for the next to the second most prevalent autoimmune disorder: Hashimito's disease (an autoimmune thyroid disorder).
www.thyroidbook.com

The Truth about Soy: Exhaustively referenced and detailed throughout.
www.soyonlineservice.co.nz

Recommended Reading

▪▪▪▪▪▪▪▪▪▪▪▪

Note: Please also see the References chapter for studies that were cited by the author in the text.

Paleolithic Diet/Protein/mTOR

Books

Audette, R., and T. Gilchrist. 1999. Foreword to *NeanderThin,* by M. Eades. New York: St. Martin's Press.

Bronowski, J. 1974. *Ascent of Man.* Boston: Little Brown and Co.

Crawford, M., and M. David. 1995. *Nutrition and Evolution.* New Canaan, Conn.: Keats Publishing.

———. 1994. *Nutrition Made Simple.* New York: M. Evans and Company, Inc.

Diamond, J. 1992. *The Third Chimpanzee: The Evolution and Future of the Human Animal.* New York: HarperCollins.

Harris, M., and E. B. Ross, eds. 1987. *Food and Evolution: Toward a Theory of Human Food Habits.* Philadelphia: Temple University Press.

Eades, Michael R., and Mary Dan Eades. 1999. Foreword to *Charles Hunt's Diet Evolution: Eat Right and Get Fit,* by Charles Hunt. Maximum Human Potential Productions.

Leakey, R. E., and L. Roger. 1977. *Origins: The Emergence and Evolution of Our Species and Its Possible Future.* New York: E. P. Dutton.

Peskin, B. 2001. *Peak Performance—Radiant Health: Moving Beyond the Zone.* Houston: Noble Publishing.

Schmid, R. F., ND. 1997. *Traditional Foods Are Your Best Medicine: Improving Health and Longevity with Native Nutrition.* Rochester, Vt.: Healing Arts

Press. Originally published in 1987 under the title *Native Nutrition: Eating According to Ancestral Wisdom* and reprinted in 1994.

Simopoulos, A. P., ed. 1999. *Evolutionary Aspects of Nutrition and Health: Diet, Exercise and Chronic Disease.* Vol. 84. Washington, D.C.: *World Review of Nutrition and Dietetics.*

Stanford, Craig B. 1999. *The Hunting Apes: Meat Eating and the Origins of Human Behavior.* Princeton, N.J.: Princeton University Press.

Stefansson, V. 1956. Foreword to *The Fat of the Land,* by P. D. White. New York: The Macmillan Company. Enlarged edition of *Not by Bread Alone,* published in 1946.

———. 1922. *Hunters of the Great North.* New York: Harcourt, Brace and Company.

Articles

Abrams, H. L., Jr. 1987. "The Preference for Animal Protein and Fat: A Cross Cultural Survey." In *Food and Evolution: Toward a Theory of Human Food Habits,* edited by Marvin Harris and Eric Ross. Philadelphia: Temple University Press.

Billings, Thomas E. "Rationalizations in Response to the Evolutionary and Hunter-Gatherer Evidence for Omnivorous Diets." *Beyond Vegetarianism.* www.beyondveg.com

Bogin, Barry. 1997. "The Evolution of Human Nutrition." In *The Anthropology of Medicine,* edited by Lola Romanucci-Ross, Daniel E. Moerman, and Laurence R. Tancredi. Westport, Conn.: Bergin & Garvey.

Byrnes, S., ND, RNCP. July 2000. "The Myth of Vegetarianism." *Townsend Letter,* no. 204.

Carper, J. May 1–3, 1998. "Modern Stone Age Food: Your Body Craves Nutrients Caveman Ate." *USA Weekend.*

Challem, J. April 1997. "Paleolithic Nutrition: Your Future Is in Your Dietary Past." *Nutrition Science News.*

Cordain, L. 1999. "Are Higher Protein Intakes Responsible for Excessive Calcium Excretion?" Active Low-Carber Forums. http://forum.lowcarber.org/archive/index/php/t-52311.

———. "Dietary Macronutrient Ratios and Their Effect on Biochemical Indicators of Risk of Heart Disease: Comparing High-Protein/Low-Carbohydrate Diets vs. High-Carbohydrate/Low-Fat Diets." www.karlloren.com/diet/p41.htm.

———. February 23, 2002. "Metabolic Evidence of Human Adaptation to Increased Carnivory." *Mercola Newsletter*.

———. November 1998. "The Paleolithic Diet and Its Modern Implications." Interview by R. Crayhon, MS. *Townsend Letter*, no. 184.

Day, C. July 14, 2000. "Strict Vegan Diets May Be Dangerous, Especially for Expectant Mothers and Children." *Chet Day's Health and Beyond Weekly Newsletter*.

Eaton, S. B., and S. B. Eaton III. "Evolution, Diet and Health." Emory University, Departments of Anthropology and Radiology. http://cast.uark.edu/ local/icaes/conferences/wburg/posters/sboydeaton/eaton.htm.

Fallon, S., and M. Enig. 1999. "Caveman Cuisine." *Price-Pottenger Nutrition Foundation Health Journal* 21, no. 2. http://curezone.com/art/read.asp?ID= 126&db=7&C0=77.

Grant, Bob. July 8, 2009. "Immune Drug Boosts Lifespan." *The Scientist*. www .the-scientist.com/blog/display/55816.

———. June 24, 2009. "Proteins Link Diet to Longevity." *The Scientist*. www .the-scientist.com/blog/display/55798.

Isaac, G. February 1971. "The Diet of Early Man." *World Archaeology* 2, no. 3: 278–99.

Larsen, C. S. June 2000. "Reading the Bones of La Florida: New Approaches Are Offering Insight into the Lives of Native Americans after the Europeans Arrived. Their Health Declined, Not Only Because of Disease but Because of Their Altered Diet and Living Circumstances." *Scientific American*, 80–85.

Lewin, R. July 5, 1997. "Ancestral Echoes: Were the Forebears of Today's Europeans Ancient Hunter-Gatherers or Late Arrivals Armed with Agricultural Know-how? New Genetic Research Suggests That Europeans May Be Less Modern than They Think." *New Scientist*.

Lindeberg, S. "On the Benefits of Ancient Diets." PaleoDiet.com—The Paleolithic Diet Nutrition Page. www.paleodiet.com.

Mercola, J. 2008. "Auditory: Interview with Ron Rosedale." Compact disc.

———. February 2, 2002. "The Naïve Vegetarian, Part I." *Mercola Newsletter*.

———. February 9, 2002. "The Naïve Vegetarian, Part II." *Mercola Newsletter*.

———. February 13, 2002. "The Naïve Vegetarian, Part III." *Mercola Newsletter*.

———. February 16, 2002. "The Naïve Vegetarian, Part IV." *Mercola Newsletter*.

News-Medical.Net. August 12, 2004. "Investigation into mTOR Protein Function Is Far from Over." www.news-medical.net/news/2004/08/12/4022.aspx. Also referenced at http://wi.mit.edu.

Nicholson, W. 1998. "Paleolithic Diet vs. Vegetarianism: What Was Humanity's Original, Natural Diet?" Interview. *Beyond Vegetarianism.* www.beyondveg.com/nicholson-w/hb/hb-interview1a.shtml.

————. 1997, 1999. "Longevity and Health in Ancient Paleolithic vs. Neolithic Peoples: Not What You Have Been Told." *Beyond Vegetarianism.* www.beyondveg.com/nicholson-w/angel-1984/angel-1984-1a.shtml.

Stefansson, V. December 1935. "Adventures in Diet, Part I." *Harper's Monthly Magazine,* 668–75.

————. January 1936. "Adventures in Diet, Part II." *Harper's Monthly Magazine,* 46–54.

————. February 1936. "Adventures in Diet, Part III." *Harper's Monthly Magazine,* 178–89.

Withers, M. L. April 29, 2003. "Researchers Find New Piece of Cell Growth Puzzle." Whitehead Institute for Biomedical Research. www.wi.mit.edu/news/archives/2003/ds_0429.html.

Technical

Abraham, R. T., and J. J. Gibbons. 2007. "The Mammalian Target of Rapamycin Signaling Pathway: Twists and Turns in the Road to Cancer Therapy." *Clinical Cancer Research* 13, no. 11: 3109–14.

Abrams, H. L., Jr. 1980. "Vegetarianism: An Anthropological/Nutritional Evaluation." *Journal of Applied Nutrition* 32: 2.

Asnaghi, L., et al. December 2004. "mTOR: A Protein Kinase Switching Between Life and Death." *Pharmacological Research* 50, no. 6: 545–49.

Blum, M., et al. January 1989. "Protein Intake and Kidney Function in Humans: Its Effect on 'Normal Aging.'" *Archives of Internal Medicine* 149, no. 1: 211–12.

Bower, B. January 3, 1987. "The 2-Million-Year-Old Meat and Marrow Diet Resurfaces." *Science News,* 7.

Cordain, L., et al. March 2000. "Plant-Animal Subsistence Ratios and Macronutrient Energy Estimations in Worldwide Hunter-Gatherer Diets." *American Journal of Clinical Nutrition* 1, no. 3: 682–92.

De, A. K. 1983. "Some Biochemical Parameters of Aging in Relation to Dietary Protein." *Mechanisms of Ageing and Development* 21: 37–48.

Deldicque, L., et al. 2005. "Regulation of mTOR by Amino Acids and Resistance Exercise in Skeletal Muscle." *European Journal of Applied Physiology* 94, no. 1–2: 1–10.

Easton, J. B., and P. J. Houghton. 2006. "mTOR and Cancer Therapy." *Oncogene* 25, no. 48: 6436–46.

Gannon, M. C. "Effect of Protein Ingestion on the Glucose Appearance Rate in People with Type 2 Diabetes." *Journal of Clinical Endocrinology & Metabolism* 86, no. 3: 1040–47.

Harrison, David E., et al., July 16, 2009. "Rapamycin Fed Late in Life Extends Lifespan in Genetically Heterogenous Mice." *Nature* 460: 392–95. www .nature.com/nature/journal/v460/n7253/full/nature08221.html.

Inoki, K., et al. 2005. "Dysregulation of the TSC-mTOR Pathway in Human Disease." *Nature Genetics* 37: 19–24.

Jia, K., et al. 2004. "The TOR Pathway Interacts with the Insulin Signaling Pathway to Regulate *C. elegans* Larval Development, Metabolism and Life Span." *Development* 131: 3897–3906.

Kapahi, P., et al. 2004. "Regulation of Lifespan in *Drosophila* by Modulation of Genes in the mTOR Signaling Pathway." *Current Biology* 14: 885–90.

Kerstetter, J. E., et al. 1998. "Dietary Protein Affects Intestinal Calcium Absorption." *American Journal of Clinical Nutrition* 68: 859–65.

Lariviere, F. 1994. "Effect of Dietary Protein Restriction on Glucose and Insulin Metabolism in Normal and Diabetic Humans." *Metabolism* 43, no. 4: 462–67.

Leonard, W. R., and M. L. Robertson. 1994. "Evolutionary Perspectives on Human Nutrition: The Influence of Brain and Body Size on Diet and Metabolism." *American Journal of Human Biology* 6: 77–88.

Leopold, A. C., and R. Ardrey. May 5, 1972. "Toxic Substances in Plants and the Food Habits of Early Man." *Science* 176, no. 4034: 512–14.

Lieb, C. W. July 3, 1926. "The Effects of an Exclusive Long-Continued Meat Diet, Based on the History, Experience and Clinical Survey of Vilhjalmur Stefansson, Arctic Explorer." *Journal of the American Medical Association.*

———. July 6, 1929. "The Effects on Human Beings of a Twelve-Months' Exclusive Meat Diet." *Journal of the American Medical Association.*

Lindeberg, S. 2005. "Palaeolithic Diet." *Scandinavian Journal of Food and Nutrition* 49, no. 2: 75–77.

MacLennan, A. 2001. "Women's Risk of Intraparenchymal Hemorrhage Linked to Low Meat and Saturated Fat Intake." *Circulation* 103: 856.

Powers, R. W., III, et al. 2006. "Extension of Chronological Life Span in Yeast by Decreased TOR Pathway Signaling." *Genes and Development* 20, 174–84.

Receveur, O., et al. "Variance in Food Use in Dene/Métis Communities." Center for Indigenous Peoples' Nutrition and Environment, Ste. Anne de Bellevue, QC, Canada. Research report.

———. "Yukon First Nations' Assessment of Dietary Benefit Risk." Center for Indigenous Peoples' Nutrition and Environment, Ste.Anne de Bellevue, QC, Canada. Research report.

Semela, David, et al. May 2007. "Vascular Remodeling and Antitumoral Effects of mTOR Inhibition in a Rat Model of Hepatocellular Carcinoma." *Journal of Hepatology* 46, no. 5: 840–48.

Spencer, H. 1998. "Do Protein and Phospholipids Cause Calcium Loss?" *Journal of Nutrition* 118: 657–60.

Stahl, A. B. April 1984. "Hominid Dietary Selection before Fire." *Current Anthropology* 25, no. 2: 151–68.

Tokunaga, C., et al. 2004. "mTOR Integrates Amino Acid- and Energy-Sensing Pathways." *Biochemical and Biophysical Research Communications* 313, no. 2: 443–46.

Wheat, J. B. January 1972. "The Olsen-Chubbuck Site: A Paleo-Indian Bison Kill." *American Antiquity* 37, no. 1, part 2.

Wullschleger, S., et al. 2006. "TOR Signaling in Growth and Metabolism." *Cell* 124, no. 3: 471–84.

Wolfe, B. M. October 1995. "Potential Role of Raising Dietary Protein Intake for Reducing Risk of Atherosclerosis." *Canadian Journal of Cardiology* 11, suppl. G.

Grains/Gluten/Carbohydrates/Insulin

Books and Medical Journals

Allan, C. B., and W. Lutz. 2000. *Life without Bread: Excess Carbohydrates as the Underlying Cause of Disease.* Los Angeles: Keats Publishing.

Braly, J., and R. Hoggan. 2002. *Dangerous Grains.* New York: Penguin Putnam, Inc.

Case, S. 2006. *Gluten-Free Diet.* Regina, Sask.: Case Nutrition Consulting. Originally printed in 2001.

Cohen, M. N. 1989. *Health and the Rise of Civilization.* New Haven, Conn.: Yale University Press.

Haffner, S. M. May 2006. "Risk Constellations in Patients with the Metabolic Syndrome: Epidemiology, Diagnosis, and Treatment Patterns." *American Journal of Medicine* 119, no. 5, suppl. 1: S3–9.

Hadjivassiliou, M, A. K., et al. 1997. "Neuromuscular Disorder as a Presenting Feature of Coeliac Disease." *Journal of Neurology, Neurosurgery & Psychiatry* 63: 770–75.

Lakka, H. M., et al. December 4, 2002. "The Metabolic Syndrome and Total and Cardiovascular Disease Mortality in Middle-aged Men." *Journal of the American Medical Association* 288, no. 21: 2709–16.

Lieberman, S. 2007. *The Gluten Connection: How Gluten Sensitivity May Be Sabotaging Your Health.* New York: Rodale Books.

Manrique, C., et al. August 2005. "Hypertension and the Cardiometabolic Syndrome." *Journal of Clinical Hypertension* 7, no. 8: 471–76.

Messier, C., and K. Teutenberg. 2005. "The Role of Insulin, Insulin Growth Factor, and Insulin-Degrading Enzyme in Brain Aging and Alzheimer's Disease." *Neural Plasticity* 12, no. 4: 311–28.

Peskin, B. S. 2001. *Peak Performance—Radiant Health: Moving beyond the Zone.* Houston: Noble Publishing.

Reaven, G., et al. 2000. *Syndrome X.* New York: Simon & Schuster.

Simontacchi, C. 2000. *The Crazy Makers.* New York: Mast Tarcher/Putnam Books.

Articles

Brasco, J., February 20, 2000. "Low Grain Diets." *Mercola Newsletter.*

———. February 20, 2000. "Low Grain and Carbohydrate Diets Treat Hypoglycemia, Heart Disease, Diabetes, Cancer and Nearly All Chronic Illness." *Mercola Newsletter.*

Cerami, A., et al. May 1987. "Glucose and Aging." *Scientific American,* 90–96.

Coleman, J. "Opioids in Common Food Products." www.karlloren.com/diet/p18.htm.

Cordain, L. "The Late Role of Grains and Legumes in the Human Diet, and Biochemical Evidence of Their Evolutionary Discordance." *Beyond Vegetarianism.* www.beyondveg.com.

Fox, D. March 18, 2000. "Cut the Carbs." *New Scientist,* no. 2230.

Petersen, K. F., and G. I. Shulman. May 2006. "Etiology of Insulin Resistance." *American Journal of Medicine* 119, no. 5, suppl. 1: S10–16.

Rosedale, R., "Diabetes Is Not a Disease of Blood Sugar!" http://life-enthusiast .com/index/Articles/Rosedale/Diabetes_Is_Not_a_Disease_of_Blood_ Sugar.

Stobbe, M. July 17, 2008. "Study: Low-carb Diet Best for Weight, Cholesterol." *Associated Press.* www.washingtonpost.com/wp-dyn/content/article/2008/ 07/17/AR2008071701058.html.

Technical

Abrams, H. L. Fall 1975. "Sugar—A Cultural Complex and Its Impact on Modern Society." *Journal of Applied Nutrition* 27: 2.

Calle, E. E., and R. Kaaks. 2004. "Overweight, Obesity and Cancer: Epidemiological Evidence and Proposed Mechanisms." *Nature Reviews Cancer* 4, no. 8: 579–91.

Capeau, J. December 21, 2005. "Insulin Signaling: Mechanisms Altered in Insulin Resistance" [in French]. *Med Sci* (Paris) 21, spec. no.: 34–39.

Chari, S. T., et al. 2008. "Pancreatic Cancer-Associated Diabetes Mellitus: Prevalence and Temporal Association with Diagnosis of Cancer." *Gastroenterology* 134, no. 1: 95–101.

Cordain, L. 1999. "Cereal Grains: Humanity's Double-Edged Sword." *World Review of Nutrition and Dietetics* 84: 19–73.

Feighery, C. "Coeliac Disease." July 1999. *British Medical Journal* 319: 236–39.

Flood, A., et al. August 2010. "Diabetes and Risk of Incident Colorectal Cancer in a Prospective Cohort of Women." *Cancer Causes Control* 21, no. 8: 1277–84.

Foster, G. D., et al. 2003. "A Randomized Trial of a Low-Carbohydrate Diet for Obesity. *New England Journal of Medicine* 348, no. 21: 2082–90.

Freed, D. J. April 17, 1999. "Do Dietary Lectins Cause Disease?" Editorial. *British Medical Journal* 318: 1023–24.

Gapstur, S. M., et al. May 17, 2000. "Abnormal Glucose Metabolism and Pancreatic Cancer Mortality." *Journal of the American Medical Association* 283, no. 19: 2552–58.

Ginsberg, Henry, et al., 1976. "Induction of Hypertriglyceridemia by a Low-Fat Diet." *Journal of Clinical Endocrinology & Metabolism* 42: 729.

Halton, T. L., et al. 2006. "Low-Carbohydrate-Diet Score and the Risk of Coronary Heart Disease in Women. *New England Journal of Medicine* 355, no. 19: 1991–2002.

Heller, R. F. 1994. "Hyperinsulinemic Obesity and Carbohydrate Addiction: The Missing Link Is the Carbohydrate Frequency Factor." *Medical Hypotheses* 42: 307–12.

———. May 18, 1996. "Intake of Macronutrients and Risk of Breast Cancer." *Lancet* 347, no. 9012: 1351–56.

Ho, et al. August 23, 2007. "AGFD 232—Food Bioactives and Neutraceuticals: Production, Chemistry, Analysis and Health Effects." Paper regarding the biological effects of high fructose corn syrup presented at the symposium of the American Chemical Society, Boston.

Huxley R., et al. 2005. "Type-II Diabetes and Pancreatic Cancer: A Meta-analysis of 36 Studies." *British Journal of Cancer* 92, no. 11: 95–101.

Jeppsen, J., et al. 1997. "Effect of Low-Fat, High Carbohydrate Diets on Risk Factors for Ischemic Heart Disease in Postmenopausal Women." *American Journal of Clinical Nutrition* 65: 1027–33.

Lajous, M., et al. 2005. "Glycemic Load, Glycemic Index, and the Risk of Breast Cancer Among Mexican Women." *Cancer Causes Control* 16, no. 10: 1165–69.

Michaud, D. S., et al. 2005. "Dietary Glycemic Load, Carbohydrate, Sugar, and Colorectal Cancer Risk in Men and Women. *Cancer Epidemiology, Biomarkers & Prevention* 14, no. 1: 138–47.

Noto, H., et al. September–October 2010. "Substantially Increased Risk of Cancer in Patients with Diabetes Mellitus: A Systematic Review and Meta-analysis of Epidemiologic Evidence in Japan." *Journal of Diabetes and Its Complications* 24, no. 5: 345–53.

Reaven, G. M. July 1995. "Pathophysiology of Insulin Resistance in Human Disease." *Physiological Reviews* 75: 473–86.

Wadley, G., et al. June 1993. "The Origins of Agriculture—A Biological Perspective and a New Hypothesis." *Australian Biologist* 6: 96–105.

Willet, W., et al. 1999. "Dietary Fiber and the Risk of Colorectal Cancer and Adenoma in Women." *New England Journal of Medicine* 340: 169–76.

Yudkin, J. July 4, 1964. "Dietary Fat and Dietary Sugar in Relation to Ischemic Heart Disease and Diabetes." *Lancet* 2, no. 7349: 4–5.

———. 1969. "Sucrose and Heart Disease." *Lancet* 14: 16–20.

———. 1971. "Sugar Consumption and Myocardial Infarction." *Lancet* 1, no. 7693: 296–97.

———. 1967. "Sugar Intake and Myocardial Infarction." *American Journal of Clinical Nutrition* 20: 503.

Yudkin, J., and J. Roddy. July 4, 1964. "Levels of Dietary Sucrose in Patients with Occlusive Atherosclerotic Disease." *Lancet* 2, no. 7349: 6–8.

Soy

Books

Daniel, K. T. 2005. *The Whole Soy Story: The Dark Side of America's Favorite Health Food.* Washington, D.C.: New Trends Publishing.

———. 2005. *Facts about Soy the Industry Doesn't Want You to Know: An Interview with Dr. Kaayla Daniel,* Author of "The Whole Story." Adobe Reader PDF. E-doc, Innovative Healing, Inc., www.Amazon.com.

Fallon, S., and M. Enig. 1999. *Nourishing Traditions: The Cookbook That Challenges Politically Correct Nutrition and the Diet Dictocrats*. San Diego, Calif.: ProMotion Publishing.

Articles

Altonn, H. November 19, 1999. "Too Much Tofu Induces 'Brain Aging,' Study Shows." *Honolulu Star Bulletin*.

Fagan, J. "Toxicity from Genetically Engineered Foods." *Holistic Healing*. www .holisticmed.com/ge/toxicity.html.

Fallon, S., and M. Enig. January 2, 2008. "Concerns Regarding Soybeans." *Mercola Newsletter*. http://articles.mercola.com/sites/articles/archive/2008/01/02/ soybean-concerns.aspx.

———. 1995. "The Ploy of Soy." The Weston A. Price Foundation. www .WestonAPrice.org (search for article title).

———. April–May 2000. "Tragedy and Hype: The Third International Soy Symposium." *Nexus*, 17–22; 73–74.

Finucan, B., and C. Gerson. February 7, 2001. "Soy: Too Good to Be True." *Mercola Newsletter*.

Fitzpatrick, M. "Soy Isoflavones: Panacea or Poison?" The Weston A. Price Foundation. www.WestonAPrice.org (search for article title).

Goddard, I. W. "Soy-Dementia in Men?" www.lewrockwell.com/orig4/goddard1 .htm.

———. April–May 1997. "Soybean Products: A Recipe for Disaster?" *Nexus*.

Goodwin, B., et al. October 1997. "Monsanto Genetically Engineered Soya Has Elevated Hormone Levels: Public Health Threat." *Holistic Healing*. www .holisticmed.com/ge/warning.html.

Hanson, M., and J. Halloran. "Jeopardizing the Future? Genetic Engineering, Food and the Environment." *Pest Management at the Crossroads*. www.pmac .net/jeopardy.html.

Liebovitz, B. December 1995. "Soy Protein: Sorting Out the Science." *Muscular Development, Fitness and Health*.

MacArthur, J. D. September 17, 2000. "Soy and Brain Damage." *Mercola Newsletter*. http://articles.mercola.com/sites/articles/archive/2000/09/17/soy-brain.aspx.

Mercola, J. January 2, 2008. "Link between High Soy Diet during Pregnancy and Nursing and Eventual Developmental Changes in Children." *Mercola Newsletter*. http://articles.mercola.com/sites/articles/archive/2008/01/02/ soy-and-children.aspx.

————. April 9, 2000. "New Avoid Soy Update." *Mercola Newsletter.* http://articles.mercola.com/sites/articles/archive/2000/04/09/soy-research-update.aspx.

————. January 2, 2008. "Soy Supplements Fail to Help Menopausal Symptoms." *Mercola Newsletter.* http://articles.mercola.com/sites/articles/archive/2008/01/02/soy-fails-to-help-menapause.aspx.

————. September 18, 2010. "This 'Miracle Health Food' Has Been Linked to Brain Damage and Breast Cancer." *Mercola Newsletter.* http://articles.mercola.com/sites/articles/archive/2010/09/18/soy-can-damage-your-health.aspx.

Schardt, David. January/February 2000. "Phytoestrogens for Menopause." *Nutrition Action Newsletter.* Center for Science in the Public Interest—U.S. edition.

Technical

Ardies, C. M., et al. June 1998. "Xenoestrogens Significantly Enhance Risk for Breast Cancer during Growth and Adolescence." *Medical Hypotheses* 50, no. 6: 457–64.

Atluru, S., and D. Atluru. February 1991. "Evidence That Genistein, a Protein-Tyrosine Kinase Inhibitor, Inhibits CD28 Monoclonal Antibody-Stimulated Human T-Cell Proliferation." *Transplantation* 51, no. 2: 448–50.

Canaris, G. J., et al. 2000. "The Colorado Thyroid Disease Prevalence Study." *Archives of Internal Medicine* 160: 526–34.

Connolly, J. M., et al. 1997. "Effects of Dietary Menhaden Oil, Soy and a Cyclooxygenase Inhibitor on Human Breast Cancer Cell Growth and Metastasis in Nude Mice." *Nutrition and Cancer* 29, no. 1: 48–54.

Farr, G. 1999. "Soy Can Cause Severe Allergic Reactions." *Allergy* 54: 261–65.

Fitzpatrick, M. February 11, 2000. "Soy Formulas and the Effects of Isoflavones on the Thyroid." *New Zealand Medical Journal* 113: 24–26.

Hsieh, C., et al. September 1, 1998. "Estrogenic Effects of Genistein on the Growth of Estrogen Receptor–Positive Human Breast Cancer (MCF-7) Cells In Vitro and In Vivo." *Cancer Research* 58, no. 17: 3833–38.

Ishizuki, Y., et al. May 20, 1991. "The Effects on the Thyroid Gland of Soybeans Administered Experimentally in Healthy Subjects" [in Japanese]. *Nippon Naibunpi Gakkai Zasshi* 67, no. 5: 622–29.

Lawrence, F. July 25, 2006. "Should We Worry about Soya in Our Food?" *The Guardian.* See quote by M. Fitzpatrick. www.guardian.co.uk/technology/blog/2006/jul/26/shouldweworry.

McMichael-Phillips, D. F., et al. December 1998. "Effects of Soy Protein Supplementation on Epithelial Proliferation in the Histologically Normal Human Breast." *American Journal of Clinical Nutrition* 68, no. 6 suppl.: 1431S–35S.

Metzler, M., et al. 1998. "Genotoxicity of Estrogens." *Zeitschrift für Lebensmitteluntersuchung und -Forschung A* 206: 367–73.

Morris, S. M. August 31, 1998. "P53, Mutations and Apoptosis in Genistein-Exposed Human Lymphoblastoid Cells." *Mutation Research* 405, no. 1: 41–56.

———. September–October 1999. "Pregnant Women Should Not Eat Soy Products." *Oncology Reports* 6, no. 5: 1089–95.

Nestor, J. August 13, 2006. "Too Much of a Good Thing? Controversy Rages over the World's Most Regaled Legume." *San Francisco Chronicle*. See quote by D. Kaayla. www.SFGate.com (search for article title).

Rackis, J. J., et al. 1985. "The USDA Trypsin Inhibitor Study. I. Background, Objectives and Procedural Details." *Qualification of Plant Foods in Human Nutrition* 35: 232.

Sacks, Frank M., et al. 2006. "Soy Protein, Isoflavones, and Cardiovascular Health. An American Heart Association Science Advisory for Professionals from the Nutrition Committee." *Circulation* 113: 1034–44.

Setchell, K. D., et al. July 5, 1997. "Exposure of Infants to Phyto-oestrogens from Soy-Based Infant Formula." *Lancet* 350, no. 9070: 23–27.

Wang, C., et al. 1997. "Phytoestrogen Concentration Determines Effects on DNA Synthesis in Human Breast Cancer Cells." *Nutrition and Cancer* 28, no. 3: 236–47.

Dietary Fat/Heart Disease . . . Etc.

Books

Enig, M. 2000. *Know Your Fats: The Complete Primer for Understanding the Nutrition of Fats, Oils and Cholesterol.* Silver Spring, Md.: Bethesda Press.

Enig, M., and S. Fallon. 2005. *Eat Fat Lose Fat.* New York: Hudson Street Press.

Erasmus, U. 1993. *Fats That Heal, Fats That Kill.* Burnaby, B.C.: Alive Books.

Frankel, P., and C. Kim. 1996. Preface of *Beyond Antioxidants: Methylation, Homocysteine and Nutrition,* by C. Cooney. The Research Corner.

Koga, Y., et al. 1994. "Recent Trends in Cardiovascular Disease and Risk Factors in the Seven Countries." In *Lessons for Science from the Seven Countries Study,* edited by H. Toshima, Y. Koga, and H. Blackburn, 63–74. New York: Springer.

Mann, G. V., ed. 1993. *Coronary Heart Disease: The Dietary Sense and Non-sense.* London: Janus.

Murray, M., ND, and J. Beutler, RRT, RCP. 1996. *Understanding Fats and Oils: Your Guide to Healing with Essential Fatty Acids.* Encinitas, Calif.: Progressive Health Publishing.

Peskin, B. S., 2001. *Peak Performance—Radiant Health: Moving beyond the Zone.* Houston: Noble Publishing.

Pollan, M. 2006. *The Omnivore's Dilemma: A Natural History of Four Meals.* New York: The Penguin Press.

Ravnskov, U. 2000. *The Cholesterol Myths: Exposing the Fallacy That Saturated Fat and Cholesterol Cause Heart Disease.* Washington, D.C.: New Trends Publishing.

Robinson, Jo. 2004. *Pasture Perfect: The Far Reaching Benefits of Choosing Meat, Eggs and Dairy Products from Grass-Fed Animals.* Vashon, Wash.: Vashon Island Press.

Saynor, R., and F. Ryan. 1990. *The Eskimo Diet: How to Avoid a Heart Attack.* London: Ebury Press.

Schmidt, M. A. 1997. Foreword to *Smart Fats: How Dietary Fats and Oils Affect Mental, Physical and Emotional Intelligence,* by J. S. Bland. Berkeley, Calif.: Frog, Ltd.

Taubes, G. 2007. *Good Calories, Bad Calories: Challenging the Conventional Wisdom on Diet, Weight Control and Disease.* New York: Alfred A. Knopf.

Willett, W. C., 1990. *Nutritional Epidemiology.* New York: Oxford University Press.

Articles

Ainsworth, C. September 16, 2000. "Love That Fat." *New Scientist.*

American Heart Association. March 1, 2001. "Fatty Fish Cuts Risk of Death from Heart Attack in Elderly." *Health News.*

Associated Press. October 30, 2007. "Cholesterol Drug Use Rising Rapidly in Young: Experts Cite Higher Rates of Obesity, Increased Preventive Treatments." www.msnbc.msn.com/id/21534447.

Byrnes, S., ND, RNCP. "Why Butter Is Better." *Mercola Newsletter.*

Bulkeley, W. M. July 17, 2008. "Study Fuels Low-Fat vs. Low-Carb Debate." The *Wall Street Journal,* D1.

Conner, W. March 13, 2002. "Importance of Omega Three Fats in Health and Disease." *Mercola Newsletter.*

Fallon, S., and M. Enig. "The Oiling of America." www.westonaprice.org/know-your-fats/525-the-oiling-of-america.html.

Hubbard, S. B. 2010. "Statin Drug Weakens Immune System." *Newsmax Health.* www.newsmaxhealth.com/health_stories/statin_drug_resistance/2010/03/25/313907.html.

Mercola, J. February 23, 2002. "Breakthrough Updates You Need to Know on Vitamin D." *Mercola Newsletter.*

———. November 24, 2001. "Cholesterol Is Needed to Help Your Brain Cells Communicate." *Mercola Newsletter.* www.mercola.com/2001/nov/24/cholesterol.htm.

———. September 17, 2000. "Lipoprotein(a) Increases Heart Disease Risk." *Mercola Newsletter.* www.mercola.com/2000/sept/17/lipoprotein_a.htm. Originally appeared in *Circulation,* September 5, 2000: 102.

Moore, T. J. September 1989. "The Cholesterol Myth." *The Atlantic.*

O'Neill, M. November 17, 1991. "Can Fois Gras Aid the Heart? A French Scientist Says 'Yes.'" The *New York Times.*

Passwater, R. A. June 10, 2000. "Health Risks of Processed Foods and the Dangers of Trans Fats." Interview of M. Enig. *Mercola Newsletter,* no. 157.

Peat, R. "Coconut Oil." *Mercola Newsletter,* no. 205.

Raloff, J. May 4, 1996. "High Fat Diets Help Athletes Perform." *Science News* 149, no. 18: 287.

Taubes, G. March 30, 2001. "The Soft Science of Dietary Fat." *Science,* 291.

———. July 7, 2002. "What If It's All Been a Big Fat Lie?" The *New York Times Magazine.*

Technical

Abrams, H. L., Jr. 1987. "The Preference for Animal Protein and Fat: A Cross Cultural Survey." In *Food and Evolution,* edited by Marvin Harris and Eric B. Ross. Philadelphia: Temple University Press.

Ascherio, A., and W. C. Willett. 1997. "Health Effects of Trans Fatty Acids." *American Journal of Clinical Nutrition* 66, suppl. 4: 1006S–10S.

Beane-Rogers, J. September 1995. "Are Saturated Fatty Acids Essential in the Diet?" Letter to the editor. *Nutrition Reviews* 53, no. 9: 269.

Broadhurst, C. L. 1997. "Balanced Intakes of Natural Triglycerides for Optimum Nutrition: An Evolutionary and Phytochemical Perspective." *Medical Hypotheses* 49: 247–61.

Carlson, B. A., and J. D. Kingston. January/February 2007. "Docosahexaenoic Acid, the Aquatic Diet, and Hominin Encephalization: Difficulties in Establishing Evolutionary Links." *American Journal of Human Biology* 19, no. 1: 132–41.

Carrol, K. K., and H. T. Khan. 1971. "Lipids: Effect of Level and Type of Dietary Fat on Incidence of Mammary Tumors Induced in Female Sprague-Dawley Rats by 7, 12-dimethybenz(a)anthracene." *Lipids* 6: 415–20.

Caso, G., et al. May 15, 2007. "Effect of Coenzyme Q10 on Myopathic Symptoms in Patients Treated with Statins." *American Journal of Cardiology* 99, no. 10: 1409–12.

Castilli, W. July 1992. "Concerning the Possibility of a Nut . . ." *Archives of Internal Medicine* 152, no. 7: 1371–72.

Corr, L. A., and M. F. Oliver. January 1997. "The Low Fat/Low Cholesterol Diet Is Ineffective." *European Heart Journal* 18: 18–22.

Dhingra R., et al. 2007. "Soft Drink Consumption and Risk of Developing Cardiometabolic Risk Factors and the Metabolic Syndrome in Middle-Aged Adults in the Community." *Circulation* 116: 480–88.

Dhiman, T. October 10, 1998. "Detailed Fatty Acid Composition Report of Organic Pasture-Fed Beef from River Run Farm in Clatskanie, OR." Research done at Skaggs Nutrition Laboratory, Utah State University.

Elias, P. K., et al. 2005. "Serum Cholesterol and Cognitive Performance in the Framingham Heart Study." *Psychosomatic Medicine* 67, no. 1: 24–30.

Felton, C. V., et al. 1994. "Dietary Polyunsaturated Fatty Acids and Composition of Human Aortic Plaques." *Lancet* 344: 1195.

Folkers, et al. 1990. "Lovastatin Decreases Coenzyme Q Levels in Humans." *Proceedings of the National Academy of Sciences* 87, no. 22: 8931–34.

Garrett, H. E., et al. August 31, 1964. "Serum Cholesterol Values in Patients Treated Surgically for Atherosclerosis." *Journal of the American Medical Association* 189, no. 9: 655–59.

Gillman, M. W., et al. December 24–31, 1997. "Inverse Association of Dietary Fat with Development of Ischemic Stroke in Men." *Journal of the American Medical Association* 278, no. 24: 2145–50.

Golomb, B. A. 2005. "Impact of Statin Adverse Events in the Elderly." *Expert Opinion on Drug Safety* 4, no. 3:389–97.

Iribarren, C., et al. 2000. "Cohort Study of Serum Cholesterol and In-Hospital Incidence of Infectious Diseases." *Epidemiology and Infection* 121, no. 2: 335–47.

Jacobs, D., et al. 1992. "Report of the Conference on Low Blood Cholesterol: Mortality Association." *Circulation* 86: 1046–60.

Kabera, J. J. 1978. *The Pharmacological Effects of Lipids.* Champaign, Ill.: *The American Oil Chemists Society,* 1–14.

Knopp, Robert H., and Barbara M. Retzlaf. 2004. "Saturated Fats Prevent Coronary Artery Disease? An American Paradox." *American Journal of Clinical Nutrition* 80, no. 5: 1102–3.

Krumholz, H. M., et al. 1994. "Lack of Association between Cholesterol and Coronary Heart Disease Mortality and Morbidity and All-Cause Mortality in Persons Older Than 70 Years." *Journal of the American Medical Association* 272: 1334–40.

Lourdes, Ribas, et al. 1995. "How Could Changes in Diet Explain Changes in Coronary Heart Disease Mortality in Spain? The Spanish Paradox." *American Journal of Clinical Nutrition* 61, suppl. 6: 1351S–59S.

Lutsey, P., et al. 2008. "Dietary Intake and the Development of the Metabolic Syndrome: The Atherosclerosis Risk in Communities Study." *Circulation* 117: 754–61.

MacLennan, A. 2001. "Women's Risk of Intraparenchymal Hemorrhage Linked to Low Meat and Saturated Fat Intake." *Circulation* 103: 856.

Mann, G., et al. 1994. "Metabolic Consequences of Dietary Trans Fatty Acids." *Lancet* 343: 1268–71.

Nelson, G. J. 1998. "Dietary Fat, *Trans* Fatty Acids, and Risk of Coronary Heart Disease." *Nutrition Reviews* 56: 250–52.

Newbold, H. L. January 1988. "Reducing Serum Cholesterol with a Diet High in Animal Fat." *Southern Medical Journal* 81, no. 1: 61–63.

Newman, T. B., et al. January 3, 1996. "Carcinogenicity of Lipid-Lowering Drugs." *Journal of the American Medical Association* 275, no. 1.

Okuyama, H., et al. 1997. "Dietary Fatty Acids: The N-6/N-3 Balance and Chronic Elderly Diseases. Excess Linoleic Acid and Relative N-3 Deficiency Syndrome Seen in Japan." *Progress in Lipid Research* 35, no. 4: 409–57.

Oliver, M. F. 1997. "It Is More Important to Increase the Intake of Saturated Fats than to Decrease the Intake of Saturated Fats: Evidence from Clinical Trials Relating to Ischemic Heart Disease." *American Journal of Clinical Nutrition* 66, suppl. 4: 980S–86S.

Olsen, R. E. 1998. "Evolution of Ideas about the Nutritional Value of Dietary Fat." *Journal of Nutrition* 128, suppl. 2: 421S.

Pan, D. A., et al. 1994. "Critical Review: Dietary Fats, Membrane Phospholipids and Obesity." *Journal of Nutrition* 124, no. 9: 1555–65. http://jn.nutrition.org/content/124/9/1555.full.pdf.

———. 1988. "Re: Golomb's Dissent." *Journal of Clinical Epidemiology* 51, no. 6: 465.

Rodney A. H., et al. October 3, 2006. "Narrative Review: Lack of Evidence for Recommended Low-Density Lipoprotein Treatment Targets: A Solvable Problem." *Annals of Internal Medicine* 145, no. 7: 520–30.

Salmond, C., MSc. August 1981. "Cholesterol, Coconuts and Diet on Polynesian Atolls: A Natural Experiment: The Pukapuka and Tokelau Island Studies." *The American Journal of Clinical Nutrition* 34: 1552–61.

Schatz, I. J., et al. August 4, 2001. "Cholesterol and All-Cause Mortality in Elderly People from the Honolulu Heart Program: A Cohort Study." *Lancet* 358, no 9279: 351–55.

Shai, I., and D. Schwarzfuchs, et al. July 17, 2008. "Weight Loss with a Low-Carbohydrate, Mediterranean, or Low-Fat Diet." *New England Journal of Medicine* 359, no. 3: 229–41.

Shestov, D. B., et al. 1993. "Increased Risk of Coronary Heart Disease Death in Men with Low Total and Low-Density-Lipoprotein Cholesterol in the Russian Lipid Research Clinics Prevalence Follow-up Study." *Circulation* 88: 846–53.

Stender, S., and J. Dyerberg. 2001. "The Importance of Trans-fatty Acids for Health." Ugeskr Laeger (Denmark) 163: 2349–53.

Tavani, A., et al. 1997. "Margarine Intake and Risk of Nonfatal Acute Myocardial Infarction in Italian Women." *European Journal of Clinical Nutrition* 51: 30–32.

Watkins, B. A., and M. F. Seifert. 1996. "Food Lipids and Bone Health." In *Food Lipids and Health,* edited by R. E. McDonald and D. B. Min, 101. New York: Marcel Dekker, Inc.

Yam, D., et al. 1996. "Diet and Disease—the Israeli Paradox: Possible Dangers of a High Omega-6 Polyunsaturated Fatty Acid Diet." *Israeli Journal of Medical Sciences* 32: 1134–43.

Vitamin D

Books

Hobday, R. 1999. *The Healing Sun: Sunlight and Health in the 21st Century.* Scotland: Findhorn Press, 67.

Sears, A., and J. Herring. 2007. *Your Best Health under the Sun.* Self-published; available by request from: 12794 Forest Hill Blvd., Suite 16, Wellington, FL 33414.

Articles/information

Byrnes, S. February 6, 2002. "Most of Us Need Supplemental Vitamin D." *Mercola Newsletter.* http://articles.mercola.com/sites/articles/archive/2002/02/06/vegetarianism-myths-03.aspx.

Cannell, J. J. February 28, 2004. "Vitamin D Lowers Inflammation." *Mercola Newsletter.* http://articles.mercola.com/sites/articles/archive/2004/02/28/vitamin-d-part-twenty.aspx.

Cannell, J. J., and A. Vasquez. July 3, 2004. "Measuring Your Vitamin D Levels: Your Most Important Blood Test?" *Mercola Newsletter.* http://articles.mercola.com/sites/articles/archive/2004/07/03/vitamin-d-levels.aspx.

Kotz, D. June 23, 2008. "Time in the Sun: How Much Is Needed for Vitamin D?" *U.S. News and World Report.* http://health.usnews.com/health-news/family-health/heart/articles/2008/06/23/time-in-the-sun-how-much-is-needed-for-vitamin-d.html.

Marshall, Trevor G., et al. "Vitamin D: The Alternative Hypothesis." PDF download. http://autoimmunityresearch.org/transcripts/AR-Albert-VitD.pdf.

Mercola, J. April 23, 2002. "Vitamin D Decreases Heart Disease Death Risk." Paper presented at the 42nd Annual Conference on Cardiovascular Disease and Epidemiology Prevention in Honolulu. http://articles.mercola.com/2002/may/11/vitamin_d.htm.

Prevent Disease.com. February 13, 2007. "More Evidence Vitamin D Prevents Cancer." http://preventdisease.com/news/articles/021307_vit_D_cancer.shtml.

Stein, R. July 4, 2008. "Some Seek Guidelines to Reflect Vitamin D's Benefits." The *Washington Post.*

———. May 21, 2004. "Vitamin D Deficiency Is Major Health Risk." The *Washington Post.*

Technical

Bodnar, L. M., et al. 2007. "High Prevalence of Vitamin D Insufficiency in Black and White Pregnant Women Residing in the Northern United States and Their Neonates." *Journal of Nutrition* 137: 447–52.

Garland, C. F., et al. 2005. "Vitamin D and Prevention of Breast Cancer: Pooled Analysis." *Journal of Steroid Biochemistry and Molecular Biology* 97, nos. 1–2: 179–94.

Giovannucci, E., et al. 2006. "A Prospective Study of Predictors of Vitamin D

Status and Cancer Incidence and Mortality in Men." *Journal of the National Cancer Institute* 98: 451–59.

Gorham, E. D., et al. "Optimal Vitamin D Status for Colorectal Cancer Prevention: A Quantitative Meta-analysis." *American Journal of Preventive Medicine* 32, no. 3: 210–16.

Grant, W. B., et al. 2006. "The Association of Solar Ultraviolet B (UVB) with Reducing Risk of Cancer: Multifactorial Ecologic Analysis of Geographic Variation in Age-Adjusted Cancer Mortality Rates." *Anticancer Research* 26: 2687–2700.

Holick, M. F. March 2004. "Vitamin D: Importance in the Prevention of Cancers, Type 1 Diabetes, Heart Disease, and Osteoporosis." *American Journal of Clinical Nutrition* 79, no. 3: 362–71.

Houghton, L. A., and V. Reinhold. October 2006. "The Case against Ergocalciferol (Vitamin D$_2$) as a Vitamin Supplement." *American Journal of Clinical Nutrition* 84, no. 4: 694–97.

Lappe, et al. 2006. "Vitamin D Status in a Rural Postmenopausal Female Population." *Journal of the American College of Nutrition* 25, no. 5: 395–402.

Marshall, T. G. January 15, 2008. "Vitamin D Discovery Outpaces FDA Decision Making." *Bioessays* 30, no. 2: 173–82.

Munger, K. L., et al. January 13, 2004. "Vitamin D Intake and Incidence of Multiple Sclerosis." *Neurology* 62, no. 1: 60–65.

Whitworth, A., 2006. "Low Vitamin D Levels Associated with Increased Total Cancer Incidence" [press release]. *Journal of the National Cancer Institute* 98, no. 7: 425.

Wilkins, C. H., et al. December 2006. "Vitamin D Deficiency Is Associated with Low Mood and Worse Cognitive Performance in Older Adults." *American Journal of Geriatric Psychiatry* 14: 1032–40.

Genetic Influence

Books

Dawkins, R. 1976. *The Selfish Gene.* New York: Oxford University Press, Inc.

Lipton, B. 2005. *The Biology of Belief.* Santa Rosa, Calif.: Elite Books.

Pert, C. 1997. *Molecules of Emotion: The Science behind Mind-Body Medicine.* New York: Scribner.

Articles

Pearson, H. 2003. "Geneticists Play the Numbers Game in Vain." *Nature* 423: 576.

Silverman, P. H. 2004. "Re-thinking Genetic Determinism: With Only 30,000

Genes, What Is It That Makes Humans Human?" *The Scientist* 18, no. 10: 32–33.

Willet, W. C. 2002. "Balancing Lifestyle and Genomics Research for Disease Prevention." *Science* 296: 695–98.

Technical

Nijout, H. F. 1990. "Metaphors and the Role of Genes in Development." *Bioessays* 12, no. 9: 441–46.

Waterland, R. A., and R. L. Jirtle. 2003. "Transposable Elements: Targets for Early Nutritional Effects on Epigenic Gene Regulation." *Molecular and Cell Biology* 23, no. 15: 5293–5300.

Digestion

Books

Campbell-McBride, N. 2004. *Gut and Psychology Syndrome: Natural Treatment for Autism, Dyspraxia, Dyslexia, ADD/ADHD, Depression and Schizophrenia.* Cambridge, Mass.: Medinform Publishing.

Lipski, E. 2005. *Digestive Wellness: How to Strengthen the Immune System and Prevent Disease through Healthy Digestion.* 3rd ed. New York: McGraw-Hill Companies.

Wright, J., and L. Lenard. 2001. *Why Stomach Acid Is Good for You: Natural Relief from Heartburn, Indigestion, Reflux and GERD.* Brooklyn, N.Y.: M. Evans and Company.

Technical

Bested, A. C., et al. 2001. "Chronic Fatigue Syndrome: Neurological Findings May Be Related to Blood–Brain Barrier Permeability." *Medical Hypotheses* 57: 231–37.

Liu, Z., et al. 2005. "Tight Junctions, Leaky Intestines, and Pediatric Diseases." *Acta Paediatrica* 94: 386.

Little, T. J., et al. November 2005. "Role of Cholecystokinin in Appetite Control and Body Weight Regulation." *Obesity Reviews* 6, no. 4: 297–306.

Macdonald, T. T., and G. Monteleone. 2005. "Immunity, Inflammation, and Allergy in the Gut." *Science* 307: 1920–25.

Meddings, J. 2008. "The Significance of the Gut Barrier in Disease." *Gut* 57: 438–40.

Sigthorsson, G., et al. 1998. "Intestinal Permeability and Inflammation in Patients on NSAIDs." *Gut* 43: 506–11.

White, J. F. 2003. "Intestinal Pathophysiology in Autism." *Experimental Biology and Medicine* 228: 639–49.

Miscellaneous Dietary Topics
Books

Batmanghelidj, F. 1995. *Your Body's Many Cries for Water.* 2nd ed. Falls Church, Va.: Global Health Solutions, Inc.

Bland, Jeffrey S., et al. 2004. *Clinical Nutrition: A Functional Approach.* 2nd ed. Gig Harbor, Wash.: Institute for Functional Medicine.

Fallon, S., and M. Enig. 1999. *Nourishing Traditions: The Cookbook That Challenges Politically Correct Nutrition and the Diet Dictocrats.* San Diego, Calif.: ProMotion Publishing.

Guyton, A. C., and J. E. Hall. 1996. *Textbook of Medical Physiology.* 9th ed. Philadelphia: W. B. Saunders Company.

Haas, E. M., with B. Levin. 2006. *Staying Healthy with Nutrition.* Berkeley, Calif.: Celestial Arts.

Hendler, Sheldon S. 2001. *PDR for Nutritional Supplements.* 2nd ed. Montvale, N.J.: Physicians Desk Reference Inc.

Moynihan, R., and A. Cassels. 2005. *Selling Sickness: How the World's Biggest Pharmaceutical Companies Are Turning Us All into Patients.* New York: Nation Books.

Passwater, R. A., and E. M. Cranton. 1983. *Trace Elements, Hair Analysis and Nutrition.* New Canaan, Conn.: Keats Publishing.

Peat, R. 1997. *From PMS to Menopause.* Eugene, Ore.: Raymond Peat.

Pfeiffer, C. C., and the Publications Committee of the Brain Bio Center. 1975. *Mental and Elemental Nutrients: A Physician's Guide to Nutrition and Healthcare.* New Canaan, Conn.: Keats Publishing.

Rapp, D. J. 1979. *Allergies and the Hyperactive Child.* New York: Simon & Schuster.

———. 1991. *Is This Your Child? Discovering and Treating Unrecognized Allergies in Children and Adults.* New York: William Morrow and Company.

Ross, J. 1999. *The Diet Cure.* New York: Penguin Putnam.

Schauss, A. 1995. *Minerals and Human Health: The Rationale for Optimal and Balanced Trace Element Levels.* Tacoma, Wash.: AIBR.

Schauss, A. G., 1981. Introduction to *Diet, Crime and Delinquency,* by Michael Lesser. Mira Loma, Calif.: Parker House Publishing.

Segala, Melanie. 2003. *Disease Prevention and Treatment.* 4th ed. Gig Harbor, Wash.: Life Extension Media.

Simontacchi, C. 2000. *The Crazy Makers: How the Food Industry Is Destroying Our Brains and Harming Our Children*. New York: Jeremy Tarcher/Putnam Books.

Timon, M. S. 1979. *Mineral Logic: Understanding the Mineral Transporting System*. San Francisco: Benjamin/Cummings Publishing Co. Reviewed by J. S. Bland, Ph.D.

Tortora, Gerard J., and Sandra R. Grabowski. 2004. *Introduction to the Human Body: The Essentials of Anatomy and Physiology*. 6th ed. Old Tappan, N.J.: Biological Sciences Textbooks, Inc.

Werbach, M. R. 1996. *Nutritional Influences on Illness: A Sourcebook of Clinical Research*. 2nd ed. Tarzana, Calif.: Third Line Press.

Wiley, T. S. 2000. *Lights Out: Sleep, Sugar and Survival*. New York: Pocket Books.

Articles

Anderson, F. "The Thesis of Body Mineral Balancing." *Trace Minerals Research*. Summary of research. www.health-enz.com/minerals/minerals5.shtml.

Ashmead, D. April 1981. "What a Zinc Deficiency Can Do to You." *Bestways Magazine*.

Bushman, J. September/October 1998. "ADD: Attention Deficit Disorder: Natural Therapies May Offer Improvement without the Side Effects of Conventional Drugs." *Consumer News*.

Dean, W., 2004. "DMAE: Cognitive-Enhancing, Life-Extending Nutrient." *Vitamin Research News* 18, no. 8: 1–4.

"Doctors Say, Raise the RDAs Now." October 30, 2007. *Orthomolecular Medicine News Service*.

Ethridge, E., September 1997. "Brain Food." *Energy Times*.

Freedman, David H., November 2010. "Lies, Damned Lies, and Medical Science." *The Atlantic*. www.theatlantic.com/magazine/archive/2010/11/lies-damned-lies-and-medical-science/8269.

Heinerman, J., March/April 1997. "Mineral Nutrition of Coastal Cultures in Prehistoric Times." *The Source Newsletter*.

Hill, A. August 16, 2009. "Healthy Food Obsession Sparks Rise in New Eating Disorder: Fixation with Healthy Eating Can Be a Sign of a Serious Psychological Disorder." *The Observer/Guardian*. www.guardian.co.uk/society/2009/aug/16/orthorexia-mental-health-eating-disorder.

Nielsen, M. T. "Ions: The Body's Electrical Energy Source." *Trace Minerals*

Research. www.ionique.com/docs/Ions%20and%20Electrical%20Energy .pdf.

Osborne, S. E. "Book Review: Eat Right for Your Type Hype." Price-Pottenger Foundation, *Health and Healing Wisdom Journal* 22, no. 4. http://editor .nourishedmagazine.com.au/articles/book-review-eat-right-for-your-type-hype.

Sahley, B. J. 2000. "Natural Control of ADD and ADHD." *Vitamin Research News* 14, no. 10.

Saul, S., and G. Harris. 2007. "Diabetes Drug Still Has Heart Risks, Doctors Warn." The *New York Times.*

Singh, et al. 2007. "Rosiglitazone and Cardiovascular Risk." *New England Journal of Medicine* 30, no. 24: 2148–53.

Stitt, B. R. October/November 1997. "Healing the Delinquent Mind: A Complementary Approach." *Nature's Impact.*

"Trade Secrets, Moyer's Report Confidential: Chemical Body Burden." Public Broadcasting Service. www.pbs.org/tradesecrets/problem/bodyburden .html.

Technical

Adriani, W., et al. November 2004. "Acetyl-l-carnitine Reduces Impulsive Behaviour in Adolescent Rats." *Psychopharmacology* 176, nos. 3–4: 296–304.

"Body Burden—the Pollution in Newborns." July 14, 2005. Environmental Working Group. www.ewg.org (search for article title).

Heini, A. F., and R. L. Weinsier. March 1997. "Divergent Trends in Obesity and Fat Intake Patterns: The American Paradox." *American Journal of Medicine* 102, no. 3: 259–64.

McConnell, H., et al. 1985. "Catecholamine Metabolism in Attention Deficit Disorder." *Medical Hypotheses* 17, no. 4: 305–11.

Mitchell, A. E., et al. 2007. "Ten-Year Comparison on the Content of Flavonoids in Tomatoes." *The Journal of Agriculture and Food Chemistry* 55, no. 15: 6154–59.

Tankova, T., et al. 2004. "Alpha Lipoic Acid in the Treatment of Autonomic Diabetic Neuropathy," *Romanian Journal of Internal Medicine* 42, no. 4: 457–64.

Wang, S. 2001. "Effects of Chromium and Fish Oil on Insulin Resistance and Leptin Resistance in Obese Developing Rats" [in Chinese]. *Wei Sheng Yan Jiu* 30, no. 5: 284–86.

Endocrine/Leptin

Books

Richards, B. J. 2009. *Mastering Leptin: The Leptin Diet, Solving Obesity and Preventing Disease.* Minneapolis: Wellness Resources Books.

Talbott, S. 2002. *The Cortisol Connection: Why Stress Makes You Fat and Ruins Your Health—and What You Can Do about It.* Alameda, Calif.: Hunter House Publishers.

Wilson, J. L. 2001. *Adrenal Fatigue: The 21st Century Stress Syndrome.* Petaluma, Calif.: Smart Publications.

Articles

Rosedale, R. January 13, 2008. "Insulin, Leptin, Diabetes, and Aging: Not So Strange Bedfellows." *Diabetes Health.* www.diabeteshealth.com/read/2008/01/13/5617.html.

Technical

Agus, M. S. 2000. "Dietary Composition and Physiologic Adaptations to Energy Restriction." *American Journal of Clinical Nutrition* 71, no. 4: 901–7.

Ahima, R. S. 1996. "Role of Leptin in the Neuroendocrine Response to Fasting." *Nature* 382: 250–52.

Aida, J., et al. January 2010. "Telomere Lengths in the Oral Epithelia with and without Carcinoma." *European Journal of Cancer* 46, no. 2: 430–38.

Ainslie, D. A. 2000. "Short Term, High Fat Diets Lower Circulating Leptin Concentrations in Rats." *American Journal of Clinical Nutrition* 71: 438–42.

Baile, C. A. 2000. "Regulation of Metabolism and Body Fat Mass by Leptin." *Annual Review of Nutrition* 20: 105–27.

Blum, M., et al. July 2003. "Leptin, Body Composition and Bone Mineral Density in Premenopausal Women." *Calcified Tissue International* 73, no. 1: 27–32.

Cleare, A. J. April 2003. "The Neuroendocrinology of Chronic Fatigue Syndrome." *Endocrine Reviews* 24, no. 2: 236–52.

Diehl, M. C., et al. July 13, 2010. "Elevated TRF2 in Advanced Breast Cancers with Short Telomeres," *Breast Cancer Research and Treatment.*

Ducy, P. 2000. "The Osteoblast: A Sophisticated Fibroblast under Central Surveillance." *Science* 289: 1502–4.

Figlewicz, D. P. 2003. "Adiposity Signals and Food Reward: Expanding the CNS Roles of Insulin and Leptin." *American Journal of Physiology—Regulatory, Integrative and Comparative Physiology* 284: R882–92.

Harris, R. B. 2000. "Leptin—Much More Than a Satiety Signal." *Annual Review of Nutrition* 20: 45–75.

Hauner, H. May 2005. "Secretory Factors from Human Adipose Tissue and Their Functional Role." *Proceedings of the Nutrition Society* 64, no. 2: 163–69.

Karsenty, G. 2000. "The Central Regulation of Bone Remodeling." *Trends in Endocrinology and Metabolism* 11, no. 10: 437–39.

Kharrazian, D., D.H.Sc., D.C., M.S. September 2007. Course, "Functional Endocrinology." Sponsored by Apex Energetics and the University of Bridgeport College of Chiropractic. Course #PG 952/NCCAOM, course #ACHB 404-007. Portland, Ore.

Lafafe-Poust, M. H., et al. March 2003. "Glucocorticoid-Induced Osteoporosis: Pathophysiology Data and Recent Treatments." *Joint Bone Spine* 70, no. 2: 109–18.

Lang, Janet R., DC. May 2007. Course, "Thyroid, Adrenals and Blood Sugar." Sponsored by Standard Process and Lang Integrative Health Seminars. Portland, Ore.

McGrath, M., et al. April 2007. "Telomere Length, Cigarette Smoking and Bladder Cancer Risk in Men and Women." *Cancer Epidemiology, Biomarkers & Prevention* 16, no. 4: 815–19.

Rampazzo, E., et al. April 13, 2010. "Relationship between Telomere Shortening, Genetic Instability and Site of Tumour Origin in Colorectal Cancers." *British Journal of Cancer* 102, no. 8: 1300–5.

Roberts, A. D., et al. February 2004. "Salivary Cortisol Response to Awakening in Chronic Fatigue Syndrome." *British Journal of Psychiatry* 184: 136–41.

Trayhurn, P. August 2005. "Endocrine and Signalling Role of Adipose Tissue: New Perspectives on Fat." *Acta Physiologica Scandinavica* 184, no. 4: 285–93.

Wadden, T. A. 1998. "Short and Long Term Changes in Serum Leptin in Dieting Obese Women: Effects of Caloric Restriction and Weight Loss." *Journal of Clinical Endocrinology & Metabolism* 83, no. 1: 214–18.

Wust, S., et al. February 2004. "Common Polymorphisms in the Glucocorticoid Receptor Gene Are Associated with Adrenocorticoid Responses to Psychosocial Stresses." *Journal of Clinical Endocrinology & Metabolism* 89, no. 2: 565–73.

Zarković, M., et al., September–October 2003. "Disorder of Adrenal Gland Function in Chronic Fatigue Syndrome" [article in Serbian]. *Srpski Arhiv za Celokupno Lekarstvo* 131, no. 9–10: 370–74.131.

Exercise

Books

Lee, R. 2007. *The Millionaire Workout*. New Canaan, Conn.: Okenzie Publishing.

Sears, A. 2006. *PACE: Rediscover Your Native Fitness*. Wellington, Fla.: Wellness Research Consulting, Inc.

Tsatsouline, P. 2003. *The Naked Warrior*. Little Canada, Minn.: Dragon Door Publications, Inc.

———. 1999. *Power to the People*. Little Canada, Minn.: Dragon Door Publications, Inc.

Articles

Lee, R. "Everything You've Been Told about Exercise Might Be Wrong." *Mercola Newsletter*. www.selfgrowth.com/articles/Mercola59.html.

Mercola, J. May 2007. "If You Aren't Using This Type of Exercise You Are Missing Out Big Time." *Mercola Newsletter*.

Technical

Deldicque, L., D. Theisen, and M. Francaux. 2005. "Regulation of mTOR by Amino Acids and Resistance Exercise in Skeletal Muscle." *European Journal of Applied Physiology* 94, nos. 1–2: 1–10

Long, B. C., and R. van Stavel. 1995. "Effects of Exercise Training on Anxiety: A Meta-analysis." *Journal of Applied Sport Psychology* 7: 167–89.

Martinsen, E. W. 1994. "Physical Activity and Depression: Clinical Experience." *Acta Psychiatrica Scandinavica* 377: 23–27.

Miller, W. C., et al. 1997. "A Meta-analysis of the Past 25 Years of Weight Loss Research Using Diet, Exercise, or Diet Plus Exercise Intervention." *International Journal of Obesity and Related Metabolic Disorders* 21, no. 10: 941–47.

Neilan, T. G., et al. 2006. "Myocardial Injury and Ventricular Dysfunction Related to Training Levels among Non-elite Participants in the Boston Marathon." *Circulation* 114: 2325–33.

North, T. C., et al. 1990. "Effect of Exercise on Depression." *Exercise and Sport Science Reviews* 18: 379–415.

O'Connor, P. J., and M. A. Youngstedt. 1995. "Influence of Exercise on Human Sleep." *Exercise and Sport Science Reviews* 23: 105–34.

Petruzzello, S. J., et al. 1991. "A Meta-analysis of the Anxiety-Reducing Effects of Acute and Chronic Exercise." *Sports Medicine* 11, no. 3: 143–82.

Schlicht, W. 1994. "Does Physical Exercise Reduce Anxious Emotions? A Meta-analysis." *Anxiety, Stress, and Coping* 6: 275–88.

Tabata, I., et al. October 1996. "Effects of Moderate-Intensity Endurance and High-Intensity Intermittent Training on Anaerobic Capacity and VO2max." *Medicine & Science in Sports and Exercise* 28, no. 10:1327–30.

Talanian, J. L., et al. 2007. "Two Weeks of High-Intensity Aerobic Interval Training Increases the Capacity for Fat Oxidation during Exercise in Women." *Journal of Applied Physiology* 102: 1439–47. doi:10.1152/japplphysiol.01098 .2006 8750-7587/07.

Primal Mind: Nutrition and Mental Health
Books

Braverman, E. R. 1997. *The Healing Nutrients Within: Facts, Findings and New Research on Amino Acids.* New Canaan, Conn.: Keats Publishing.

Breggin, P. R. 2001. *The Anti-depressant Fact Book.* Cambridge, Mass.: Perseus Publishing.

Cozolino, L. 2002. *The Neuroscience of Psychotherapy: Building and Rebuilding the Human Brain.* New York: W. W. Norton & Company, Inc.

Kolb, B., and I. Q. Whishaw. 2001. *An Introduction to Brain and Behavior.* New York: Worth Publishers.

LeDoux, J. *The Emotional Brain.* New York: Touchstone.

Pert, C., *Molecules of Emotion.* New York: Scribner.

Pfeiffer, C. C. 1975. *Mental and Elemental Nutrients.* New Canaan, Conn.: Keats Publishing.

Ross, J., 2002. *The Mood Cure.* New York: Penguin Putnam Inc.

Technical

Ahlbom, A. 2001. "Neurodegenerative Diseases, Suicide and Depressive Symptoms in Relation to EMF." *Bioelectromagnetics* suppl. 5: S132–43.

Balestreri, R., et al. May 1987. "A Double-Blind Placebo Controlled Evaluation of the Safety and Efficacy of Vinpocetine in the Treatment of Patients with Chronic Vascular Senile Cerebral Dysfunction." *Journal of the American Geriatrics Society* 35, no. 5: 425–30.

Blumenthal, J. A., et al. 2007. "Exercise and Pharmacotherapy in the Treatment of Major Depressive Disorder." *Psychosomatic Medicine* 69, no. 7: 587–96.

Boukje, M., et al. 2007. "Fish Consumption, n-3 Fatty Acids, and Subsequent 5-y Cognitive Decline in Elderly Men." *American Journal of Clinical Nutrition* 85, no. 4, 1142–47.

Crook, T. H., et al. 1997. "Effects of Phosphatidylserine in Age-Associated Memory Impairment." *Neurology* 41, no. 5: 644–49.

Ehninger, D., and G. Kempermann. 2008. "Neurogenesis in the Adult Hippocampus." *Cell and Tissue Research* 331, no. 1: 243–50.

Feychting, M. F., et al. 2003. "Occupational Magnetic Field Exposure and Neurodegenerative Disease." *Epidemiology* 14, no. 4: 413–19; discussion, 427–28.

Flint, B. M. July 17–22, 2004. "Oxidative Mechanisms, Inflammation, and Alzheimer's Disease Pathogenesis." Paper presented at the Ninth International Conference on Alzheimer's Disease, Philadelphia.

Helisalmi, S., et al. 2006. "Association of CYP46 Intron 2 Polymorphism in Finnish Alzheimer's Disease." *Journal of Neurology, Neurosurgery, and Psychiatry* 77: 421–42.

Kharrazian, D., D.H.Sc., D.C., M.S. September 2008. Course, "Neurotransmitters and the Brain." Sponsored by Apex Energetics and the University of Bridgeport College of Chiropractic, course #PG 952/NCCAOM, course #ACHB 404-009. Portland, Ore.

Kirsch, I., et al. February 2008. "Initial Severity and Antidepressant Benefits: A Meta-analysis of Data Submitted to the Food and Drug Administration." *PLoS Medicine* 5, no. 2: e45. www.plosmedicine.org (search for title).

Krewski, D., et al. 2007. "Recent Advances in Research on Radiofrequency Fields and Health: 2001–2003." *Journal of Toxicology and Environmental Health, Part B: Critical Reviews* 10, no. 4: 287–318.

Mattson, Mark P. 2003. "Gene–Diet Interactions in Brain Aging and Neurodegenerative Disorders." *Annals of Internal Medicine* 139, no. 5: 441–44.

May, A., et al. 2007. "Plasma n-3 Fatty Acids and the Risk of Cognitive Decline in Older Adults." *American Journal of Clinical Nutrition* 85, no. 4: 1103–11.

Messier, C., and K. Teutenberg. 2005. "The Role of Insulin, Insulin Growth Factor, and Insulin-Degrading Enzyme in Brain Aging and Alzheimer's Disease." *Neural Plasticity* 12, no. 4: 311–28.

Millward, C., et al. 2004. "Gluten- and Casein-Free Diets for Autistic Spectrum Disorder" [review]. *Cochrane Database of Systematic Reviews* 2: CD003498.

Morris, M. C., et al. 2003. "Dietary Fats and the Risk of Incident Alzheimer Disease." *Archives of Neurology* 60, no. 2: 194–202.

Mousain-Bosc, M., et al. 2006. "Improvement of Neurobehavioral Disorders in Children Supplemented with Magnesium-Vitamin B6. I. Attention Deficit Hyperactivity Disorders." *Magnesium Research* 19, no. 1: 46–52.

Papakostas, G. I. 2007. "Limitations of Contemporary Antidepressants: Tolerability." *Journal of Clinical Psychiatry* 68, suppl. 10: 11–7.

Paulose-Ram, R., et al. 2007. "Trends in Psychotropic Medication Use among U.S. Adults." *Pharmacoepidemiology and Drug Safety* 16, no. 5: 560–70.

Sinn, N. 2007. "Physical Fatty Acid Deficiency Signs in Children with ADHD Symptoms." *Prostaglandins, Leukotrienes and Essential Fatty Acids* 77, no. 2: 109–15.

Stevenson, J. 2006. "Dietary Influences on Cognitive Development and Behaviour in Children." *Proceedings of the Nutrition Society* 65, no. 4: 361–65.

Tiemeir, H., et al. 2002. "Vitamin B_{12}, Folate, and Homocysteine in Depression: The Rotterdam Study." *American Journal of Psychiatry* 159, no. 12: 2099–101.

Turner, E. H., et al. 2008. "Selective Publication of Antidepressant Trials and Its Influence on Apparent Efficacy." *New England Journal of Medicine* 358, no. 3: 252–60.

Whitmer, R., et al. April 29, 2005. "Obesity in Middle Age and Future Risk of Dementia." *British Medical Journal* 330, no. 7504: 1360.

Wu, A., et al. 2004. "Dietary Omega-3 Fatty Acids Normalize BDNF Levels, Reduce Oxidative Damage, and Counteract Learning Disability after Traumatic Brain Injury in Rats." *Journal of Neurotrauma* 21, no. 10: 1457–67.

Yaffe, K., et al. 2004. "The Metabolic Syndrome, Inflammation, and Risk of Cognitive Decline." *Journal of the American Medical Association* 292, no. 18: 2237–42.

Pyroluria

Books

Pfeiffer, C. C. 1988. *Nutrition and Mental Illness: An Orthomolecular Approach to Balancing Body Chemistry*. Rochester, Vt.: Healing Arts Press.

Ross, J. 2002. *The Mood Cure*. New York: Penguin Putnam Inc.

Articles

Graham, Blake, BSc (Honours), AACNEM. "Pyroluria." *The Analyst*. www.diagnose-me.com/cond/C372380.html.

McGinnis, W. May 21, 2004. "Pyroluria: Hidden Cause of Schizophrenia, Bipolar, Depression, and Anxiety Symptoms." *Safe Harbor*. www.alternativementalhealth.com/articles/pyroluria.htm.

"Pyroluria." DrKaslow.com. www.drkaslow.com/html/pyroluria.html.

"Pyroluria." *Nutritional Healing*. www.nutritional-healing.com.au/content/articles-content.php?heading=Pyroluria.

Technical

Bibus, D. M., et al. April 25–28, 2000. "Fatty Acid Profiles of Schizophrenic Phenotypes." Paper presented at the 91st AOCS Annual Meeting and Expo, San Diego, Calif. www.biobalance.org.au/articles/15.

Hoffer, A., et al. 1961. "The Presence of Unidentified Substances in the Urine of Psychiatric Patients." *Journal of Neuropsychiatry and Clinical Neurosciences* 2: 331–62.

Hoffer, A., and H. Osmond. 1963. "Malvaria: A New Psychiatric Disease." *Acta Psychiatrica Scandinavica* 39: 335–66.

Jackson, J. A., and H. D. Riordan, et al. 1997. "Urinary Pyrrole in Health and Disease." *The Journal of Orthomolecular Medicine.* 12 (2nd quarter): 96–98.

Pfeiffer, Carl, "Twenty-Nine Medical Causes of 'Schizophrenia'" (under heading: "Pyroluria"). *Safe Harbor.* www.alternativementalhealth.com/articles/causesofschizophrenia.htm#Pyroluria.

Pfeiffer, C., et al. 1973. "Biochemical Relationship between Kryptopyrrole (Mauve Factor and Trans-3-methyl-2-hexenoic Acid Schizophrenia Odor)." *Research Communications in Chemical Pathology and Pharmacology.*

———. 1988. "Pyroluria—Zinc and B6 Deficiencies." *International Clinical Nutrition Review.*

Pfeiffer, C., and A. Sohler. 1974. "Treatment of Pyroluric Schizophrenia (Malvaria) with Large Doses of Pyridoxine and a Dietary Supplement of Zinc." *Journal of Orthomolecular Psychiatry* 3, no. 4: 292.

Riordan, et al. 1997. "Urinary Pyrrole in Health and Disease." *Journal of Orthomolecular Medicine* 12: 96–98.

Sohler, A. 1974. "A Rapid Screening Test for Pyroluria; Useful in Distinguishing a Schizophrenic Subpopulation." *Journal of Orthomolecular Psychiatry* 3, no. 4: 273.

Walker, J. L. March–April 1975. "Neurological and Behavioral Toxicity of Kryptopyrrole in the Rat." *Pharmacology Biochemistry and Behavior* 3, no. 2: 243–50.

Walsh, William. "Commentary on Nutritional Treatment of Mental Disorders" ("Pyrroles" heading). *Safe Harbor.* www.alternativementalhealth.com/articles/walshMP.htm#Py.

Walsh, W. J., et al. 2004. "Reduced Violent Behavior Following Biochemical Therapy." *Physiology & Behavior* 82, no. 5: 835–59.

Aging/Antiaging
Books

Pearson, D., and S. Shaw. 1982. *Life Extension: A Practical and Scientific Approach.* New York: Warner Books, Inc.

———. Life Extension Companion. New York: Warner Books, Inc.

Walford, R. L. 1983. *Maximum Life Span.* New York: Avon Books.

Weindruch, R., and R. L. Walford. 1988. *The Retardation of Aging and Disease by Dietary Restriction.* Springfield, Ill.: Charles C. Thomas.

Technical

Apfeld, J. K. October 16, 1998. "Cell Nonautonomy of *C. elegans* daf-2 Function in the Regulation of Diapause and Life Span." *Cell* 95, no. 2: 199–210.

Aziz, M. H., et al. 2005. "Chemoprevention of Skin Cancer by Grape Constituent Resveratrol: Relevance to Human Disease?" *FASEB Journal* 19, no. 9: 1193–95.

Barrows, C.H., Jr., and G. C. Kokkman. 1978. "Diet and Life Extension in Animal Model Systems." *Age* 1: 131.

Block, M. June 2002. "Discovering the Genetic Controls that Dictate Life Span: Profile of Cynthia Kenyon, Ph.D." *Life Extension Magazine.*

Bluher, M. 2003. "Extended Longevity in Mice Lacking the Insulin Receptor in Adipose Tissue." *Science* 299, no. 24: 572–74.

Carlson, A. H., and F. Hoelzel. 1946. "Apparent Prolongation of the Life Span of Rats by Intermittent Fasting." *Journal of Nutrition* 31: 363.

Civitarese, A. E., et al. March 2007. "Calorie Restriction Increases Muscle Mitochondrial Biogenesis in Healthy Humans." *PLoS Medicine* 4, no. 3: e76.

Coleman, R. J., et al. April 1998. "The Effect of Dietary Restriction on Body Composition in Adult Male and Female Rhesus Macaques." *Aging (Milano)* 10, no. 2: 83–92.

Dorman, J. B., et al. December 1995. "The age-1 and daf-2 Genes Function in a Common Pathway to Control the Life Span of *Caenorhabditis elegans.*" *Genetics* 141, no. 4: 1399–406.

Duffy, P. H. 1989. "Effect of Chronic Caloric Restriction on Physiological Variables Related to Energy Metabolism in the Male Fischer 344 Rat." *Mechanisms of Ageing and Development* 48, no. 2: 117–33.

Dye, D. "Calorie Restriction May Help Reduce the Risk of Carcinoma." Life Extension Foundation. www.lef.org/whatshot/2008_04.htm#Calorie-restriction-may-help-reduce-the-risk-of-carcinoma.

Everitt, A.V., and D. G. Le Couteur. October 2007. "Life Extension by Calorie Restriction in Humans." *Annals of the New York Academy of Sciences* 1114: 428-33.

Everitt, A. V., et al. 1980. "The Effects of Hypophysectomy and Continuous Food Restriction, Begun at Ages 70 and 400 Days, on Collagen Aging, Proteinuria, Incidence of Pathology and Longevity in the Male Rat." *Mechanics of Ageing and Development* 12, no. 2: 161.

Fernandez-Galaz, C. 2002. "Long Term Food Restriction Prevents Ageing-Associated Central Leptin Resistance in Wistar Rats." *Diabetologia* 45, no. 7: 997–1003.

Garvin, S., et al. 2006. "Resveratrol Induces Apoptosis and Inhibits Angiogenesis in Human Breast Cancer Xenografts In Vivo." *Cancer Letters* 231, no. 1: 113–22.

Genaro Pde, S., et al. July 2009. "Effect of Caloric Restriction on Longevity" [in Portuguese]. *Arq Bras Endocrinol Metabol* 53, no. 5: 667–72.

Guarente, L., and C. Kenyon. November 9, 2000. "Genetic Pathways That Regulate Ageing in Model Organisms." *Nature* 408, no. 6809: 255–62.

Hansen, B. C. 2001. "Symposium: Calorie Restriction: Effects on Body Composition, Insulin Signaling and Aging." *Journal of Nutrition* 131: 900S–2S

Harper, C. E., et al. 2007. "Resveratrol Suppresses Prostate Cancer Progression in Transgenic Mice." *Journal of Carcinogenesis* 28, no. 9: 1946–53.

Heilbronn, L. K., and E. Ravussin. September 2003. "Calorie Restriction and Aging: Review of the Literature and Implications for Studies in Humans." *American Journal of Clinical Nutrition* 78, no. 3: 361–69.

Holloszy, J. O., and L. Fontana. August 2007. "Caloric Restriction in Humans." *Experimental Gerontology* 42, no. 8: 709-12.

Howitz, K. T., et al. 2003. "Small Molecule Activators of Sirtuins Extend *Saccharomyces cerevisiae* Lifespan." *Nature* 425, no. 6954: 191–96.

Hsin, H., and C. Kenyon. February 1999. "Signals from the Reproductive System Regulate the Life Span of *C. elegans*." *Development* 126, no. 5: 1055–64.

Hursting, S. D., et al. 2003. "Calorie Restriction, Aging and Cancer Prevention: Mechanisms of Action and Applicability to Humans." *Annual Review of Medicine* 54: 131–52.

Jia, K., et al. 2004. "The TOR Pathway Interacts with the Insulin Signaling Pathway to Regulate *C. elegans* Larval Development, Metabolism and Life Span." *Development* 131: 3897–3906.

Kalant, N., et al. December 1988. "Effect of Diet Restriction on Glucose Metabolism and Insulin Responsiveness in Aging Rats." *Mechanics of Ageing and Development* 46, nos. 1–3: 89–104.

Kapahi, P., et al. 2004. "Regulation of Lifespan in *Drosophila* by Modulation of Genes in the mTOR Signaling Pathway." *Current Biology* 14: 885–90.

Kealy, R. D., et al. May 1, 2002. "Effects of Diet Restriction on Life Span and Age-Related Changes in Dogs." *Journal of the American Veterinary Medical Association* 220, no. 9: 1315–20.

Lagouge, M., et al. 2006. "Resveratrol Improves Mitochondrial Function and Protects against Metabolic Disease by Activating SIRT1 and PGC-1alpha." *Cell* 127, no. 6: 1109–22.

Lane, M. A., et al. July 1997. "Dehydroepiandrosterone Sulfate: A Biomarker of Primate Aging Slowed by Calorie Restriction." *Journal of Clinical Endocrinology & Metabolism* 82, no. 7: 2093–96.

Lin K., et al. June 2001. "Regulation of the *Caenorhabditis elegans* Longevity Protein DAF-16 by Insulin/IGF-1 and Germline Signaling." *Nature Genetics* 28, no. 2: 139–45.

Masoro, E. J. January–March 1998. "Hormesis and the Antiaging Action of Dietary Restriction." *Experimental Gerontology* 33, nos. 1–2: 61–66.

———. February 26, 2003. "Subfield History: Caloric Restriction, Slowing Aging, and Extending Life." *Science of Aging Knowledge Environment* 8: RE2.

Masoro, E. J., et al. July 1982. "Action of Food Restriction in Delaying the Aging Process." *Proceedings of the National Academy of Sciences* 79, no. 13: 4239–41.

Mattison, J. A. 2001. "Endocrine Effects of Dietary Restriction and Aging: The National Institute of Aging Study." *Journal of Anti-Aging Medicine* 4, no. 3, 215–34.

Merry, B. J. November 2002. "Molecular Mechanisms Linking Calorie Restriction and Longevity." *International Journal of Biochemistry & Cell Biology* 34, no. 11: 1340–54.

Nelson, D. W. 2003. "Insulin Worms Its Way into the Spotlight." *Genes and Development* 17: 813–18.

Partridge, L. "Mechanisms of Aging: Public or Private?" *Nature Reviews Genetics* 3, no. 3: 173.

Powers, R. W., III, et al. 2006. "Extension of Chronological Life Span in Yeast by Decreased TOR Pathway Signaling." *Genes and Development* 20: 174–84.

Rae, M. Spring 2004. "It's Never Too Late: Caloric Restriction Is Effective in Older Mammals." *Rejuvenation Research* 7, no. 1: 3–8.

Richards, J. B., et al. November 2007. "Higher Serum Vitamin D Concentrations Are Associated with Longer Leukocyte Telomere Length in Women." *Journal of Clinical Nutrition* 86, no. 5: 1420–25.

Roth, G. S. 2002. "Biomarkers of Caloric Restriction May Predict Longevity in Humans." *Science* 297, no. 2: 811.

———. 2000. "Effects of Reduced Energy Intake on the Biology of Aging: The Primate Model." *European Journal of Clinical Nutrition* 54, no. S3, S15–S20.

Salser, S. J., and C. A. Kenyon. May 1996. "*C. elegans* Hox Gene Switches On, Off, On and Off Again to Regulate Proliferation, Differentiation and Morphogenesis." *Development* 122, no. 5: 1651–61.

Shimokawa, I. 2001. "Leptin and Anti-aging Action of Caloric Restriction." *Journal of Nutrition, Health & Aging* 5: 43–48.

———. 2001. "Leptin Signaling and Aging: Insight from Caloric Restriction." *Mechanisms of Ageing and Development* 122, no. 14L: 1511–19.

Sinclair, D. A., and L. Guarente. 2006. "Unlocking the Secrets of Longevity Genes." *Scientific American* 294, no. 3: 48–57.

Song, Z., et al. August 2010. "Lifestyle Impacts on the Aging-Associated Expression of Biomarkers of DNA Damage and Telomere Dysfunction in Human Blood." *Aging Cell* 9, no. 4: 607–15.

Subbiah, M. T. R., and R. G. Siekert Jr. 1979. "Dietary Restriction and the Development of Atherosclerosis." *Journal of Nutrition* 41: 1.

Tannenbaum, A. 1945. "The Dependence of Tumor Formation on the Composition of the Calorie-Restricted Diet as Well as on the Degree of Restriction." *Cancer Research* 5: 616–25.

Wang, Z., et al. 2007. "Effects of Red Wine and Wine Polyphenol Resveratrol on Platelet Aggregation In Vivo and In Vitro." *International Journal of Molecular Medicine* 9, no. 1: 77–79.

Weindruch, R. H., et al. 1979. "The Influence of Controlled Dietary Restriction on Immunologic Function and Aging." *Federation Proceedings* 38, no. 6: 2007–16.

———. 1982. "Modification of Age-Related Immune Decline in Mice Dietarily Restricted from or after Midadulthood." *Proceedings of the National Academy of Sciences* 79: 898–902.

Werner, C., et al. 2009. "Physical Exercise Prevents Cellular Senescence in Circulating Leukocytes and in the Vessel Wall." *Circulation* 120: 2438–47.

Willeit, P., et al. 2010. "Telomere Length and Risk of Incident Cancer and Cancer Mortality." *Journal of the American Medical Association* 304, no. 1: 69–75.

Wolkow, C. A., et al. October 6, 2000. "Regulation of *C. elegans* Life Span by Insulinlike Signaling in the Nervous System." *Science* 290, no. 5489: 147–50.

Xia, L., et al. January 29, 2009. "Resveratrol Reduces Endothelial Progenitor Cells Senescence through Augmentation of Telomerase Activity by Akt-Dependent Mechanisms." *British Journal of Pharmacology* 155, no. 3: 387–94.

Xu, Q., et al. March 11, 2009. "Multivitamin Use and Telomere Length in Women." *American Journal of Clinical Nutrition* 89, no. 6: 1857–63.

Yu, B. P. 1996. "Aging and Oxidative Stress: Modulation by Dietary Restriction." *Free Radical Biology & Medicine* 21, no. 5: 651–68.

Yu, B. P., and H. Y. Chung. April 2001. "Stress Resistance by Caloric Restriction for Longevity." *Annals of the New York Academy of Sciences* 928: 39–47.

Zern, T. L., et al. 2005. "Grape Polyphenols Exert a Cardioprotective Effect in Pre- and Postmenopausal Women by Lowering Plasma Lipids and Reducing Oxidative Stress." *Journal of Nutrition* 135, no. 8: 1911–17.

References

Aarsland, A., and R. R. Wolfe. 1998. "Hepatic Secretion of VLDL Fatty Acids during Stimulated Lipogenesis in Men." *Journal of Lipid Research* 39: 1280–86.

Abenavoli, L., et al. 2004. "Neurologic Disorders in Patients with Celiac Disease: Are They Mediated by Brain Perfusion Changes?" *Pediatrics* 114: 1734.

Abou-Donia, M. B., et al. 2008. "Splenda Alters Gut Microflora and Increases Intestinal p-Glycoprotein and Cytochrome p-450 in Male Rats." *Journal of Toxicology and Environmental Health, Part A* 71, no. 21: 1415–29.

Addolorato, G., et al. 2004. "Regional Cerebral Hypoperfusion in Patients with Celiac Disease." *The American Journal of Medicine* 116, no. 5: 312–17.

Aiello, L. C., et al. 1995. "The Relationship of Dietary Quality and Gut Efficiency to Brain Size/the Expensive-Tissue Hypothesis: The Brain and the Digestive System in Human and Primate Evolution." *Current Anthropology* 36, no. 2: 199–221.

Alawi, A., et al. 2007. "Effect of the Magnitude of Lipid Lowering on Cancer." *Journal of the American College of Cardiology* 50: 409–18.

Ardrey, R. 1976. *The Hunting Hypothesis.* New York: Bantam.

Armanios, M., et al. December 11, 2009. "Short Telomeres Are Sufficient to Cause the Degenerative Defects Associated with Aging." *American Journal of Human Genetics* 85, no. 6: 823–32.

Aro, A. March 10, 2001. "Complexity of Issue of Dietary Trans Fatty Acids." *Lancet* 357, no. 9258: 732–33.

Bjornholt, J. V., et al. 1999. "Fasting Blood Glucose: An Underestimated Risk Factor for Cardiovascular Death. Results from a 22-Year Follow-up of Healthy Nondiabetic Men." *Diabetes Care* 22, no. 1: 45–49.

Block, M. A., DO. October/November 1997. "Treating Attention Deficit Disorder Naturally." *Nature's Impact.*

Brown, A. M., et al. 1987. "Pathogenesis of the Impaired Gallbladder Contraction of Coeliac Disease." *Gut* 28: 1426–32.

Brownstein, D. 2008. *Iodine: Why You Need It, Why You Can't Live Without It.* 3rd ed. West Bloomfield, Mich.: Medical Alternatives Press.

Bryant, V. M., Jr., and G. Williams-Dean. January 1975. "The Coprolites of Man." *Scientific American,* 100–109.

Bures, J., J. Cyrany, D. Kohoutova, et al. 2010. "Small Intestinal Bacterial Overgrowth Syndrome." *World J. Gastroenterology* 16, no. 24: 2978–90.

Calvin, W. H. 2002. *A Brain for All Seasons.* London: University of Chicago Press.

Cassidy, A., S. Bingham, and K. D. Setchell. 1994. "Biological Effects of a Diet of Soy Protein Rich in Isoflavons on the Menstrual Cycle of Premenopausal Women." *The American Journal of Clinical Nutrition* 60: 333–40.

Coffey, Rebecca. October 2009. "20 Things You Didn't Know About . . . Sugar." *Discover Magazine.*

Coleman, R. J., et al. July 10, 2009. "Caloric Restriction Delays Disease Onset and Mortality in Rhesus Monkeys." *Science* 325, no. 5937; 201–4.

Cordain, L. February 23, 2002. "Cave Men Diets Offer Insights to Today's Health Problems." *Mercola Newsletter.*

———. 2002. *The Paleo Diet.* New York: John Wiley & Sons, Inc.

Corrao, G., et al. August 2001. "Mortality in Patients with Coeliac Disease and Their Relatives: A Cohort Study." *Lancet* 358, no. 9279: 356–61.

Crayhon, R., MS. 1998. *The Carnitine Miracle.* New York: M. Evans and Company, Inc.

Dees, C., et al. April 5, 1997. "Dietary Estrogens Stimulate Human Breast Cells to Enter the Cell Cycle." *Environmental Health Perspectives,* suppl. 3: 633–36.

Czap, A. L. 1999. "T-helper Cells Become the Target of Stearic Acid." *Townsend Letter for Doctors and Patients* 192: 117–19.

Dekker, J. M., et al. August 2, 2005. "Metabolic Syndrome and 10-Year Cardiovascular Disease Risk in the Hoorn Study." *Circulation* 112, no. 5: 666–73.

Dell'Amore, C. February 26, 2010. "Cocaine, Spices, Hormones Found in Drinking Water." *National Geographic News.*

Divi, Rao L., and Daniel R. Doerge. January 15, 1996. "Inhibition of Thyroid Peroxidase by Dietary Flavonoids." *Chemical Research in Toxicology* 9, no. 1: 16–23.

Divi, R. L., et al. November 15, 1997. "Anti-thyroid Isoflavones from Soybean: Isolation, Characterization, and Mechanisms of Action." *Biochemical Pharmacology* 54, no. 10: 1087–96.

Dolinoy, D. C., et al. 2007. "Epigenetic Gene Regulation: Linking Early Developmental Environment to Adult Disease." *Reproductive Toxicology* 23: 297–307.

Duerksen, D. R., et al. 2010. "A Comparison of Antibody Testing, Permeability Testing, and Zonulin Levels with Small-Bowel Biopsy in Celiac Disease Patients on a Gluten-Free Diet." *Digestive Diseases and Sciences* 55: 1026–31.

Eades, M. R., and M. D. Eades. 2000. *The Protein Power Lifeplan: A New Comprehensive Blueprint for Optimal Health.* New York: Warner Books, Inc.

Eaton, S. B., et al. 1997. "Paleolithic Nutrition Revisited: A Twelve-Year Retrospective on Its Nature and Implications." *European Journal of Clinical Nutrition* 51, no. 4: 207–16.

Enig, M. 2001. *Know Your Fats: The Complete Primer for Understanding the Nutrition of Fats, Oils, and Cholesterol.* Bethesda, Md.: Bethesda Press.

Erdmann, R., and M. Jones. 1995. *Fats that Can Save Your Life: The Critical Role of Fats and Oils in Health and Disease.* London: Thorsons Publishing Limited.

Faber, K. A., and C. L. Hughes. 1991. "The Effect of Neonatal Exposure to Diethylstylbestrol, Genistein, and Zearalenone on Pituitary Responsiveness and Sexually Dimorphic Nucleus Volume in the Castrated Adult Rat." *Biology of Reproduction* 45: 649–53.

Fallon, S., and M. G. Enig. 1996. "Diet and Heart Disease—Not What You Think." *Consumers' Research* 53: 15–19.

Farrell, R. J., and C. P. Kelly. January 17, 2002. "Current Concepts: Celiac Sprue." *New England Journal of Medicine* 346, no. 3: 180–88.

Fasano, A. May 2000. "ANTIBODIES: Zonulin Elevated in Celiac Disease." *Applied Genetics News.*

———. 2003. "Celiac Disease—How to Handle a Clinical Chameleon." *New England Journal of Medicine* 348: 2568–70.

Fasano, A., and C. Catassi. February 2001. "Current Approaches to Diagnosis and Treatment of Celiac Disease: An Evolving Spectrum." *Gastroenterology* 120, no. 3: 636–51.

Fasano, A., and T. Shea-Donohue. 2005. "Mechanisms of Disease: The Role of Intestinal Barrier Function in the Pathogenesis of Gastrointestinal Autoimmune Diseases." *Nature Clinical Practice Gastroenterology & Hepatology* 2, no. 9: 416–22.

Fasano, A., et al. 2003. "Prevalence of Celiac Disease in At-Risk and Not-At-Risk Groups in the United States: A Large Multicenter Study." *Archives of Internal Medicine* 163: 286–92.

Feighery, C. "Coeliac Disease." July 1999. *British Medical Journal* 319: 236–39.

Fields, M. 1984. *Proceedings of the Society of Experimental Biology and Medicine* 175: 530–37.

Fontana, L., et al. October 2008. "Long-term Effects of Calorie or Protein

Restriction on Serum IGF-1 and IGFBP-3 Concentration in Humans." *Aging Cell* 7, no. 5: 681–87.

Forette, B., et al. 1989. "Cholesterol as Risk Factor for Mortality in Elderly Women." *Lancet* 1: 868–70.

Gallagher, T. "ADDers Are More Likely to Have Fatty Acid Deficiencies." *Mercola Newsletter.* http://www.mercola.com/beef/adhd.htm.

Gerstein, H. C., et al. June 12, 2008. "Effects of Intensive Glucose Lowering in Type 2 Diabetes." *New England Journal of Medicine* 358, no. 24: 2545–59.

Godfrey, K., et al. 1996. "Maternal Nutrition in Early and Late Pregnancy in Relation to Placental and Fetal Growth." *British Medical Journal* 42: 243–51.

Godfrey, R. J., et al. 2003. "The Exercise-Induced Growth Hormone Response in Athletes." *Sports Medicine* 33, no. 8: 599–613.

Gopinath, B., et al. December 1, 2010. "Dietary Glycemic Load Is a Predictor of Age-Related Hearing Loss in Older Adults." *Journal of Nutrition* 140, no. 12: 2207–12.

Green, P. H., et al. 2005. "Mechanisms Underlying Celiac Disease and Its Neurologic Manifestations." *Cellular and Molecular Life Sciences* 62: 791–99.

Gurr, M., et al. 2002. *Lipid Biochemistry.* 5th ed. Blackwell Science.

Hadjivassiliou, M. February 13, 2001. "Headache and CNS White Matter Abnormalities Associated with Gluten Sensitivity." *Neurology* 56, no. 3.

Hadjivassiliou, M., et al. 1997. "Neuromuscular Disorder as a Presenting Feature of Coeliac Disease." *Journal of Neurology, Neurosurgery & Psychiatry* 63: 770–75.

———. 2010. "Gluten Sensitivity from Gut to Brain." *Lancet Neurology* 9: 318–30.

Hallert, C., et al. July 2002. "Evidence of Poor Vitamin Status in Coeliac Patients on a Gluten-Free Diet for 10 Years." *Alimentary Pharmacology & Therapeutics* 16, no. 7: 1333–39.

Heilbronn, L. K., et al. April 5, 2006. "Effect of 6-Month Calorie Restriction on Biomarkers of Longevity, Metabolic Adaptation, and Oxidative Stress in Overweight Individuals: A Randomized Controlled Trial." *Journal of the American Medical Association* 295, no 13: 1539–48.

Herman-Giddens, M. E., et al. April 1997. "Secondary Sexual Characteristics and Menses in Young Girls Seen in Office Practice: A Study from the Pediatric Research in Office Settings Network." *Pediatrics* 99, no. 4: 505–12.

Hoffer, A. 1995. "The Discovery of Kryptopyrrole and Its Importance in Diagnosis of Biochemical Imbalances in Schizophrenia and in Criminal Behavior." *Journal of Orthomolecular Medicine* 10, no. 1: 3.

Holman, P. 1996. "Treating the Ectomorphic Constitution." *Journal of Nutritional and Environmental Medicine* 6: 359–70.

Hulley, S. B., et al. 1992. "Health Policy on Blood Cholesterol. Time to Change Directions." *Circulation* 86: 1026–29.

Irvine, C. H., et al. March 1998. "Phytoestrogens in Soy-Based Infant Foods: Concentration, Daily Intake, and Possible Biological Effects." *Proceedings of the Society for Experimental Biology and Medicine* 217, no. 3: 247–53.

Kekwick, A., and G. Pawan. July 28, 1956. "Calorie Intake in Relation to Body Weight Changes in the Obese," *Lancet* 271, no. 6935: 155–61.

Kemper, Kathi J., 2007. "Lifestyle and Complementary Therapies for ADHD: How Health Professionals Can Approach Patients." *Medscape.*

Kenyon, C., et al. December 2, 1993. "A *C. elegans* Mutant That Lives Twice as Long as Wild Type." *Nature* 366, no. 6454: 461–64. *Comment in Nature* 366, no. 6454: 404–5.

Kleslich, M., et al. August 2001. "Brain White-Matter Lesions in Celiac Disease: A Prospective Study of 75 Diet-Treated Patients." *Pediatrics* 108, no. 2: e21.

Klinghardt, D., 2008. "Special Inner Circle Audio Interview by Dr. Joseph Mercola."

Kozanoglu, E., et al. 2005. "Proximal Myopathy as an Unusual Presenting Feature of Celiac Disease." *Clinical Rheumatology* 24: 76–78.

Kristjánsson, G., et al. 2007. "Mucosal Reactivity to Cow's Milk Protein in Coeliac Disease." *Clinical & Experimental Immunology* 147, no. 3: 449–55.

Krumholz, H. M. 1990. "Lack of Association between Cholesterol and Coronary Heart Disease Mortality and Morbidity and All-cause Mortality in Persons Older than 70 Years." *Journal of the American Medical Association* 272: 1335–40.

LaRocca, T. J., et al. February 2010. "Leukocyte Telomere Length Is Preserved with Aging in Endurance Exercise-Trained Adults and Related to Maximal Aerobic Capacity." *Mechanisms of Ageing and Development* 131, no. 2: 165–57.

Layton, L. December 19, 2010. "Probable Carcinogen Hexavalent Chromium Found in Drinking Water of 31 U.S. Cities." *Washington Post.*

Lemon, J. A., et al. March 2005. "A Complex Dietary Supplement Extends Longevity of Mice." *Journals of Gerontology, Series A: Biological Sciences and Medical Sciences* 60, no. 3: 275–79.

Leonard, W. R., et al. 2003. "Metabolic Correlates of Hominid Brain Evolution." *Comparative Biochemistry and Physiology Part A: Molecular & Integrative Physiology* 136: 5–15.

Linder, M. 1991. *Nutritional Biochemistry and Metabolism.* 2nd ed. Norwalk, Conn.: Appleton & Lange.

Long, T. C., et al. November 2007. "Nanosize Titanium Dioxide Stimulates Reactive Oxygen Species in Brain Microglia and Damages Neurons In Vitro." *Environmental Health Perspectives* 115, no. 11: 1631–37.

Ludvigsson, J. F., et al. 2009. "Small-Intestinal Histopathology and Mortality Risk in Celiac Disease." *Journal of the American Medical Association* 302, no. 11: 1171–78.

Lustig, R. H. 2009. "The Bitter Truth." www.youtube.com/watch?v=dBnnivab -oM (accessed May 6, 2011).

Marshall, T. G. "Vitamin D Discovery Outpaces FDA Decision Making." *Bioessays* 30, no. 2 (2008): 173–82.

Masoro, E. J. 2003. *Calorie Restriction: A Key to Understanding and Modulating Aging* (Research Profiles in Aging). Burlington, Mass.: Elsevier.

Matthews, A. W. December 28, 2010. "So Young and So Many Pills." The *Wall Street Journal*.

Matthews, C. E., et al. August 2010. "Metabolic Syndrome and Risk of Death from Cancers of the Digestive System." *Metabolism* 59, no. 8: 1231–39.

McGowan, K. E., et al. 2009. "The Changing Face of Childhood Celiac Disease in North America: Impact of Serological Testing." *Pediatrics* 124: 1572–78.

Mercola, J. 2002. "Omega-3 Is Essential to the Human Body." http://articles .mercola.com/sites/articles/archive/2002/03/16/omega3-part-one.aspx. Accessed April 1, 2011.

Morehouse, L. E., and L. Gross. 1977. *Maximum Performance.* New York: Pocket Books.

Nicolas, A. S., et al. 1999. "Caloric Restriction and Aging." *Journal of Nutrition, Health & Aging* 3, no. 2: 77–83.

Niederhofer, H., and K. Pittschieler. November 2006. "A Preliminary Investigation of ADHD Symptoms in Persons with Celiac Disease." *Journal of Attention Disorders* 10, no. 2: 200–204.

Osterberg, K. L., and C. L. Melby. March 2000. "Effect of Acute Resistance Exercise on Postexercise Oxygen Consumption and Resting Metabolic Rate in Young Women." *International Journal of Sport Nutrition and Exercise Metabolism* 10, no. 1: 71–81.

Petrakis, N. L., et al. October 1996. "Stimulatory Influence of Soy Protein Isolate on Breast Secretion in Pre- and Post-menopausal Women." *Cancer Epidemiology, Biomarkers & Prevention* 5, no. 10: 785–94.

Phinney, S. D. 2004. "Ketogenic Diets and Physical Performance." *Nutrition & Metabolism* 1:2. doi:10.1186/1743-7075-1-2.

Pollack, G. H. 2001. *Cells, Gels and the Engines of Life.* Seattle: Ebner and Sons Publishing.

———. 2011. "The Single Most Important Element for Your Health." http://articles.mercola.com/sites/articles/archive/2011/01/29/dr=pollack =on=structured=water.aspx. Accessed May 6, 2011.

Prasad, A. N., et al. 1996. "Alternative Epilepsy Therapies: The Ketogenic Diet, Immunoglobulins and Steroids." *Epilepsia* 37, suppl. 1: S81–S95.

Price, W., DDS. 1989. *Nutrition and Physical Degeneration.* New Canaan, Conn.: Keats Publishing. Previously published in 1939, 1945, and 1970.

Puterman, E., et al. May 2010. "The Power of Exercise: Buffering the Effect of Chronic Stress on Telomere Length." *PLoS ONE* 5, no. 5: e10837.

Ravnskov, U. 1998. "The Questionable Role of Saturated and Polyunsaturated Fatty Acids in Cardiovascular Disease." *Journal of Clinical Epidemiology* 51, no. 6: 443–60.

Rosedale, R. August 1999. "Insulin and Its Metabolic Effects." Paper presented at the Designs for Health Institute's BoulderFest seminar, Boulder, Colorado.

Rosedale, R., and C. Coleman. 2004. *The Rosedale Diet.* New York: Harper Resource/HarperCollins.

Rosedale, R., et al. 2009. "Clinical Experience of a Diet Designed to Reduce Aging." *Journal of Applied Research* 9, no. 4: 159–65.

Ross, R. K., et al., May 15, 1983. "Effect of In-Utero Exposure to Diethylstilbestrol on Age at Onset of Puberty and on Post Pubertal Hormone Levels in Boys." *Canadian Medical Association Journal* 128, no. 10: 1197–98.

Rubio-Tapia, A., and J. A. Murray. 2007. "The Liver in Celiac Disease." *Hepatology* 46, no. 5.

Rubio-Tapia, A., et al. July 2009. "Increased Prevalence and Mortality in Undiagnosed Celiac Disease." *Gastroenterology* 137, no. 1: 88–93.

Said, S. "Study: Neanderthals Cooked, Ate Vegetables." www.cnn.com/2010/HEALTH/12/29/neanderthals.diet/index.html?hpt=C2. Accessed May 6, 2011.

Sapone, A., et al. May 2006. "Zonulin Upregulation Is Associated with Increased Gut Permeability in Subjects with Type 1 Diabetes and Their Relatives." *Diabetes* 55: 1443–49.

Schauss, A. 1997. "An Analysis of Colloidal Mineral Claims." *Health Counselor Magazine.* http://khup.com/download/4_keyword-analysis-minerals/an-analysis-of-colloidal-mineral-claims.pdf.

Schunemann, et al. 2000. "Pulmonary Function Is a Long-term Predictor of Mortality in the General Population: 29-Year Follow-up of the Buffalo Health Study." *Chest* 118: 656–64.

Schwarzbein, D., and N. Deville. 1999. *The Schwarzbein Principle.* Deerfield Beach, Fla.: Health Communications, Inc.

Sears, A. "PACE: The 12-Minute Fitness Revolution." www.pacerevolution.com.

Sheehan, D. M., and D. R. Doerge. 1998. "FDA Scientists Protest Soy Approval." Letter to U.S. Food and Drug Administration regarding opposition to health claims for soy products, fully referenced. SoyOnline Service. www .soyonlineservice.co.nz/downloads/nctrpti.pdf.

Siegell, G. J., et al. 1999. *Basic Neurochemistry: Molecular, Cellular and Medical Aspects.* 6th ed. American Society for Neurochemistry.

Sijbrands. E. J., et al. April 28, 2001. "Mortality over Two Centuries in Large Pedigree with Familial Hypercholesterolaemia: Family Tree Mortality Study." *BMJ* 322:1019–23.

Siri-Torino, P. W., et al. 2010. "Meta-analysis of Prospective Cohort Studies Evaluating the Association of Saturated Fat With Cardiovascular Disease." *American Journal of Clinical Nutrition* 91, no. 3: 535–46. doi:10.3945/ ajcn.2009.27725.

Sparagna, G. C., and D. L. Hickson-Bick. 1999. "Cardiac Fatty Acid Metabolism and the Induction of Apoptosis." *Am J Med Sci* 318: 15–21.

Stolberg, S. G. January 21, 1999. "Fiber Does Not Help Prevent Colon Cancer, Study Finds." The *New York Times.*

Stoll, W. 1998. "Sugar and Immunity: Leukocytic Index Proves the Devastating Effect of Refined Carbohydrates on Immunity." http://askwaltstollmd.com/ articles/sugarimm.php.

Sullivan, K., CN. 2006. *Naked at Noon: Understanding Sunlight and Vitamin D.* Laguna Beach, Calif: Basic Health Publications.

———. "Magnesium." www.krispin.com/magnes.html. Accessed March 17, 2011.

Taubes, Gary. April 13, 2011. "Is Sugar Toxic?" *New York Times* www.nytimes .com/2011/04/17/magazine/mag-17Sugar-t.html?ref=magazine (accessed May 6, 2011).

———. July 7, 2002. "What If It's All Been a Big Fat Lie?" *The New York Times Magazine.*

Tebbey, P. W., and T. M. Buttke. 1990. "Molecular Basis for the Immunosuppressive Action of Stearic Acid on T Cells." *Immunology* 70, no. 3: 379–86.

Thomas, K. E., et al. 2006. "Gliadin Stimulation of Murine Macrophage Inflammatory Gene Expression and Intestinal Permeability Are MyD88-Dependent: Role of the Innate Immune Response in Celiac Disease." *Journal of Immunology* 176: 2512–21.

Toney, Jeffrey H. 2011. "The Two Ton Sugar Burden." At http://scienceblogs
.com/deanscorner/2011/04/the_two_ton_sugar_burden.php (accessed May
6, 2011).

Tremblay. A., et al. 1994. "Impact of Exercise Intensity on Body Fatness and
Skeletal Muscle Metabolism." *Metabolism* 43, no. 7: 814–18.

Ulloth J. E., et al. 2003. "Palmitic and Stearic Fatty Acids Induce Caspase-
dependent and -independent Cell Death in Nerve Growth Factor Differentiated PC12 Cells." *Journal of Neurochemistry* 84, no. 4: 655–68.

Vallejo, et al. 2003. "Phenolic Compound Contents in Edible Parts of Broccoli
Inflorescences after Domestic Cooking." *Journal of the Science of Food and
Agriculture* 83, no. 14: 1511–16.

Verkasalo, M. 2005. "Undiagnosed Silent Celiac Disease: A Risk for Underachievement." *Scandinavian Journal of Gastroenterology*, 40: 1407–12.

Vasquez, A. 2005. "Reducing Pain and Inflammation Naturally. Part II: New
Insights into Fatty Acid Supplementation and Its Effects on Eicosanoid Production and Genetic Expression." *Nutritional Perspectives* 28, no. 1: 5–16.

Vermiglio, F., et al. 2004. "Attention Deficit and Hyperactivity Disorders in the
Offspring of Mothers Exposed to Mild–Moderate Iodine Deficiency: A Pos-
sible Novel Iodine Deficiency Disorder in Developed Countries." *Journal of
Clinical Endocrinology & Metabolism* 89: 6054–60.

Wadoa, R. S., et al. 2004. "Hyperhomocysteinaemia and Vitamin B$_{12}$ Deficiency
in Ischaemic Strokes in India." *Annals of Indian Academy of Neurology* 7, no.
2: 387–92.

White, L., et al. July 27, 1996. "Association of Mid-life Consumption of Tofu
with Late Life Cognitive Impairment and Dementia: The Honolulu-Asia
Aging Study." Paper presented at the Fifth International Conference on
Alzheimer's Disease, Osaka, Japan.

Witte, J., et al. 1997. "Diet and Premenopausal Bilateral Breast Cancer: A Case
Control Study." *Breast Cancer Research and Treatment* 42: 243–51.

Woodruff, T. J., et al. January 14, 2011. "Environmental Chemicals in Pregnant
Women in the US: NHANES 2003-2004." *Environmental Health Perspectives.* doi:10.1289/ehp.1002727.

Xu, D., et al. 2000. "Homocysteine Accelerates Endothelial Cell Senescence."
FEBS Letters 470: 20–24.

Yang, H. T., J. Baur, et al. 2007. "Nutrient-Sensitive Mitochondrial NAD$^+$ Levels Dictate Cell Survival." *Cell* 130, no. 6: 1095–1107.

About the Author

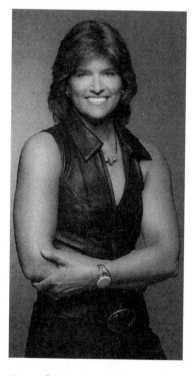

Raised in a prominent Minnesota medical family, Nora Gedgaudas, C.N.S., C.N.T., has a background in diet and nutrition spanning twenty-five years and is a respected and sought-after expert and teacher in the field. She is recognized by the Nutritional Therapy Association as a certified nutritional therapist/ nutritional therapy practitioner and is board certified in holistic nutrition through the National Association of Nutritional Professionals. Nora has appeared as a guest lecturer, as a trainer for the State of Washington Institute of Mental Health—illuminating nutrition's impact on mental health—and as a radio and television guest. Nora has also been the host of her own popular Internet radio program, *Primal Body– Primal Mind Radio,* on VoiceAmerica's Health and Wellness channel. She maintains a private practice as a certified nutritional therapist and board-certified clinical neurofeedback specialist in Portland, Oregon.

Index

■ ■ ■ ■ ■ ■ ■ ■ ■ ■ ■

Page numbers in *italics* refer to illustrations.

BOOKS OF RELATED INTEREST

Primal Cuisine
Cooking for the Paleo Diet
by Pauli Halstead

Primal Nutrition
Paleolithic and Ancestral Diets for Optimal Health
by Ronald F. Schmid, N.D.

Natural Remedies for Inflammation
by Christopher Vasey, N.D.

Radical Medicine
Cutting-Edge Natural Therapies That
Treat the Root Causes of Disease
by Louisa L. Williams, M.S., D.C., N.D.

Food Allergies and Food Intolerance
The Complete Guide to Their Identification and Treatment
by Jonathan Brostoff, M.D., and Linda Gamlin

Nutrition and Mental Illness
An Orthomolecular Approach to Balancing Body Chemistry
by Carl C. Pfeiffer, Ph.D., M.D.

The Transformational Power of Fasting
The Way to Spiritual, Physical, and Emotional Rejuvenation
by Stephen Harrod Buhner

Food Energetics
The Spiritual, Emotional,
and Nutritional Power of What We Eat
by Steve Gagné

Inner Traditions • Bear & Company
P.O. Box 388
Rochester, VT 05767
1-800-246-8648
www.InnerTraditions.com

Or contact your local bookseller